# Healthcare Solutions Using Machine Learning and Informatics

*Healthcare Solutions Using Machine Learning and Informatics* covers novel and innovative solutions for healthcare that apply machine learning and biomedical informatics technology. The healthcare sector is one of the most critical in society. This book presents a series of artificial intelligence, machine learning, and intelligent IoT-based solutions for medical image analysis, medical big-data processing, and disease predictions. Machine learning and artificial intelligence use cases in healthcare presented in the book give researchers, practitioners, and students a wide range of practical examples of cross-domain convergence.

The wide variety of topics covered include:

- Artificial Intelligence in healthcare
- Machine learning solutions for such disease as diabetes, arthritis, cardiovascular disease, and COVID-19
- Big data analytics solutions for healthcare data processing
- Reliable biomedical applications using AI models
- Intelligent IoT in healthcare

The book explains fundamental concepts as well as advanced use cases, illustrating how to apply emerging technologies such as machine learning, AI models, and data informatics in practice to tackle challenges in the field of healthcare with real-world scenarios. Chapters contributed by noted academics and professionals examine various solutions, frameworks, applications, case studies, and best practices in the healthcare domain.

**Dr. Punit Gupta** is an Associate Professor in the Department of Computer and Communication Engineering at Manipal University, Jaipur, India.

**Dr. Dinesh Kumar Saini** is a Professor in the Department of Computer and Communication Engineering at Manipal University, Jaipur, India.

**Dr. Rohit Verma** is affiliated with the INSIGHT Research Lab SFI, Dublin City University, Dublin, Ireland.

# Healthcare Solutions Using Machine Learning and Informatics

Edited by
Punit Gupta
Dinesh Kumar Saini
Rohit Verma

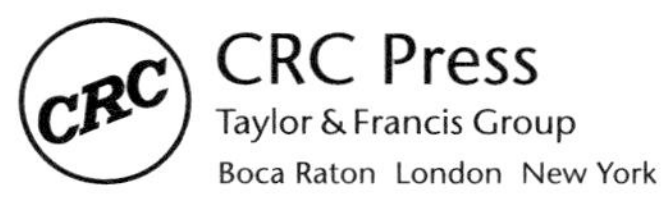


CRC Press is an imprint of the
Taylor & Francis Group, an **informa** business

First edition published 2023
by CRC Press
6000 Broken Sound Parkway NW, Suite 300, Boca Raton, FL 33487-2742

and by CRC Press
4 Park Square, Milton Park, Abingdon, Oxon, OX14 4RN

CRC Press is an imprint of Taylor & Francis Group, LLC



ISBN: 978-1-032-20198-6 (hbk)
ISBN: 978-1-032-34522-2 (pbk)
ISBN: 978-1-003-32259-7 (ebk)

DOI: 10.1201/9781003322597

Typeset in Adobe Garamond Pro
by SPi Technologies India Pvt Ltd (Straive)

# Contents

Preface ........................................................................................ vii
Acknowledgments ........................................................................................ xi

1 Introduction to Artificial Intelligence in Healthcare ........................ 1
DIVYANI JIGYASU, SUNIL KUMAR, RAJVEER SINGH SHEKHAWAT AND SHALLY VATS

2 Machine Learning in Radio Imaging ........................ 25
NITESH PRADHAN, PUNIT GUPTA AND ANITA SHROTRIYA

3 Solutions Using Machine Learning for Diabetes ........................ 39
JABAR H. YOUSIF, KASHIF ZIA AND DURGESH SRIVASTAVA

4 A Highly Reliable Machine Learning Algorithm for Cardiovascular Disease Prediction ........................ 61
HORESH KUMAR, TARUN JAIN, KARTIK SONI, AMISHA GUPTA, RISHI GUPTA, ARJUN SINGH AND ADITYA SINHA

5 Machine Learning Algorithms for Industry Using Image Sensing ......... 75
AAKASH DHALL, HEMANT K UPADHYAY, SAPNA JUNEJA AND ABHINAV JUNEJA

6 Solutions Using Machine Learning for COVID-19 ........................ 99
MUHAMMAD SHAFI, KASHIF ZIA AND JABAR H. YOUSIF

7 Big Data Analytics in Healthcare Data Processing ........................ 123
TANVEER AHMED, RISHAV SINGH AND RITIKA SINGH

8 Reliable Biomedical Applications Using AI Models ........................ 147
SHAMBHAVI MISHRA, TANVEER AHMED AND VIPUL MISHRA

9 Plant Disease Detection Using Imaging Sensors, Deep Learning and Machine Learning for Smart Farming ........................ 173
CHANCHAL UPADHYAY, HEMANT K UPADHYAY, SAPNA JUNEJA AND ABHINAV JUNEJA

**10** **IoT Application for Healthcare** ........................................ 187
MONIKA SHARMA, HEMANT K UPADHYAY, SAPNA JUNEJA AND ABHINAV JUNEJA

**11** **Machine Learning Techniques for Prediction of Diabetes** ........................................ 205
TARUN JAIN, PAYAL GARG, JALAK YOGESH PATEL, DIV CHAUDHARY, HORESH KUMAR, VIVEK K. VERMA AND RISHI GUPTA

**12** **Use of Machine Learning in Healthcare** ........................................ 237
ISHITA MEHTA AND ARNAAV ANAND

**Index** ........................................ 251

# Preface

*Healthcare Solutions using Machine Learning and Informatics* covers novel and innovative solutions for the healthcare domain with machine learning and informatics-based technological solutions. The healthcare sector is one of the most critical sectors in human society. This book presents a series of artificial intelligence, machine learning, intelligent IoT-based solutions for medical image analysis, medical big-data processing, and disease prediction. Machine learning and artificial intelligence use cases in healthcare presented in the book give researchers, practitioners, and students a wide range of practical examples of cross-domain convergence.

A wide variety of topics is offered to readers:

- Artificial Intelligence in healthcare
- Machine learning solutions for diabetes, arthritis, cardiovascular disease, COVID-19
- Big data analytics solutions for healthcare data processing
- Reliable biomedical applications using AI models
- Intelligent IoT in healthcare

Readers will learn the fundamental concepts as well as the advanced use cases to learn how to apply emerging technologies such as machine learning, AI models, and data informatics in practice to tackle challenges in the field of healthcare with real-world scenarios. High-quality chapters contributed by academics and professionals from organizations of repute provide and describe various solutions, frameworks, applications, case studies, and best practices in the healthcare domain.

***Chapter 1*** is a general introduction to healthcare as one of the most critical sectors in modern human society. Human-friendly and intelligent systems are the need of the hour. Artificial intelligence has made inroads into almost every aspect of human life, and is used in disease diagnosis, disease treatment, drug development, and patient monitoring.

***Chapter 2*** covers the three-dimensional geometry of a bone, which is important for the correct diagnosis of disease, arthritis, or other bone deformities. Modalities such as CT scan and MRI are used for a three-dimensional view of a bone. Both the above modalities are associated with high costs and expose the patient to strong cancer-causing radiation. Computed tomography captures a large number of images to gather the necessary information from a bone.

***Chapter 3*** reviews the most important studies about diabetes and methods to prevent it using machine learning techniques. The chapter further elaborates on analytical models and technologies for simulating and predicting the incidence of diabetes efficiently. These models help find the disease early to reduce medical costs and prevent more complicated health problems.

***Chapter 4*** shows AI's consistent growth in healthcare niches like dermatology and radiology, and its recent growth in cardiology, where it is imperative that reliable deep learning algorithms exist for detection of the presence of disease in the heart. The chapter discusses some of the commonly known machine learning algorithms: the random forest algorithm, which yielded 86.8% accuracy, naïve Bayes, which yielded 85.2% accuracy, XGBoost algorithm, which yielded 87.91% accuracy, and finally, the most reliable algorithm, the majority voting ensemble classifier, yielding a staggering 99.3% accuracy.

***Chapter 5*** examines the role of AI and image sensing in industry. The industrial internet of things (IIoT), also known as Industry 4.0, is a sub-segment of the IoT market. Industry 4.0, also known as I4.0, is the fourth industrial revolution, and it emphasizes interconnectedness, automation, artificial intelligence, autonomy, internet of things, machine learning, deep learning and real-time data.

***Chapter 6*** considers the various challenges pertaining to the containment and treatment of the COVID-19 pandemic. The role of machine learning in screening and diagnosis of COVID-19 is discussed. Different images such as X-rays and CT scans, and different blood tests coupled with different machine learning techniques have been investigated by a number of researchers in the literature

***Chapter 7*** covers the healthcare sector which is one of the largest sectors in India in terms of revenue. With the spread of the unpredictable and devastating COVID-19 pandemic, it has become imperative for the healthcare industry, especially in a country like India, to adopt modern-day tools and techniques to handle the increasing burden on the sector. The digitization and virtual mode of conducting business for healthcare-related services, hospital management, medical equipment manufacturing, and medicines supply chains have resulted in the generation of huge data.

***Chapter 8*** covers the role of AI and image sensing in prediction of diseases in plants. The identification of plant diseases is an important step for the protection of plants. In the last decade, considerable research has been conducted to develop new technical optical methodologies for plant disease detection.

***Chapter 9*** covers the AI domain, including biomedicine. Nowadays, an enormous amount of data is being generated in the biomedical field, creating numerous opportunities for real-time decision making and learning. It would not be wrong to say that AI methods have also brought significant improvements in various biomedical applications such as medical imaging, drug discovery, protein, and genetic sequence analysis.

***Chapter 10*** covers the highlights and research gaps in the internet of things and its application in healthcare. It also examines the influence of artificial intelligence and machine learning on (i) healthcare servicing-based apps and (ii) social applications.

***Chapter 11*** covers the study of prediction of diabetes through various machine learning algorithms. There are several approaches in the area of medical science research, and machine learning is one of the most important approaches. The algorithms used are SVM, ANN, random forest, and XG Boost.

***Chapter 12*** provides a general introduction to machine learning, the simplest definition of which is a form of artificial intelligence where computers can be programmed in such a way that they can learn information and process data without the intervention of any human.

We hope that the research published in this book will be of service to both machine learning and healthcare communities.

# Acknowledgments

The editors are thankful to the authors and reviewers of the chapters, who contributed to this book with their scientific work and useful comments, respectively.

# Chapter 1

# Introduction to Artificial Intelligence in Healthcare

Divyani Jigyasu, Sunil Kumar, Rajveer Singh Shekhawat and Shally Vats

*SCIT, Manipal University, Jaipur, India*

## Contents

1.1 Introduction ........ 2
1.1.1 Major Activities in Medical Image Analysis ........ 2
1.1.2 The Role of ML in Medical Image Analysis ........ 2
1.2 Medical Imaging Types ........ 2
1.2.1 Pre-Processing Using ML ........ 2
1.2.1.1 Introduction to Pre-processing ........ 3
1.2.2 Segmentation Using ML ........ 7
1.2.2.1 Introduction to Segmentation ........ 7
1.2.3 Registration Using ML ........ 12
1.2.3.1 Introduction ........ 12
1.3 Deep Learning in Medical Imaging ........ 12
1.4 Conclusion ........ 22
References ........ 22

DOI: 10.1201/9781003322597-1

# 1.1 Introduction

## 1.1.1 Major Activities in Medical Image Analysis

Machine learning, a research field in computer science engineering, is a branch of artificial intelligence. It enables the extraction of patterns from knowledge that are available and are the part of human intelligence.

Machine learning is a powerful tool for the identification of patterns. The application of ML algorithms in the medical images field is significant for prediction and diagnosis.

## 1.1.2 The Role of ML in Medical Image Analysis

Machine learning plays an important role in computer vision and medical image analysis, which is a growing field in deep learning.

In recent years machine learning and artificial intelligence have played a major role in such aspects of medicine as computer-aided diagnosis, image processing, interpretation and fusion, and in the registration, segmentation and retrieval of images. ML extracts information and represents it effectively and efficiently. Together, machine learning and artificial intelligence can predict, prevent and diagnose diseases faster and more accurately. These techniques help doctors and researchers to understand and analyze the variations that will lead to disease. These techniques consist of algorithms without learning such as the support vector machine and neural network approaches, K-nearest neighbor and deep learning approaches such as convolutional neural network, recurrent neural network approach, long- and short-term memory and extreme learning model approaches.

# 1.2 Medical Imaging Types

Medical imaging is a process that obtains pictures of the human body. It can help in the diagnosis and treatment of patients. It may also be used to track many clinical issues and may help in treatment planning. Medical imaging modalities incorporate magnetic resonance imaging (MRI), computed tomography (CT), X-ray and positron emission tomography (PET), single photon emission computed tomography (SPECT). Research in medical image processing mainly targets the extraction of important features that might be difficult to assess with the naked eye.

## 1.2.1 Pre-Processing Using ML

In data pre-processing, raw data is prepared in a form that is more appropriate for a machine learning model. It is the first and critical step in the machine learning model.

Data for a machine learning project is not always clean and appropriately formatted. Real-world data may be noisy, or have missing values or contain data in unusable formats. Data pre-processing is required to clean such data and make it suitable for a machine learning model, which increases the accuracy and efficiency of the model. In this step, data is modified and encrypted so that the machine can easily monitor it.

#### *1.2.1.1 Introduction to Pre-processing*

There are various types of pre-processing: linear, non-linear, fixed, adaptive, pixel-based or multi-scale. These techniques are relevant for different conditions. The difference between abnormal and normal tissue can be confused by objects and noisy data, causing difficulty in the analysis of medical images where high-quality images are required for clarification by a medical specialist. Enhancement techniques are the key to pre-processing for automatic analysis. CT and MRI include patient-specific and equipment-based objects, all of which are removed during pre-processing (Tables 1.1 and 1.2).

Various denoising techniques are available:

1. *Gabor Filter*, a type of linear filter used in edge detection which is similar to the human vision system. It is appropriate for texture differentiation and characterization.
2. *Adaptive Median Filter* is used for reducing impetuous noise in images without affecting the original image. It is used to cancel unknown interference contained in a primary signal, which is the desired response of the adaptive filter. The reference signal is employed as an input to the filter.
3. *Morphological Operations* explore an image with a small template called a "structuring element". These elements are positioned at all possible locations in the image and are compared with the neighborhoods of pixels. The two morphological operations are called erosion and dilation. Erosion reduces the size of the region of interest (ROI) and removes small details from an image. Dilation expands shapes that contain an input image.
4. *Filter or Average Filter* is used to replace every pixel value in an image, using the average value of its neighbors. It is also used to remove pixel values that are unrepresentative of their surroundings.
5. *Image Normalization* improves the range of pixel intensity values. It is also called contrast stretching or histogram stretching. The main objective is to achieve consistency for a set of data.
6. *Histogram Equalization*, in which dilation expands the shapes contained by the input images. The global variance of various images is usually increased by histogram equalization, and intensities can be better distributed as a result of these types of adjustment.

**Table 1.1 Pre-Processing Techniques Compared**

| *S. No.* | *Pre-Processing Techniques* | *Advantage* | *Disadvantage* |
|---|---|---|---|
| 1 | Gabor Filter | Uniqueness.<br>Fourier analysis is fast.<br>Useful for determining magnitude of stationary signals. | Necessitates an image of around a power of two in size.<br>After segmentation, the zone can be easily identified, but there are no clear border restrictions.<br>A signal's time domain and frequency domain descriptions are mutually exclusive. |
| 2 | Adaptive Median Filter | Used to smooth non-repulsive noise without causing edge blurring.<br>Retains edge information in the event of high-density impulse sounds | When the impulse noise is more than 0.2, it does not perform properly. |
| 3 | Morphological Operations | Allows for the detection of lesions of different sizes and shapes. | Morphological operators rely on the concepts of infimum and supremum, which necessitates a proper color order. |
| 4 | Mean Filter (or) Average filter | Simple to implement and decreases variance. | Image blurring occurs as a result of averaging procedures, which has an impact on feature localization and does not totally eliminate impulse noise. |

**Table 1.1** *(Continued)* **Pre-Processing Techniques Compared**

| *S. No.* | *Pre-Processing Techniques* | *Advantage* | *Disadvantage* |
|---|---|---|---|
| 5 | Image Normalization | Size and location of endorsements consistent across different pages in the data set if images were normalized before the endorsement. If photos are printed, adopting normalized images avoids printing issues caused by page size and orientation variations. | Image normalization is a time-consuming process that can add significant time to the e-Discovery export process in large cases, and utilizing improperly designed normalization software can result in image quality degradation. |
| 6 | Histogram Equalization | Simple and effective in enhancing image contrasts. | This approach fails if the image contains gray values that are physically separated from one another. |
| 7 | Weighted Median Filter | "Salt and pepper noise" is efficiently eradicated with this method. | The most significant flaw is the inability to round corners and map texture regions to a uniform hue. |
| 8 | Weiner Filter | Minimizing mean square error is a time-saving task that can deal with both degradation and noise. | A fair degradation function estimate is ineffective. |

7. *Weighted Median Filter* removes "salt and pepper noise" from CT images. This filter has edge preservation, robustness and noise attenuation capabilities.
8. *Wiener Filter* is non-linear and is used to restore blurred and noisy images and to filter grayscale images.

**Table 1.2 Literature Review of Pre-processing in Medical Image Analysis**

| *Title* | *Author* | *Publication & Year* | *Machine Learning Techniques* | *Salient Points* | *Challenges/ Future Scope* |
|---|---|---|---|---|---|
| *Age prediction based on brain MRI images: A Survey* | Hedieh Sajedi, Nasataran Pardakhti | Springer 2019 | Neural network and deep learning-based methods, machine learning toolkits | This paper focuses on the main approaches for age prediction based on brain MRI images.<br>It includes pre-processing methods, useful tools for different research works and estimation algorithms. | Accuracy should be there in age prediction algorithms. Also, it should be fast. |
| *A Survey: Analysis on preprocessing and segmentation techniques for medical images* | R. Beaulah Jeyavathana, Dr. R.Balasubramanian, A. Anbarasa Pandian | IJRSI 2016 | Clustering, fuzzy methods, genetic algorithms | In this paper various techniques of preprocessing and segmentation are discussed. | Automated segmentation methods should be improved. |
| *A Survey on Image Preprocessing Techniques for Diverse Fields of Medical Imagery* | P. Vasuki, J. Kanimozhi, M. Balkis Devi | ICEICE 2017 | Enhancement, mammogram imagery | This paper summarizes various pre-processing techniques, enhancement tasks and mammogram imagery. | Image enhancement techniques should be improved. |

### 1.2.2 Segmentation Using ML

Image segmentation is a method for separating images into different components to make analysis and interpretation easier while maintaining quality. Within the photos, segmentation is also employed to detect objects and object borders. It categorizes the pixels based on their strength and quality. Those elements represent the actual image and are responsible for its attributes and resemblances. For clinical applications, image segmentation is also utilized to construct a 3-D contour of the body. Machine perception, malignant disease analysis, tissue volumes, anatomical and functional analyses, 3-D-rendered approach, virtual reality visualization, anomaly analysis, and object definition and detection are all examples of when segmentation is applied.

Segmentation can take place at the local level or on a global scale. In local segmentation the image is subdivided. This technique uses far fewer pixels than global segmentation, which works as a single unit throughout the entire image.

The three segmentation methods are region, boundary, and edge.

#### 1.2.2.1 Introduction to Segmentation

Accepting all the pixels that belong to an object allows for segmentation. Previously, pixel intensity was employed, and later, picture gradients with high values at the edges were used. Segmentation is a pattern recognition challenge since it includes pixel classification. Hybrid techniques in segmentation serve a critical role in medical image analysis, as these processes are time-consuming and very complicated techniques. Thresholding, histogram analysis, deformable templates, and non-linear anisotropic diffusion are examples of hybrid methods used in brain MRI segmentation (Figure 1.1).

Image segmentation is a technique for separating photos into many parts in order to identify specific objects or extract information from them. This process is influenced by the characteristics of the region of interest or by objects such as color, pixel intensity, shape, and size. There are a number of different segmentation techniques (Tables 1.3 and 1.4).

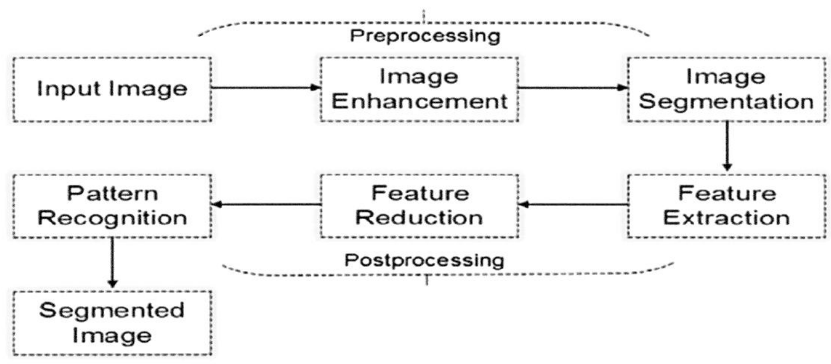


**Figure 1.1 Segmentation steps.**

**Table 1.3 Comparison of Segmentation Techniques**

| *S. No* | *Segmentation Technique* | *Advantages* | *Disadvantages* |
|---|---|---|---|
| 1. | Pixel Based | A collection of strategies that are used to simulate human thinking capacities in order to solve real-world problems. | 1) Costly in terms of computational time and memory.<br>2) In photos, there may be under-and over-segmentations, as well as gaps in the region. |
| 2. | Edge Based | 1) No prior knowledge of image content required.<br>2) Computationally fast. | Large process if there are too many edges. |
| 3. | Region Based | Simple to categorize and execute. | 1) Difficult to calculate the number of clusters.<br>2) Difficult to make use of spatial data.<br>3) Feature selection is difficult to grasp. |
| 4. | Deformable Models Approach | 1) Strong approach for noise and spurious edges.<br>2) Able to generate surface from images | 1) Manual approach required for initial model.<br>2) Difficult to choose parameters. |
| 5. | Texture based | 1) Easy technique to solve complex problems using training data.<br>2) Error detection is an easier task. | 1) Training procedure is expensive and prone to human error.<br>2) Analysis of many image kinds is required. |
| 6. | Artificial neural network Based | 1) Does not require writing of monotonous programs.<br>2) Could make use of parallel nature of neural net. | 1) Extended training period.<br>2) Initialization may affect the outcome. |

**Table 1.3** *(Continued)* **Comparison of Segmentation Techniques**

| *S. No* | *Segmentation Technique* | *Advantages* | *Disadvantages* |
|---|---|---|---|
| 7. | Fuzzy theory based | 1) A single fuzzy rule was used to emphasize the value of the image's feature-based and spatial information.<br>2) Structure of membership functions and associated parameters examined and derived automatically. | 1) Noise sensitive.<br>2) Computer resources are limited.<br>3) Difficult to resolve ambiguous membership. |
| 8. | Genetic algorithm based | 1) Demonstrate that you can get out of local optima.<br>2) Provides a lot of versatility.<br>3) Works well for enhancing contrast and producing images with realistic contrast.<br>4) Offers a simple and generic approach to solving difficult optimization problems | In complex design, a simple genetic algorithm may converge very slowly or fail due to convergence to an unsatisfactory local optimum. |

1. **Clustering:** an unsupervised learning approach for categorizing a set of things into a variety of different classes. It is used in a variety of industries, including geology, engineering, machine learning, statistics, and medicine. It is similar to picture segmentation. There are many different types of clustering algorithms. Algorithms that are both fuzzy and non-fuzzy, such as k-means clustering, are particularly common.
2. **Region-based segmentation:** groups regions with similar values together, while regions with differing values are grouped together. The center of objects is where this process begins. It continues to grow until it hits the limit.
3. **Edge-based segmentation:** Filters are used to identify edges and non-edges based on the filter output. Pixels that are not separated by edges fall into the same category.
4. **Image enhancement:** improves photos to make them easier to analyze so that further research can be done. Values such as brightness, contrast, sharpness, and noise removal are manipulated to achieve this.
5. **Feature**: a property of an object that includes its color, form, and size.

**Table 1.4 Literature Review: Segmentation Techniques**

| *Title* | *Author* | *Publication & Year* | *Machine Learning Techniques* | *Salient Points* | *Challenges/ Future Scope* |
|---|---|---|---|---|---|
| *Soft computing approaches for image segmentation: a survey.* | Siddharth Singh Chouhan, Ajay Kaul & Uday Pratap Singh | Springer 2018 | Fuzzy logic, ANN, genetic algorithms. | Presents image segmentation applications using soft computing methods. | New methods of performing segmentation must be developed. |
| *Deep Learning Techniques for medical Image Segmentation: Achievements and Challenges.* | Mohammad Hesam Hesamian, Wenjing Jia, Xiangjian He, Paul Kennedy | Springer 2019 | Deep learning, convolutional neural network (CNN). | Network structure approaches, training techniques and challenges. | Increasing size of training dataset may help to solve overfitting problem. |
| *A Review: Deep Learning for medical image segmentation using multi-modality fusion.* | Tongxue Zhou, Su Ruan, Stephane Canu | Elsevier 2017 | Network architecture – CNN, fusion strategies, morphological techniques. | Deep learning-based approaches in multimodal medical image segmentation tasks. | Overfitting, class imbalance. |

| *Title* | *Author* | *Publication & Year* | *Machine Learning Techniques* | *Salient Points* | *Challenges/ Future Scope* |
|---|---|---|---|---|---|
| *Segmentation and feature extraction in medical imaging: A systematic review* | Chiranji Lal Choudhary, D.P. Acharjya | Elsevier 2019 | Fuzzy segmentation techniques, clustering-based segmentation. | Various segmentation and feature extraction methods in medical images for pre-processing. | Hybridization algorithms must be designed. |
| *A Comparative Analysis of Medical Image Segmentation* | Neeraj Shrivastava, Jyoti Bharti | Springer 2019 | Segmentation techniques, mammograms 98% accuracy. | Various segmentation techniques for mammograms and various positive/ negative factor parameters. | Automatic seed point selection algorithm must be designed for improved seed point analysis. |

6. **Feature extraction:** the process of lowering the dimensionality of an image by expressing the region of interest as feature vectors.
7. **Soft computing:** a collection of strategies that are used to simulate human thinking capacities in order to solve real-world problems.

### *1.2.3 Registration Using ML*

#### *1.2.3.1 Introduction*

The process of transforming several photographs into a single coordinate system is known as registration. This step is required when analyzing photographs taken from various perspectives, at various times, and with various modalities. Previously, clinicians had to perform picture registration manually, and most registration tasks can be extremely difficult. Manual alignment quality is heavily dependent on the user's expertise, which might be therapeutically detrimental. Automatic registration was created to compensate for the flaws in manual registration (see Figure 1.4).Several deep learning approaches for automatic image registration have been intensively investigated, transforming picture registration as shown in Figure 1.2.

Registering the input images is the initial step in the image fusion technique. When the mapping process contains input images and uses a referenced image, this is defined as the image registration process. The purpose of the mapping process is to match images based on features in order to help with the image fusion process (Figures 1.3 and 1.4) (Tables 1.5 and 1.6).

## 1.3 Deep Learning in Medical Imaging

Deep learning-based picture segmentation has proven to be a reliable approach for image segmentation. To separate homogeneous regions of the diagnosis and treatment pipeline, deep learning techniques have been frequently deployed.

The pixels of lesions in background CT or MRI images are identified using medical image segmentation. Delivering complex information on the forms and sizes of lesions is one of the most important challenges in medical image analysis. Many academics have proposed a variety of automated segmentation techniques

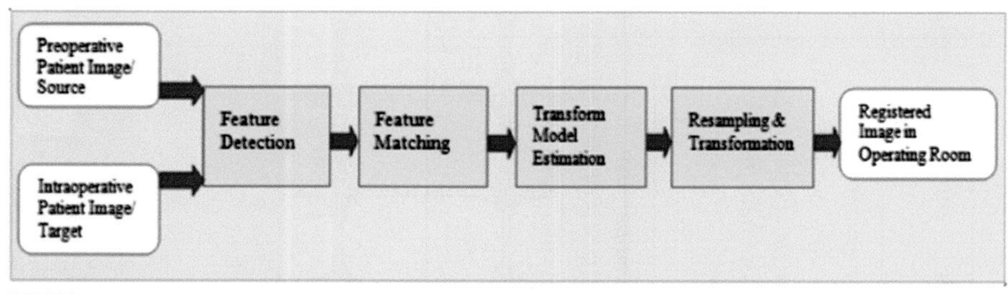


**Figure 1.2 The process of image registration.**

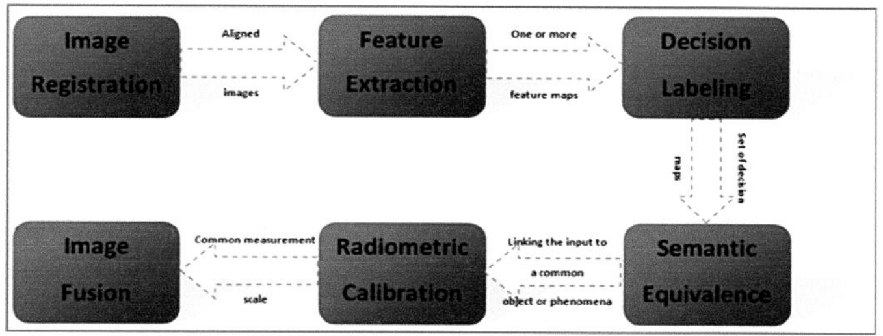


**Figure 1.3 The main steps of image fusion.**

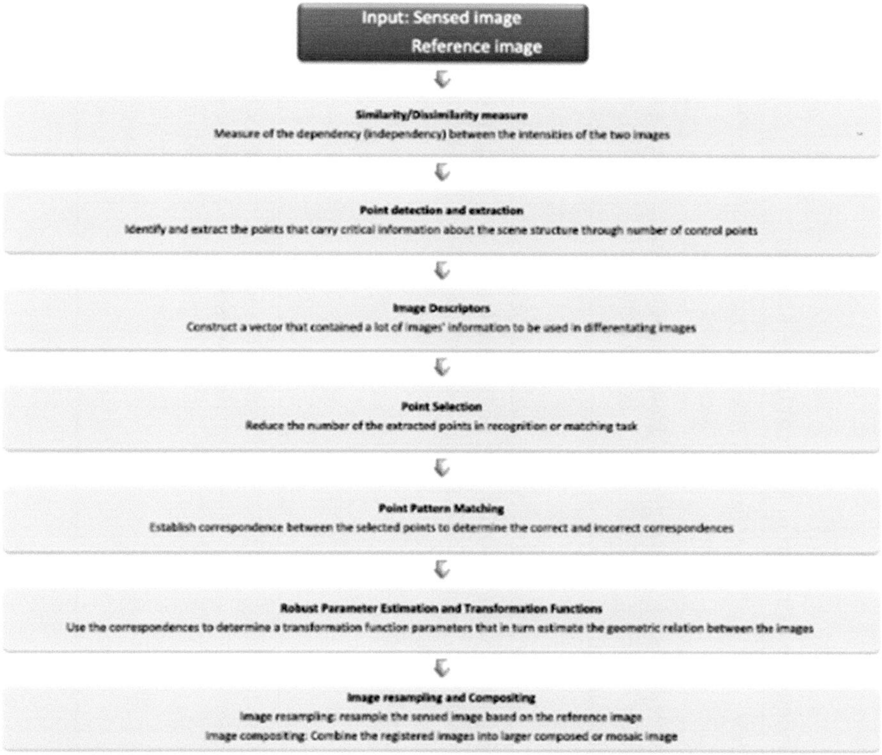

Input: Sensed image
Reference image

**Similarity/Dissimilarity measure**
Measure of the dependency (independency) between the intensities of the two images

**Point detection and extraction**
Identify and extract the points that carry critical information about the scene structure through number of control points

**Image Descriptors**
Construct a vector that contained a lot of images' information to be used in differentiating images

**Point Selection**
Reduce the number of the extracted points in recognition or matching task

**Point Pattern Matching**
Establish correspondence between the selected points to determine the correct and incorrect correspondences

**Robust Parameter Estimation and Transformation Functions**
Use the correspondences to determine a transformation function parameters that in turn estimate the geometric relation between the images

**Image resampling and Compositing**
Image resampling: resample the sensed image based on the reference image
Image compositing: Combine the registered images into larger composed or mosaic image

**Figure 1.4 Image registration steps.**

based on already available technologies. In the past, traditional technologies such as edge detection filters and mathematical methods were used to create systems. Machine learning, which now extracts individualized features, has proven to be a superior technique over time. The key concern in systems design has been to design and extract the features. The intricacies of these approaches have been cited as a major impediment to their implementation (Table 1.7).

**Table 1.5 Literature Review: Registration in Medical Image Analysis**

| *Title* | *Author* | *Publication & Year* | *Machine Learning Techniques* | *Salient Points* | *Challenges/Future Scope* |
|---|---|---|---|---|---|
| *Deep learning in medical image registration: a survey* | Grant Haskins, Uwe Kruger, Pingkun Yan1 | Springer 2020 | Deep convolutional neural network | Deep learning techniques, CNN for image registration | Better deep learning approach framework must be designed for multimodal registration of medical images. |
| *Medical image registration in image guided surgery: Issues, challenges and research opportunities* | Fakhre Alam Sami Ur Rahman, Sehat Ullah, Kamal Gulati | Elsevier 2017 | Segmentation-based registration techniques. | Popular types of image registration, process of registration, classification of registration and fusion | Feature-based registration technique and point pattern matching create difficulties when medical images contain noise and missing data. |
| *Image Registration of Medical Images* | Sehrish Jamil Gul, E Saman | IEEE 2017 | Feature-based classification, image registration techniques. | New technique proposed based on feature-based image registration using speeded-up robust features | Generic registration algorithms required that work in all cases, choice of data and optimization strategy remain highly problem specific. |

| *Title* | *Author* | *Publication & Year* | *Machine Learning Techniques* | *Salient Points* | *Challenges/Future Scope* |
|---|---|---|---|---|---|
| *Medical image registration using deep neural networks: A comprehensive review* | Hamid Reza Boveir, Raouf Khayami, Reza Javidan, Alireza Mehdizadeh | Elsevier 2020 | Deep neural network | This paper focuses on optimization-based image registration techniques and deep learning techniques for medical image registration. | Multistage and multi-resolution policy, apply spatial transformer network. |
| *Current trends in medical image registration and fusion* | Fatma El-Zahraa, Ahmed El-Gamal, Mohammed Elmogy, Ahmed Atwan | Elsevier | Hybrid-based registration techniques, segmentation-based registration techniques. | Challenges in medical image registration and fusion. | Availability of dataset and medical modality challenges. |

**Table 1.6 Combined Literature Review: Pre-processing, Segmentation and Registration in Medical Images**

| *Title* | *Author* | *Publication & Year* | *Machine Learning Techniques* | *Salient Points* | *Challenges/Future Scope* |
|---|---|---|---|---|---|
| *Deep learning in medical image registration: a survey* | Grant Haskins, Uwe Kruger, Pingkun Yan1 | Springer 2020 | Deep convolutional neural networks. | CNN for image registration techniques. | Improved deep learning-based frameworks should be designed for multimodal registration of medical images. |
| *Medical image registration in image guided surgery: Issues, challenges and research opportunities* | Fakhre Alam, Sami Ur Rahman, Sehat Ullah, Kamal Gulati | Elsevier 2017 | Segmentation-based registration techniques. | Popular types of image registration, process of registration, classification of registration and fusion. | Point pattern matching creates difficulties in feature-based registration, when medical images contain noise and missing data. |
| *Image Registration of Medical Images* | Sehrish Jamil Gul E Saman | IEEE 2017 | Feature-based classification, image registration techniques. | Proposes new feature-based image registration technique using speeded-up robust feature. | Generic registration algorithms that work in all cases required. Choice of data and optimization strategy remain highly problem specific. |

| *Title* | *Author* | *Publication & Year* | *Machine Learning Techniques* | *Salient Points* | *Challenges/Future Scope* |
|---|---|---|---|---|---|
| *Medical image registration using deep neural networks: A comprehensive review* | Hamid Reza Boveir, Raouf Khayami, Reza Javidan a, Alireza Mehdizadeh | Elsevier 2020 | Deep neural network | Optimization-based image registration techniques and deep learning techniques for medical image registration. | Multistage and multi-resolution policy, apply spatial transformer network. |
| *Current trends in medical image registration and fusion* | Fatma El-Zahraa Ahmed El-Gamal, Mohammed Elmogy, Ahmed Atwan | Elsevier | Hybrid-based and segmentation-based registration techniques. | Current challenges in medical image registration and fusion approach through analyzing process. | Availability of dataset and medical modality challenges. |
| *Deep Learning for Medical Image Processing: Overview, Challenges and the Future* | Muhammad Imran Razzak, Saeeda Naz and Ahmad Zaib | SPRINGER 2018 | Convolutional neural networks | Deep learning techniques rather than machine learning approaches. Accuracy 95.79%. | Need to capitalize on big image data advances in deep learning and use of methods black-boxes, their acceptance by health professionals. |

*(Continued)*

**Table 1.6 *(Continued)* Combined Literature Review: Pre-processing, Segmentation and Registration in Medical Images**

| *Title* | *Author* | *Publication & Year* | *Machine Learning Techniques* | *Salient Points* | *Challenges/Future Scope* |
|---|---|---|---|---|---|
| *MRI Based Medical Image Analysis: Survey on brain tumor grade classification* | Geethu Mohan, M. Monica Subashini | Elsevier 2017 | Support vector machine and artificial neural network | The focus of this paper is to include segmentation technique and tumor based classification techniques of brain magnetic resonance images. | Tumor segmentation model should be excluding contrast enhanced blood vessels and include tumor areas with con-trast enhancement. |
| *Soft computing approaches for image segmentation: a survey* | Siddharth Singh Chouhan & Ajay Kaul & Uday Pratap Singh | Springer 2018 | Fuzzy logic, artificial neural networks, and genetic algorithm for segmentation | The focus of this paper is to present the application of image segmentation using soft computing methods. | New methods to perform segmentation must be developed. |
| *Deep Learning Techniques for medical Image Segmentation: Achievements and Challenges* | Mohammad Hesam Hesamian, Wenjing Jia, Xiangjian He, Paul Kennedy | Springer 2019 | Deep learning, convolutional neural network (CNN) | Network structure approaches, training techniques and challenges. | Overfitting, Reason is the small size of the training dataset. So, increase in the size of data may help to solve the overfitting problem as well. |

| *Title* | *Author* | *Publication & Year* | *Machine Learning Techniques* | *Salient Points* | *Challenges/Future Scope* |
|---|---|---|---|---|---|
| *A Review: Deep Learning for medical image segmentation using multi-modality fusion.* | Tongxue Zhou Su Ruan, St ephane Canu | Elsevier 2017 | Netwok architecture – CNN, fusion strategies, morphological techniques. | In this paper the main focus is on the deep learning techniques approaches in multi modal medical image segmentation tasks. | Overfitting, class imbalance. |
| *Segmentation and feature extraction in medical imaging: A systematic review* | Chiranji Lal Choudhary, D.P. Acharjya | Elsevier 2019 | Fuzzy segmentation techniques, clustering-based segmentation. | The main focus is on the various segmentation and feature extraction methods in medical images for pre-processing. | Hybridization algorithms must be designed. |
| *A Comparative Analysis of Medical Image Segmentation* | Neeraj Shrivastava and Jyoti Bharti | Springer 2019 | Segmentation techniques, mammograms – accuracy 98%. | The focus of this paper is to use various segmentation techniques mammograms and various positive negative factors parameters. | Automatic seed point selection algorithm must be designed for analysis better seed point. |

**Table 1.7 Deep Learning Models**

| *Types of network* | *Detail of networks* | *Pros* | *Cons* |
|---|---|---|---|
| Deep neural network (DNN) | Has more than two layers, which allows for complicated non-linear relationships and can be used for both classification and regression. | Mostly used with great accuracy and precision. | Training procedure is not simple since errors are propagated back to previous individual layers, resulting in extremely minor errors, and the model's learning process is also far too slow. |
| Convolutional neural network (CNN) | Ideal for two-dimensional data. Convolutional filters are also included, which convert 2D to 3D. | Excellent performance, and the model learns quickly. | Data that has been labeled is required for classification. |
| Recurrent neural network (RNN) | Capacity to memorize sequences in a large number of ways.<br>All steps and neurons share the same weights. | Can learn sequential events and model time dependencies. | Many challenges arise as a result of the diminishing gradient and the requirement for large datasets. |
| Deep conventional extreme learning machine (DC-ELM) | Uses a Gaussian probability function for sampling of local connections. | Sampling of local connection is improved by using probability function. | If the amount of labeled data is small and learning function is simple then initialization can possibly be effective. |

| *Types of network* | *Detail of networks* | *Pros* | *Cons* |
| --- | --- | --- | --- |
| Deep Boltzmann machine (DBM) | DBM is based on Boltzmann machines and comprises one-way connections between all hidden Layers. | For robust inference, top-down feedback incorporates ambiguous data. | For big datasets, parameter optimization is not possible. |
| Deep belief network (DBN) | Has a one-way link. Utilized in both supervised and unsupervised machine learning, and each sub-hidden network's layers serve as a detectable layer for the next layer. | Is a one-way network. Each sub-hidden network's layers and learning serve as a detectable layer for the next layer. | Initialization process makes the training process computationally high cost. |

## 1.4 Conclusion

This report presented three aspects of the medical imaging system: Image pre-processing, Image segmentation and image registration. Various deep learning architectures were described. A literature review of various pre-processing techniques, comparison of various image segmentation techniques and a combined literature review of all the three aspects are included.

## References

[1] C. L. Chowdhary and D. P. Acharjya, "Segmentation and feature extraction in medical imaging: A systematic review," *Procedia Computer Science*, vol. 167, pp. 26–36, 2020, doi: 10.1016/j.procs.2020.03.179.

[2] T. Zhou, S. Ruan, and S. Canu, "A review: Deep learning for medical image segmentation using multi-modality fusion," *Array*, vol. 3–4, p. 100004, Sep. 2019, doi: 10.1016/j.array.2019.100004.

[3] S. S. Chouhan, A. Kaul, and U. P. Singh, "Soft computing approaches for image segmentation: A survey," *Multimedia Tools and Applications*, vol. 77, no. 21, pp. 28483–28537, Nov. 2018, doi: 10.1007/s11042-018-6005-6.

[4] G. Mohan and M. M. Subashini, "MRI based medical image analysis: Survey on brain tumor grade classification," *Biomedical Signal Processing and Control*, vol. 39, pp. 139–161, Jan. 2018, doi: 10.1016/j.bspc.2017.07.007.

[5] M. I. Razzak, S. Naz, and A. Zaib, "Deep learning for medical image processing: Overview, challenges and the future," in Classification in BioApps, vol. 26, N. Dey, A. S. Ashour, and S. Borra, Eds. Cham: Springer International Publishing, 2018, pp. 323–350.

[6] N. Shrivastava and J. Bharti, "A comparative analysis of medical image segmentation," in International Conference on Advanced Computing Networking and Informatics: ICANI-2018, vol. 870, R. Kamal, M. Henshaw, and P. S. Nair, Eds. Singapore: Springer Singapore, 2019, pp. 459–467.

[7] F.E.-Z. A. El-Gamal, M. Elmogy, and A. Atwan, "Current trends in medical image registration and fusion," *Egyptian Informatics Journal*, vol. 17, no. 1, pp. 99–124, Mar. 2016, doi: 10.1016/j.eij.2015.09.002.

[8] F. P. Oliveira, and J. M. R. Tavares, (2014). "Medical image registration: A review," *Computer Methods in Biomechanics and Biomedical Engineering*, vol. 17, no. 2, pp. 73–93.

[9] H. R. Boveiri, R. Khayami, R. Javidan, and A. Mehdizadeh, "Medical image registration using deep neural networks: A comprehensive review," *Computers & Electrical Engineering*, vol. 87, p. 106767, Oct. 2020, doi: 10.1016/j.compeleceng.2020.106767.

[10] S. Jamil and G. E. Saman, "Image registration of medical images," in 2017 Intelligent Systems and Computer Vision (ISCV), 2017, pp. 1–9, doi: 10.1109/ISACV.2017.8054911.

[11] G. Haskins, U. Kruger, and P. Yan, "Deep learning in medical image registration: A survey," *Machine Vision and Applications*, vol. 31, no. 1–2, p. 8, Feb. 2020, doi: 10.1007/s00138-020-01060-x.

[12] F. Alam, S. U. Rahman, S. Ullah, and K. Gulati, "Medical image registration in image guided surgery: Issues, challenges and research opportunities," Biocybernetics and Biomedical Engineering, vol. 38, no. 1, pp. 71–89, 2018, doi:10.1016/j.bbe.2017.10.001.

[13] H. Sajedi and N. Pardakhti, "Age prediction based on brain MRI image: A survey," *Journal of Medical Systems*, vol. 43, no. 8, p. 279, Jul. 2019, doi: 10.1007/s10916-019-1401-7.
[14] V. Devi, "Diverse Fields of Medical Imagery."
[15] G. T. Selvi, "Extraction of Tumor Image from MRI Images Using Gabor XOR Pattern."
[16] P. Chinmayi, L. Agilandeeswari, and M. Prabukumar, "Survey of image processing techniques in medical image analysis: Challenges and methodologies," in *Proceedings of the Eighth International Conference on Soft Computing and Pattern Recognition (socpar 2016)*, vol. 614, A. Abraham, A. K. Cherukuri, A. M. Madureira, and A. K. Muda, Eds. Cham: Springer International Publishing, 2018, pp. 460–471.
[17] R. B. Jeyavathana, R. Balasubramanian, & A. A. Pandian, "A survey: Analysis on pre-processing and segmentation techniques for medical images," *International Journal of Research and Scientific Innovation (IJRSI)*, vol. *3*, no. 6, pp. 113–120, 2016.
[18] M. Sharma, G. N. Purohit, and S. Mukherjee, "Information retrieves from brain MRI images for tumor detection using hybrid technique K-means and Artificial Neural Network (KMANN)," in Networking Communication and Data Knowledge Engineering, vol. 4, G. M. Perez, K. K. Mishra, S. Tiwari, and M. C. Trivedi, Eds. Singapore: Springer Singapore, 2018, pp. 145–157.
[19] H. Dong, G. Yang, F. Liu, Y. Mo, and Y. Guo, "Automatic brain tumor detection and segmentation using U-net based fully convolutional networks," in Medical Image Understanding and Analysis, vol. 723, M. Valdés Hernández and V. González-Castro, Eds. Cham: Springer International Publishing, 2017, pp. 506–517.
[20] M. Berahim, N. A. Samsudin, and S. S. Nathan, "A review: Image analysis techniques to improve labeling accuracy of medical image classification," in Recent Advances on Soft Computing and Data Mining, vol. 700, R. Ghazali, M. M. Deris, N. M. Nawi, and J. H. Abawajy, Eds. Cham: Springer International Publishing, 2018, pp. 298–307.
[21] S. Kumar, S. Mishra, P. Asthana, and Pragya, "Automated detection of acute leukemia using K-mean clustering algorithm," in *Advances in Computer and Computational Sciences*, vol. 554, S. K. Bhatia, K. K. Mishra, S. Tiwari, and V. K. Singh, Eds. Singapore: Springer Singapore, 2018, pp. 655–670.
[22] T. T. Ademujimi, M. P. Brundage, and V. V. Prabhu, "A review of current machine learning techniques used in manufacturing diagnosis," in *Advances in Production Management Systems. The Path to Intelligent, Collaborative and Sustainable Manufacturing*, vol. 513, H. Lödding, R. Riedel, K.-D. Thoben, G. von Cieminski, and D. Kiritsis, Eds. Cham: Springer International Publishing, 2017, pp. 407–415.
[23] Q. Wang, Y. Shi, and D. Shen, "Machine learning in medical imaging," *IEEE Journal of Biomedical and Health Informatics*, vol. 23, no. 4, pp. 1361–1362, Jul. 2019.
[24] R. J. S. Raj, S. J. Shobana, I. V. Pustokhina, D. A. Pustokhin, D. Gupta, and K. Shankar, "Optimal feature selection-based medical image classification using deep learning model in internet of medical things," *IEEE Access*, vol. 8, pp. 58006–58017, 2020.
[25] J. H. Thrall, X. Li, Q. Li, C. Cruz, S. Do, K. Dreyer, and J. Brink, "Artificial intelligence and machine learning in radiology: Opportunities, challenges, pitfalls, and criteria for success," *Journal of the American College of Radiology*, vol. 15, no. 3 Pt B, pp. 504–508, Feb. 2018.
[26] G. Litjens, T. Kooi, B. E. Bejnordi, A. A. A. Setio, F. Ciompi, M. Ghafoorian, J. A. W. M. van der Laak, B. van Ginneken, and C. I. Sánchez, "A survey on deep learning in medical image analysis," *Medical Image Analysis*, vol. 42, pp. 60–88, Dec. 2017.

[27] D. Patel, Y. Shah, N. Thakkar, K. Shah, and M. Shah, "Implementation of artificial intelligence techniques for cancer detection," *Augmented Human Research*, vol. 5, no. 1, p. 6, Dec. 2020.
[28] A. Ravishankar, S. Anusha, H. K. Akshatha, A. Raj, S. Jahnavi, and J. Madhura, "A survey on noise reduction techniques in medical images," in *2017 International Conference of Electronics, Communication and Aerospace Technology (ICECA)*, 2017, pp. 385–389.
[29] M. Shukla and K. Kumar Sharma, "A comparative study to detect tumor in brain MRI images using clustering algorithms," in *2020 2nd International Conference on Innovative Mechanisms for Industry Applications (ICIMIA)*, 2020, pp. 773–777.
[30] D. D. Miller and E. W. Brown, "Artificial intelligence in medical practice: The question to the answer?" *The American Journal of Medicine*, vol. 131, no. 2, pp. 129–133, 2018.
[31] A. Maity, A. Pattanaik, S. Sagnika, and S. Pani, "A comparative study on approaches to speckle noise reduction in images," in *2015 International Conference on Computational Intelligence and Networks*, 2015, pp. 148–155.
[32] P. Kaur, G. Singh, and P. Kaur, "A review of denoising medical images using machine learning approaches," *Current Medical Imaging Reviews*, vol. 14, no. 5, pp. 675–685, Oct. 2018.
[33] A. Maier, C. Syben, T. Lasser, and C. Riess, "A gentle introduction to deep learning in medical image processing," *Zeitschrift für Medizinische Physik*, vol. 29, no. 2, pp. 86–101, May 2019.
[34] S. Huang, J. Yang, S. Fong, and Q. Zhao, "Artificial intelligence in cancer diagnosis and prognosis: Opportunities and challenges," *Cancer Letter*, vol. 471, pp. 61–71, Feb. 2020.

# Chapter 2

# Machine Learning in Radio Imaging

Nitesh Pradhan, Punit Gupta and Anita Shrotriya
*SCIT, Manipal University, Jaipur, India*

## Contents

2.1 Introduction ....................25
2.2 Analysis of Related Work ....................26
2.3 Summary ....................34
References ....................34

## 2.1 Introduction

The three-dimensional (3-D) structure of an organ illustrates its exact configuration and orientation and is therefore useful in the detection of disease in tissues or fractures in bones. This structure also gives information about chronic bone loss, such as a glenoid defect in recurrent shoulder dislocation and the extent of osteophytes in arthritic joints. Computer tomography (CT) scan and magnetic resonance imaging (MRI) provide a 3-D configuration of a bone. However, 2-dimensional (2-D) techniques are preferred due to the high cost and heavy exposure to the carcinogenic radiation incurred in 3-D techniques [1].

Dual-energy X-ray absorptiometry (DXA) images used to diagnose osteoporosis provide a T-score. A T-score value between +1 and −1 indicates healthy bone. A value between −1 and −2.5 shows that the bone has become prone to osteoporosis [2]. This state is called osteopenia. A value below 2.5 is an indication of the poor quality of a bone and a sign of osteoporosis. The decrease in bone mineral density

DOI: 10.1201/9781003322597-2

(BMD) characteristic of osteoporosis increases the risk of bone fracture. In Europe, 30% of women over the age of 50 years suffer from osteoporosis [3]. According to a 2000 report, 3.1 to 3.7 million cases of osteoporosis were recorded, with a direct treatment cost of 32 billion dollars, a cost that could rise to 76.8 billion dollars per year in 2050 if this trend continues [4].

X-ray imaging is a medical imaging technique used to capture bone deformities. This technique shows a clear demarcation between the bones and soft tissues and it is therefore easy to read information about any bone deformity. X-ray imaging is preferred over CT scan for weight-bearing imaging and dynamic imaging of joint motion (fluoroscopy) due to its high availability and low cost. A technique is required that can provide a 3-D view of a bone using 2-D imaging techniques such as DXA and X-ray. This chapter reviews 3-D and 2-D techniques used in medical imaging. Table 2.1 lists different medical imaging techniques, and ways of reconstructing 3-D images from 2-D images are shown in Figure 2.1.

## 2.2 Analysis of Related Work

Researchers have proposed various models for 3-D reconstruction of medical images from 2-D images.

Wei et al. [1] identified that X-ray imaging is preferred over CT scan due to the low intensity of exposure and low cost. They proposed a 3-D recreation system for the femoral shaft shape. They used an orthographical heading to recreate

**Table 2.1 Comparison of CT Scan, X-ray and DXA Techniques**

| *Parameters* | *CT Scan* | *X-ray* | *DXA* |
|---|---|---|---|
| Radiation vulnerability | Effective radiation dose from CT ranges from 2 to 10 millisievert (mSv) [5] | Exposure to ionizing radiation is about 0.1mSv [5] | Exposure to ionizing radiation lies in the range of 0.1μSv to 5μSv [6] |
| Cost | Cost of CT scan ranges from $1,200 to $3,200 [7] | Cost is from $1200 to $4000 [7] | Three times more costly than X-ray [8] |
| Time taken for complete scan | Takes about 5 minutes | Takes a few seconds | Takes more time than X-ray techniques but less time than CT scan technique |
| Application | Suitable for bone injuries, lung and chest imaging, cancer detection. | Useful to examine fractured bones and to diagnose diseases in tissues. | Useful to diagnose osteoporosis or measure BMD |

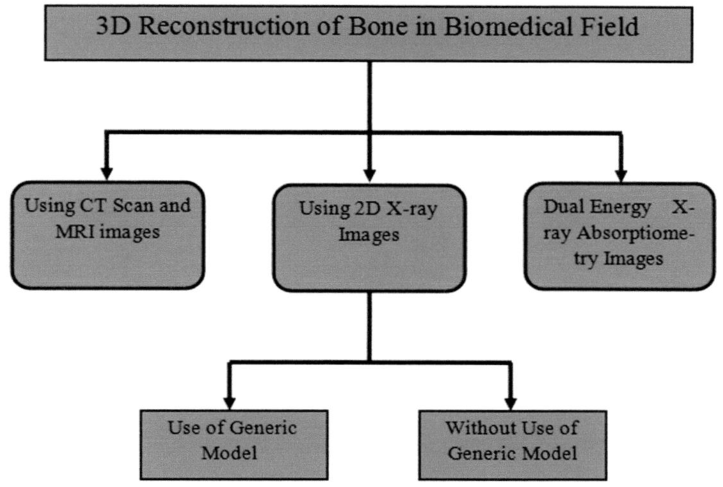


**Figure 2.1 Imaging in the biomedical field.**

a 3-D femur. They used a numerical morphology strategy for boundary detection. Further, they determined the central point of the femur shaft edge as a pole datum line. Then they computed three coordinates of the pole datum line by stamp point. Finally, their system displayed an enrolment of the 3-D layout model and state of the femur shaft by creating the boundary. This technique is useful to eliminate noise for tending to qualities of shapes but the computational time is high for the complex structure of the bone shape.

Zhang et al. proposed an effective strategy for 3-D recreation of the femur using direct linear transformation (DLT) [9]. Their strategy uses two orthogonal X-ray images – the anterior-posterior and lateral views – to reconstruct the 3-D structure. DLT does not required multiple images to calculate distortion boundaries. Therefore, its computational expense is low and it is used in various fields. The steps for 3-D reconstruction are shown in Figure 2.2.

A. Le Bras et al. performed a comparison-based examination for 3-D reconstruction of the proximal femur [10]. They used the 3-D CT scan remaking method and a 3-D stereo radiographic reconstruction method [10]. In the 3-D CT scan reconstruction they considered the following parameters: a scout view, volume, image procurement, and recreation. They input these parameters to the SliceOmatic software to obtain a 3-D reconstruction of the femur. In the 3-D stereo radiographic reconstruction method, the low-measurement computerized X-ray device performs a linear scanning of the femur in the posterior-anterior and lateral view. This method employs a non-stereo corresponding contours (NSCC) algorithm to develop 3-D reconstruction. The authors in [10]state that applying both methods on 25 proximal femora gave a low mean error value of P2S. The error reported is less than 2.0 mm. This proves the reliability of the 3-D stereo radiographic method of reconstruction.

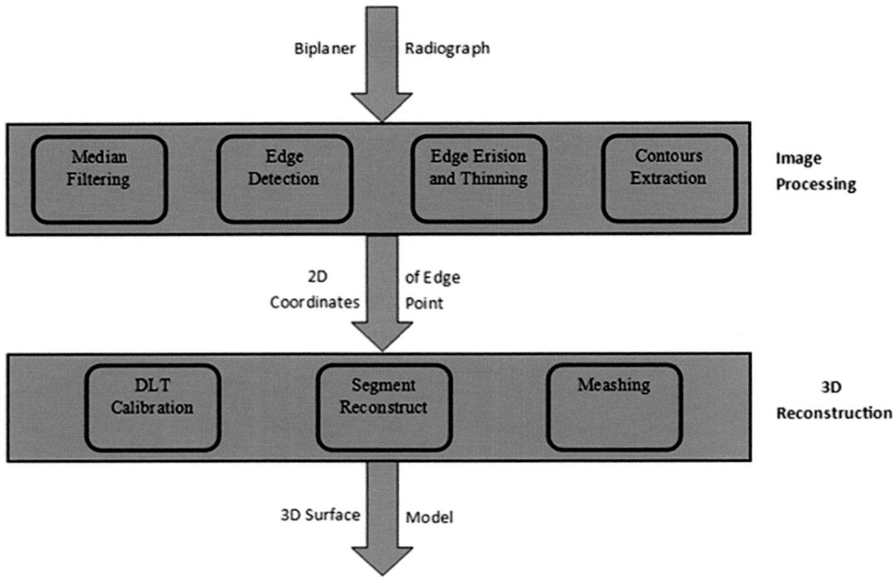


**Figure 2.2 Step-by-step 3-D reconstruction process.**

The advantage of this strategy is that it may well be utilized for hard structures with a constant shape but this technique is tedious in term of computational cost.

Kyung Koh et al. [11] built a 3-D format model of the femur from a healthy subject of ordinary height and weight. They considered two X-ray images and three CT scan images of five patients. They used a B spline free from deformation (FFD) to procure the patient-specific femur as shown in Figure 2.3. To control the deformation precision, FFD provides the facility to place the control points at variable distances. The control points are easily manipulated by FFD at lower cost. On the other hand, it is difficult to apply the FFD technique on complex structures.

Sonia Akkoul et al. [12] proposed a model for 3-D proximal femur surface recreation. The model uses pseudo-stereo matching and 3-D point from the highest quality level to decrease the non-availability of data. They used three cadaveric proximal femurs scanned with CT scans and X-ray images. They followed a set of steps for the 3-D reconstruction of the proximal femur. In the first stage, they used the projection display to discover an angle between two X-ray images of a femur. In the next stage, the system marks the boundary of the femur using active contours. In the third stage, the system finds the coordinating point between 2-D shapes using the Euclidian distance. The system then produces a 3-D point cloud. Next it applies the iterative closed point (ICP) algorithm for 3-D rigid registration. In the final stage, the system applies a meshing technique to find the 3-D shape of the proximal femur. The ICP algorithm is straightforward and simple to implement but it calculates the starting value of the iteration in the first step which should be correctly initialized; otherwise, this algorithm suffers from the local optimum problem.

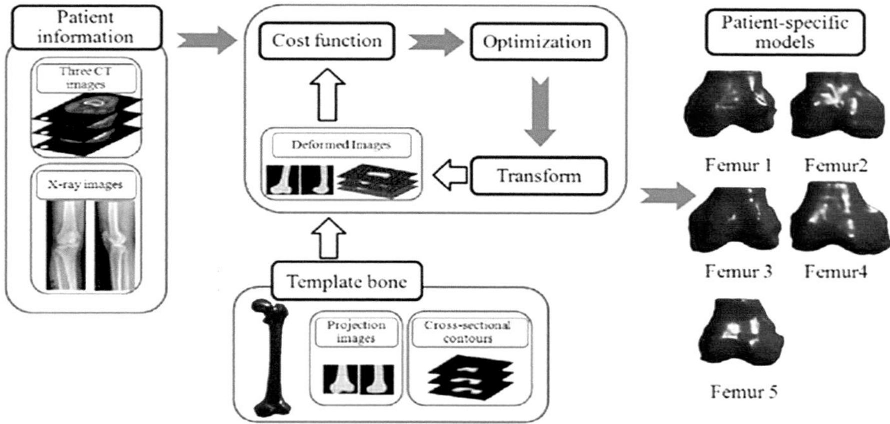


**Figure 2.3 Spine FFD.**

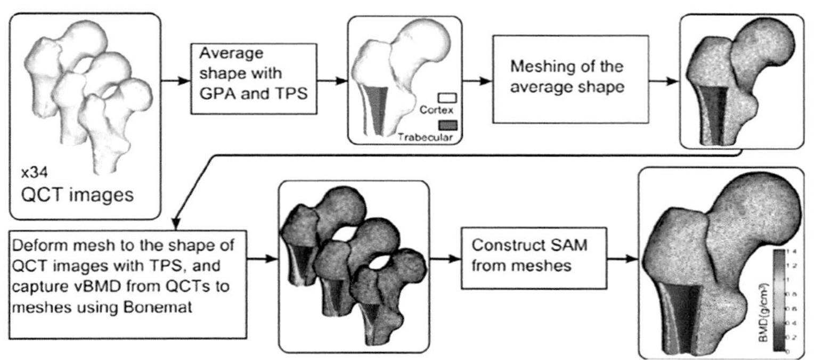


**Figure 2.4 Development of SAM model.**

Sami P. Vaananen et al. [13] proposed a programmed technique for reconstruction of a 3-D shape. They applied a structured auxiliary mesh (SAM) algorithm for this purpose as shown in Figure 2.4. The authors used three sets of bone images. The two sets of bone images were used for training the model and the remaining third set of bone images is used as a testing dataset for the model.

N. Baka et al. [14] proposed a statistical shape model (SSM)-based technique for the posture estimation and shape reconstruction of a 3-D bone surface using two X-ray images. The SSM technique captures the global shape of the surface without reducing the size of the object.

P.E. Galibarov et al. proposed a patient-specific proximal femur surface reconstruction model [15]. They applied their model to planer radiographs. The model completes the reconstruction in three steps. First, the contours of the femur are extracted from the planer radiograph. Next, a coordinating process is performed on the extracted contours. In the last step, the 3-D geometry is reconstructed.

P. Gamage et al. proposed a technique for the 3-D remaking of a patient-specific bone model from 2-D radiographs [16]. They extracted the edge points from 2-D X-ray images to determine the boundary of the femur. Then they applied a non-rigid registration between the edges recognized in the radiograph. They projected the contours point of the genetic model. The translational field then distinguishes the deformation required by the 3-D anatomical model in the anterior and lateral viewpoint. In the final step, an entire 3-D translational field is developed through a thin plate spline (TPS) based on insertion and the 3-D generic anatomical data. The TPS technique does not include surface patches in a calculation that gives robust results. On the other hand, if the data size is too large, there is an issue with edge points.

Tristan Whitmarsh et al. [17] proposed a reconstruction model for the 3-D shape of the proximal femur from a single DXA. This technique uses a statistical model applied to a large data set of quantitative computerized tomography (QCT) scans (Table 2.2).

Guoyan Zheng et al. proposed a partial least-square regression (PLSR) model for the 3-D reconstruction of volumetric intensity from 2-D X-ray images [20]. In this technique, the authors used the independent statistical shape and displacement and appearance (DA) approach. The PLSR technique can easily handle the multi-collinearity between the independent points at the time of 3-D reconstruction. On the other hand PLSR needs a large amount of data for training.

Moon Kyu Lee et al. created a 3-D model to complete a femoral bone [21]. The authors used a regular X-ray image and joined anatomical parameters such as neck length, femoral length, head offset length, anatomical axis, and sagittal radius into a referential 3-D shape. They calculated the internal position and range of the femoral head by nonlinear regression. They determined the center point of the anatomical axis by applying elliptical regression.

Haithem Boussaid et al. [22] proposed a model for the 3-D reconstruction of the proximal femur using low-dose biplanar X-ray images.

S. Laporte et al. worked on a 3-D reconstruction model by detecting the contours from biplanar radiographs [23]. They employed the DLT and non-stereoradiography corresponding points algorithms (NSCP) for the reproduction of the

**Table 2.2 Performance comparison of 3-D Reconstruction Models on Different Image Types**

| *Image used* | *Average Error* | *Root Mean Square Error (RMS)* | *Number of projections* |
|---|---|---|---|
| Single DXA image [17] | 1.1 mm | 2.6 mm | 1 |
| X-ray image [18] | 1.2 mm | 2.8 mm | 2 |
| Two DXA image [19] | 0.8 mm | 2.1 mm | 2 |

structure. NSCP fails in structures such as the knee joint. Therefore, the authors applied the NSCC algorithm to recreate the 3-D shape of the bone.

Ryo Kurazume et al. proposed a technique for the 3-D reconstruction of a femoral shape using a parametric approach [24]. They performed statistical analysis of 3-D femoral shapes obtained from CT scan images of 56 patients. They employed manual segmentation and marching cubes algorithms, and principal component analysis (PCA) [25].

S. Kolta et al. [26] proposed a model for the 3-D reconstruction of proximal femur bone from a DXA image. The model works by detecting the contours in the images.

V.H. Kim et al. used the simulated implantation system (SIS) [27] for 3-D perception and numerical investigations between the artificial hip joint and the femur [28, 29]. The architecture of 3-D reconstruction simulation systems is shown in Figure 2.5.

Vikas Karade et al. [30] proposed a Laplacian surface deformation (LSD)-based technique for 3-D femur reconstruction from biplanar X-ray images.

Moritz Ehlke et al. introduced a GPU-based method to render virtual X-ray projections of deformable tetrahedral networks for 3-D geometry reconstruction from X-ray [31].

Guoyan Zheng et al. introduced a 2-D to 3-D correspondence-building technique by a point-matching procedure in non-rigid 2-D structures [18]. They employed the adapted ICP algorithm [32] in the first stage and statistical instantiation in the second phase. The authors applied regularized shape deformation in the third stage [33].

The above discussion shows that many researchers have proposed techniques for the reconstruction of 3-D medical images [1, 9–16]. These techniques, which focus on the reconstruction of the femur, are based on a numerical morphology strategy for boundary detection [1], DLT [9], 3-D stereo radiographic reconstruction [10], B spline FFD [11], SSM [14], contour detection [15], and edge detection [16] for the reconstruction of a 3-D view of the femur from 2-D images. These techniques report low accuracy due to ineffectiveness in detecting edges or boundaries. A performance comparison of the most effective techniques is given in Table 2.3.

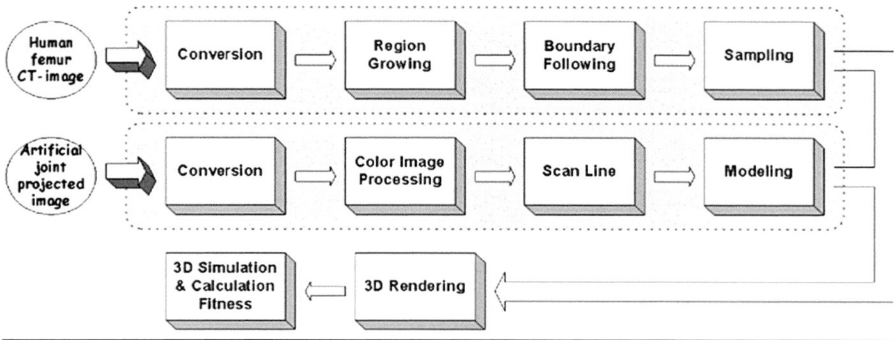


**Figure 2.5 Architecture of 3-D reconstruction simulation systems.**

**Table 2.3 Comparative Analysis of Methods of 3-D Reconstruction**

| *S. No* | *Author* | *Method* | *Shape* | *Input* | *Contour Generations* | *Number of Cases* | *Mean P2S Error* | *RMS P2S Errror* | *Computation Time (S)* | *System Configuration* |
|---|---|---|---|---|---|---|---|---|---|---|
| 1 | Karade et al. [30] | LSD-SOM | Distal femur | Real | Manual | 5 | 1.2 | 1.4 | 52 | Intel. 2.4 GHz, 8GB |
| 2 | Karade et al. [30] | LSD-SOM | Distal femur | Simulated | Automatic | 22 | 1.2 | 1.5 | 46 | Intel. 2.4 GHz, 8GB |
| 3 | Filippi et al. [34] | FFD | Full Femur | Simulated | Manual | 5 | 1.4 | — | — | — |
| 4 | Gunay et al. [35] | FFD | Tibia | Real | — | — | — | | 100 | AMD, 1GHz |
| 5 | Baka et al. [14] | SSM | Distal Femur | Real | Automatic (canny) | 10 | — | 1.68 | 300 | 2.4 GHz, 2GB |
| 6 | Zhu et al. [36] | SSM | Distal Femur | Real | Manual | 10 | 0.9 | | 178 | Intel 2.67 GHz, 9GB |
| 7 | Fleute et al. [37] | SSM | Distal Femur | Simulated | Automatic | — | — | 1.0 | 60 | — |
| 8 | Gamage et al. [38] | TPS | Full femur | Real | Automatic | 6 | 0.9 | — | — | — |
| 9 | Laporte et al. [39] | NSCC | Distal femur | Real | Semi-automatic | 8 | — | 1.4 | — | — |

| *S. No* | *Author* | *Method* | *Shape* | *Input* | *Contour Generations* | *Number of Cases* | *Mean P2S Error* | *RMS P2S Errror* | *Computation Time (S)* | *System Configuration* |
|---|---|---|---|---|---|---|---|---|---|---|
| 10 | Tang et al. [40] | Hybrid atlas | Distal Femur | Simulated | Automatic | 2 | 2.0 | – | – | – |
| 11 | Le Bras. et al. [10] | NSCC | Proximal Femur | Real | Manual | 28 | 2.0 | – | – | – |
| 12 | S. Kolta et al. [26] | NSCC | Proximal femur | Real | Manual | 25 | 0.8 | 2.1 | 600 | – |
| 13 | Ryo et al. [24] | SSM | Proximal Femur | Real | Manual | 56 | 1.1 | – | – | – |
| 14 | Gyoyan et al. [18] | SSM | Femur | Simulated | automatic | – | 1.1 | 1.4 | – | – |
| 15 | Galibarov et al. [15] | SSM | Proximal femur | Real | Manual | 32 | 3.04 | – | 300 | 4 CPU, 3GHz |
| 16 | Tristan et al. [17] | SSM | Proximal femur | Real | Automatic | 115 | 1.1 | 2.6 | – | – |
| 17 | Sonia et al. [12] | SSM | Proximal Femur | Simulated | Automatic | 3 | 0.89 | 1.37 | – | – |
| 18 | Sami et al. [13] | SAM | Proximal femur | Real | Manual | 83 | 1.42 | – | – | – |

Furthermore, existing techniques can be categorized into three classes – manual, simulated and automatic – based on the methodology used for contour detection. An analysis of these techniques clearly shows that the automatic techniques report the minimum value of root mean square (RMS) P2S error and mean square (MS) P2S error (Table 2.3). The automatic techniques also take less time for contour detection and hence are adopted for 3-D reconstruction.

However, although the automation of 3-D reconstruction has been observed in the literature, the systems are not intelligent. They do not learn from the errors generated. So, there is low scope for reducing errors. Moreover, existing techniques rely solely on the input dataset available or data generated by simulation. The techniques are incapable of generating a dataset if a small dataset is given as input. Some recent work in the fiend of medical image processing are [41–43]

## 2.3 Summary

This chapter reviewed the techniques used for 3-D reconstruction from 2-D medical imaging. The techniques may be manual, simulated, or automatic. The automatic techniques outperform the manual and simulated techniques in terms of MS P2S error, RMS P2S error, and computation time, as shown in Table 2.3. However, automatic techniques lack dataset self-generation in cases where a small dataset is available. They are also unable to learn from the errors generated, reducing scope for improvement.

Based on the above discussion, we conclude that automatic techniques can be adopted for the 3-D reconstruction of the femur from its 2-D images. However, there is huge scope for developing automatic and intelligent techniques for reconstruction of 3-D structures from 2-D medical images. The use of optimized neural network architectures such as generative adversarial networks (GAN) can resolve the challenges of manual, simulated and automatic techniques used for 3-D reconstruction. Our review of existing techniques suggests that there is scope for developing organ-specific, patient-specific, automatic, and intelligent models for 3-D reconstruction. The use of machine learning and deep learning can be game changers in this application. There is also huge scope for applying optimization algorithms for improving the efficiency and accuracy of 3-D reconstruction models.

## References

[1] Wei, W., Wang, G., and Chen, H. (2009, July). 3D reconstruction of a femur shaft using a model and two 2D X-ray images. In *2009 4th International Conference on Computer Science and Education* (pp. 720–722). IEEE.

[2] Garg, M. K., and Kharb, S. (2013). Dual energy X-ray absorptiometry: Pitfalls in measurement and interpretation of bone mineral density. *Indian Journal of Endocrinology and Metabolism, 17*(2), 203.

[3] Melton III, L. J., Chrischilles, E. A., Cooper, C., Lane, A. W., and Riggs, B. L. (2005). How many women have osteoporosis? *Journal of Bone and Mineral Research*, *20*(5), 886–892.

[4] Kanis, J. A., and Johnell, O. (2005). Requirements for DXA for the management of osteoporosis in Europe. *Osteoporosis International*, *16*(3), 229–238.

[5] Smith-Bindman, R., Lipson, J., Marcus, R., Kim, K. P., Mahesh, M., Gould, R., and Miglioretti, D. L. (2009). Radiation dose associated with common computed tomography examinations and the associated lifetime attributable risk of cancer. *Archives of Internal Medicine*, *169*(22), 2078–2086.

[6] Guggenheimer, Steve, and Butler, Susan (2019, November). Ionising Radiation Management Guidelines, The University of Melbourne.

[7] Ibrahim, Khalid (2017, August 27). Magnetic Resonance Imaging-MRI, *Health and Medicine*.

[8] Islamian, J. P., Garoosi, I., Fard, K. A., and Abdollahi, M. R. (2016). Comparison between the MDCT and the DXA scanners in the evaluation of BMD in the lumbar spine densitometry. *The Egyptian Journal of Radiology and Nuclear Medicine*, *47*(3), 961–967.

[9] Zhang, B., Sun, S., Sun, J., Chi, Z., and Xi, C. (2010, September). 3D reconstruction method from biplanar radiography using DLT algorithm: Application to the femur. In *2010 First International Conference on Pervasive Computing, Signal Processing and Applications* (pp. 251–254). IEEE.

[10] Le Bras, A., Laporte, S., Bousson, V., Mitton, D., De Guise, J. A., Laredo, J. D., and Skalli, W. (2003, June). Personalised 3D reconstruction of proximal femur from low-dose digital biplanar radiographs. *International Congress Series*, *1256*, 214–219. Elsevier.

[11] Koh, K., Kim, Y. H., Kim, K., and Park, W. M. (2011). Reconstruction of patient-specific femurs using X-ray and sparse CT images. *Computers in Biology and Medicine*, *41*(7), 421–426.

[12] Akkoul, S., Hafiane, A., Leconge, R., Harrar, K., Lespessailles, E., and Jennane, R. (2014, October). 3D reconstruction method of the proximal femur and shape correction. In *2014 4th International Conference on Image Processing Theory, Tools and Applications (IPTA)* (pp. 1–6). IEEE.

[13] Väänänen, S. P., Grassi, L., Flivik, G., Jurvelin, J. S., and Isaksson, H. (2015). Generation of 3D shape, density, cortical thickness and finite element mesh of proximal femur from a DXA image. *Medical Image Analysis*, *24*(1), 125–134.

[14] Baka, N., Kaptein, B. L., de Bruijne, M., van Walsum, T., Giphart, J. E., Niessen, W. J., and Lelieveldt, B. P. (2011). 2D–3D shape reconstruction of the distal femur from stereo X-ray imaging using statistical shape models. *Medical Image Analysis*, *15*(6), 840–850.

[15] Galibarov, P. E., Prendergast, P. J., and Lennon, A. B. (2010). A method to reconstruct patient-specific proximal femur surface models from planar pre-operative radiographs. *Medical Engineering and Physics*, *32*(10), 1180–1188.

[16] Gamage, P., Xie, S. Q., Delmas, P., and Xu, P. (2009, December). 3D reconstruction of patient specific bone models from 2D radiographs for image guided orthopedic surgery. In *2009 Digital Image Computing: Techniques and Applications* (pp. 212–216). IEEE.

[17] Whitmarsh, T., Humbert, L., De Craene, M., Barquero, L. M. D. R., and Frangi, A. F. (2011). Reconstructing the 3D shape and bone mineral density distribution of the proximal femur from dual-energy X-ray absorptiometry. *IEEE Transactions on Medical Imaging*, *30*(12), 2101–2114.

[18] Zheng, G., Gollmer, S., Schumann, S., Dong, X., Feilkas, T., and Ballester, M. A. G. (2009). A 2D/3D correspondence building method for reconstruction of a patient-specific 3D bone surface model using point distribution models and calibrated X-ray images. *Medical Image Analysis, 13*(6), 883–899.

[19] Kolta, S., Le Bras, A., Mitton, D., Bousson, V., de Guise, J. A., Fechtenbaum, J., ... Skalli, W. (2005). Three-dimensional X-ray absorptiometry (3D–XA): A method for reconstruction of human bones using a dual X-ray absorptiometry device. *Osteoporosis International, 16*(8), 969–976.

[20] Zheng, G. (2013, April). 3D volumetric intensity reconstruction from 2D x-ray images using partial least squares regression. In *2013 IEEE 10th International Symposium on Biomedical Imaging* (pp. 1268–1271). IEEE.

[21] Lee, M. K., Lee, S. H., Kim, A., Youn, I., Lee, T. S., Hur, N., and Choi, K. (2008). The study of femoral 3D reconstruction process based on anatomical parameters using a numerical method. *Journal of Biomechanical Science and Engineering, 3*(3), 443–451.

[22] Boussaid, H., Kadoury, S., Kokkinos, I., Lazennec, J. Y., Zheng, G., and Paragios, N. (2011, August). 3D Model-based reconstruction of the proximal femur from low-dose biplanar x-ray images. In *3D Model-Based Reconstruction of the Proximal Femur from Low-Dose Biplanar X-ray Images* (pp. 1–10).

[23] Laporte, S., Skalli, W., De Guise, J. A., Lavaste, F., and Mitton, D. (2003). A biplanar reconstruction method based on 2D and 3D contours: Application to the distal femur. *Computer Methods in Biomechanics and Biomedical Engineering, 6*(1), 1–6.

[24] Kurazume, R., Nakamura, K., Okada, T., Sato, Y., Sugano, N., Koyama, T., ... Hasegawa, T. (2009). 3D reconstruction of a femoral shape using a parametric model and two 2D fluoroscopic images. *Computer Vision and Image Understanding, 113*(2), 202–211.

[25] Chui, H., and Rangarajan, A. (2003). A new point matching algorithm for non-rigid registration. *Computer Vision and Image Understanding, 89*(2–3), 114–141.

[26] Kolta, S., Le Bras, A., Mitton, D., Bousson, V., de Guise, J. A., Fechtenbaum, J., ... Skalli, W. (2005). Three-dimensional X-ray absorptiometry (3D-XA): A method for reconstruction of human bones using a dual X-ray absorptiometry device. *Osteoporosis International, 16*(8), 969–976.

[27] Kim, Y. H., Kim, J. K., and Choi, K. (2004). Three-dimensional reconstruction of human femur using consecutive computer tomography images and simulated implantation system. *Journal of Medical Engineering and Technology, 28*(5), 205–210.

[28] Watt, A., and Policarpo, F. (1998). *The Computer Image* (Reading, MA: Addison-Wesley).

[29] Gonzalez, R. C., and Woods, R. E. (1992). *Digital Image Processing* (Reading, MA: Addison-Wesley).

[30] Karade, V., and Ravi, B. (2015). 3D femur model reconstruction from biplane X-ray images: A novel method based on Laplacian surface deformation. *International Journal of Computer Assisted Radiology and Surgery, 10*(4), 473–485.

[31] Ehlke, M., Ramm, H., Lamecker, H., Hege, H. C., and Zachow, S. (2013). Fast generation of virtual X-ray images for reconstruction of 3D anatomy. *IEEE Transactions on Visualization and Computer Graphics, 19*(12), 2673–2682.

[32] Guéziec, A., Kazanzides, P., Williamson, B., and Taylor, R. H. (1998). Anatomy-based registration of CT-scan and intraoperative X-ray images for guiding a surgical robot. *IEEE Transactions on Medical Imaging, 17*(5), 715–728.

[33] Rajamani, K. T., Styner, M. A., Talib, H., Zheng, G., Nolte, L. P., and Ballester, M. A. G. (2007). Statistical deformable bone models for robust 3D surface extrapolation from sparse data. *Medical Image Analysis, 11*(2), 99–109.

[34] Filippi, S., Motyl, B., and Bandera, C. (2008). Analysis of existing methods for 3D modelling of femurs starting from two orthogonal images and development of a script for a commercial software package. *Computer Methods and Programs in Biomedicine, 89*(1), 76–82.

[35] Gunay, M., Shim, M. B., and Shimada, K. (2007). Cost- and time-effective three-dimensional bone-shape reconstruction from X-ray images. *The International Journal of Medical Robotics and Computer Assisted Surgery, 3*(4), 323–335.

[36] Zhu, Z., and Li, G. (2011). Construction of 3D human distal femoral surface models using a 3D statistical deformable model. *Journal of Biomechanics, 44*(13), 2362–2368.

[37] Fleute, M., and Lavallée, S. (1999, September). Nonrigid 3-D/2-D registration of images using statistical models. In *International Conference on Medical Image Computing and Computer-Assisted Intervention* (pp. 138–147). Springer, Berlin, Heidelberg.

[38] Gamage, P., Xie, S. Q., Delmas, P., and Xu, P. (2009, December). 3D reconstruction of patient specific bone models from 2D radiographs for image guided orthopedic surgery. In *2009 Digital Image Computing: Techniques and Applications* (pp. 212–216). IEEE.

[39] Bredbenner, T. L., Eliason, T. D., Potter, R. S., Mason, R. L., Havill, L. M., and Nicolella, D. P. (2010). Statistical shape modeling describes variation in tibia and femur surface geometry between Control and Incidence groups from the osteoarthritis initiative database. *Journal of Biomechanics, 43*(9), 1780–1786.

[40] Tang, T. S., and Ellis, R. E. (2005, October). 2D/3D deformable registration using a hybrid atlas. In *International Conference on Medical Image Computing and Computer-Assisted Intervention* (pp. 223–230). Springer, Berlin, Heidelberg.

[41] Nishi, F. K., Khan, M. M., Alsufyani, A., Bourouis, S., Gupta, P., & Saini, D. K. (2022). Electronic Healthcare Data Record Security Using Blockchain and Smart Contract. *Journal of Sensors, 2022.*

[42] Sharma, S., Gupta, S., Gupta, D., Juneja, S., Gupta, P., Dhiman, G., & Kautish, S. (2022). Deep learning model for the automatic classification of white blood cells. *Computational Intelligence and Neuroscience, 2022.*

[43] Tazin, T., Sarker, S., Gupta, P., Ayaz, F. I., Islam, S., Monirujjaman Khan, M., … Alshazly, H. (2021). A robust and novel approach for brain tumor classification using convolutional neural network. *Computational Intelligence and Neuroscience, 2021.*

# Chapter 3

# Solutions Using Machine Learning for Diabetes

Jabar H. Yousif and Kashif Zia
*Sohar University, Sohar, Oman*

Durgesh Srivastava
*Chandigarh University, Mohali, India*

## Contents

3.1 Introduction ....40
3.2 Diabetes Prevalence ....41
3.3 Diabetes Risk Factors ....42
3.4 Machine Learning ....42
  3.4.1 Artificial Neural Networks ....45
  3.4.2 Support Vector Machine ....46
  3.4.3 Fuzzy Logic ....47
  3.4.4 Logistic Regression ....50
3.5 A Case Study ....51
3.6 Results and Discussion ....52
  3.6.1 Multicollinearity Test Results/ Variables ....55
  3.6.2 Multilinear Regression Test Results / Coefficients ....56
3.7 Conclusions ....57
References ....58

DOI: 10.1201/9781003322597-3

## 3.1 Introduction

Recent reports from the World Health Organization (WHO) and the International Diabetes Federation (IDF) have indicated a notable increase in the number of patients with diabetes worldwide. IDF and WHO define diabetes as the 21st century's leading healthcare and economic challenge [1]. Diabetes is a severe long-term condition with a significant influence on the lives and well-being of people and communities. The IDF reported in 2019 that 463 million adults aged 20–79 globally are living with diabetes, a number estimated to reach 700 million in 2045 [2]. More than one million children and adults have Type 1 diabetes. Around 79% of people with Type 2 diabetes live in low- and middle-income countries. Diabetes caused 4.2 million deaths and cost about US$760 billion in 2019 (Figure 3.1).

Machine learning techniques are computational paradigms intended to mimic human intelligence by acquiring knowledge from the surrounding environment and from experience. They are widely used in research studies to explore risk factors for diabetes. Machine learning can use deductive learning or inductive learning [4]. Deductive learning is deployed to acquire (predicate) innovative knowledge using present data, whereas inductive learning simplifies patterns and uses them instead of existing knowledge. Lama et al. [5] applied machine learning models in the Stockholm Diabetes Prevention Program to determine diabetes risk in middle-aged Swedish people based on testing features in glucose tolerance.

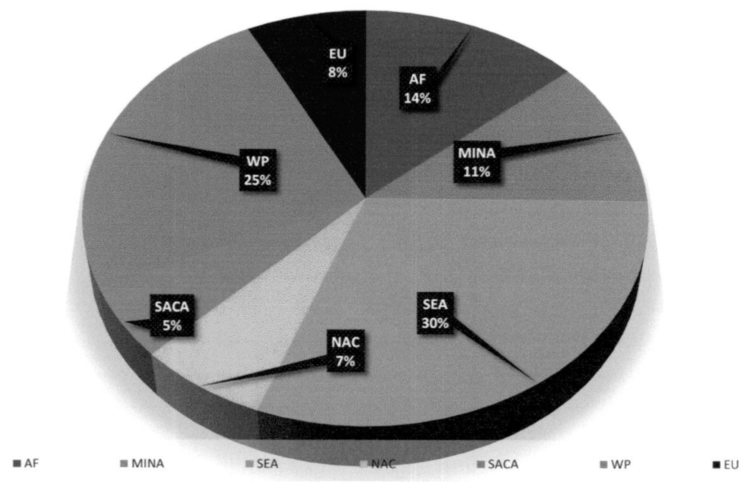


**Figure 3.1 Number of deaths due to diabetes worldwide in 2019 [2].**

*AF: Africa; MENA: Middle East & North Africa; EU: Europe; NAC: North America & Caribbean; SEA: South East Asia; SACA: South America & Central America; WP: Western Pacific.*

Jaiswal et al. [6] explored and summarized several machine learning techniques deployed in examining a rapid automatic prediction of diabetes and associated challenges. Khanam and Foo [7] implemented seven machine learning techniques to predict diabetes prevalence, including support vector machines (SVM), logistic regression (LR), and multi-layered perceptron neural network, obtaining an accuracy of about 88.6%. Khaleel and Al-Bakry [8] utilized different machine learning algorithms for the diagnosis of diabetes including LR, K-nearest neighbor (KNN), and naïve Bayes (NB). The results show that LR achieved a high accuracy level of 94%. NB obtained an accuracy of 79% and KNN 69%. Kavakiotis et al. [9] wrote a systematic review paper assessing the applications of machine learning and data mining methods to prediction and diagnosis of diabetic obstacles. They included logistic regression methods, support vector machine and decision tree (DT). Polat and Günes [10] proposed an expert system to distinguish and diagnose diabetes in ordinary patients deploying a principal component analysis (PCA) method and an adaptive neuro-fuzzy inference system.

Manikandan [11] proposed an enhanced fuzzy rule set based on a gray-wolf optimization technique for diagnosing diabetes. Mei et al. [12] deployed a prediction model using a recurrent neural network (RNN) and deep learning to deliver personalized hypoglycemic medication prediction for diabetic patients.

The discovery and prediction of diabetes are therefore of great concern and present a serious research challenge [13, 14, 15]. Some recent work in the fiend of medical image processing are [31–33]

## 3.2 Diabetes Prevalence

The National Center for Chronic Disease Prevention (CDC) in the US describes diabetes as a long-term condition in which the human body does not process food entirely for producing energy. The recent commonly known types of diabetes are Type 1 diabetes, Type 2 diabetes, and gestational diabetes. Type 1 diabetes, also called insulin-dependent, is typically caused by genetic and environmental factors. Type 2 diabetes, or non-insulin-dependent, occurs because of older age, history of gestational diabetes, and unhealthy lifestyle, including physical inactivity and obesity. Gestational diabetes develops in women during pregnancy and disappears after delivery of the baby [16].

Diabetes affects individuals, families, businesses, and society as a whole. Six Arabic countries are among the ten highest globally for the prevalence of diabetes: Egypt, United Arab Emirates (UAE), Bahrain, Kuwait, Oman, and Saudi Arabia. Dietary modifications and physical activities can prevent all types of diabetes. Typically, health care providers treat diabetes with weight management plans, exercise, self-monitoring of blood glucose, and medication if required. Gestational diabetes is associated with several risks, including hypertensive disorder, Cesarean delivery, preterm birth, and infant shoulder dystocia [17].

The IDF also states that the Middle East and North Africa had the world's highest percentage of diabetes in 2017, which led to countries in the region spending about 16.6% of their national budget on diabetes. In the same year, MENA was the second highest region for gestational diabetes in women aged 20–49, at almost 21.8%. The number of Type 1 patients under 20 was 175,800, and Saudi Arabia and Morocco were among the top ten countries globally for children and adolescents in this age group with Type 1diabetes. Moreover, 13% of adult (20–79 years) mortalities in MENA in 2017 were due to diabetes. IDF predicts a 110% increase in diabetes in MENA by 2045, rising from 39 million in 2017 to 82 million patients by 2045 [18].

## 3.3 Diabetes Risk Factors

Diabetes is of three types.

1. *Type1 diabetes*. This happens when the human immune system mistakenly attacks and destroys the β-cells, causing permanent loss of insulin. Hence, there is no insulin production in the body.
2. *Type 2 diabetes*. This occurs when tissue in the body cannot use insulin efficiently, or in medical terminology, "insulin resistance". In this there are insufficient amounts of insulin production.
3. *Gestational diabetes*. This occurs due to hormones blocking insulin production during pregnancy.

Various risk factors affect diabetes [19], including self-behavior, diabetes management and monitoring, and medication. Self-behavior is generally a reflection of the individual's way of dealing with diabetes in daily life, including lifestyle, smoking habit, excessive weight, family history, and blood sugar level (Figure 3.2). People with diabetes are usually given healthy lifestyle advice, including exercise and diet control. In other cases, medication is required.

There are three options for dealing with diabetes: (i) increasing diabetes prevention; (ii) focusing on its treatment; and (iii) improved care of diabetics to avoid complications by following the correct procedures in food and medication. Many indicators such as height, weight, blood sugar, and blood pressure can be measured by individuals in their home environments daily and shared with particular healthcare providers, reducing both cost and workload for both patients and healthcare providers.

## 3.4 Machine Learning

A learning algorithm is a computation method that applies specific functions to recognize and translate input data sets into the desired output. Machine learning is

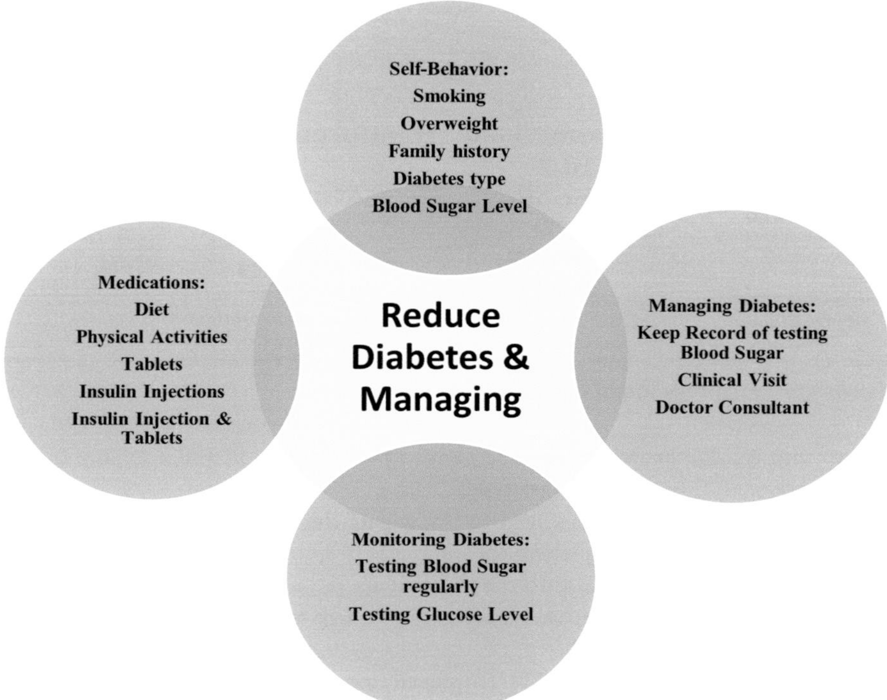


**Figure 3.2 Diabetes impact factors [19].**

a branch of artificial intelligence that emphasizes the use of data and algorithms to emulate humans, learning and thinking to improve its accuracy. It involves providing machines with the ability to learn, process data, and make decisions and future forecasts. The main learning methods, depending upon the input data and feedback, are supervised, unsupervised, semi-supervised, and reinforcement techniques (Figure 3.3).

Supervised learning is deployed when the output is known (a target pattern). The weight values will update automatically until balanced (input will lead to the desired outcome). Unsupervised learning is used to learn data behavior when the output is unknown (no target patterns). The neural cells attempt to arrange themselves in batches according to the actual input pattern. Self-organizing learning algorithms serve to discover designs that fit the real datasets by competition between neighboring nodes. Neighbors of the winner node will remain competitive iteratively until stop conditions are reached.

Analysis of diabetes is usually based on a focus group study by discussing methodological issues related to chronic diseases. Several obstacles hinder access to practical solutions, including specific definitions of risk factors and their impact on the

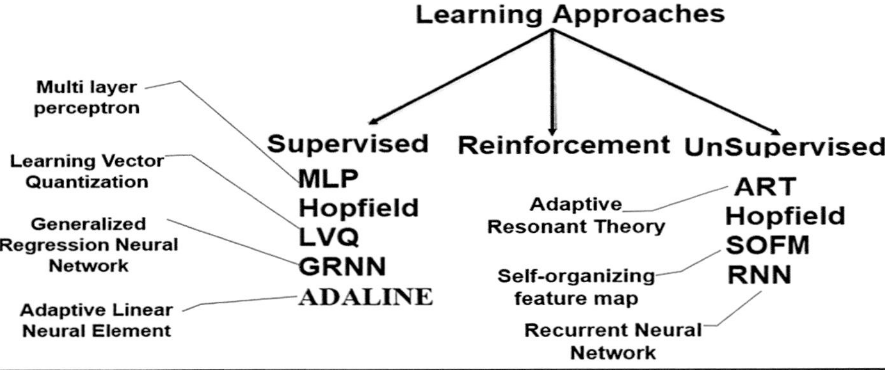


**Figure 3.3 Diabetes impact factors [19].**

patient and outcomes over time. The second problem lies in the accuracy of the collected data and the missing data types.

Many methods can be employed to investigate the missing data. The first is to examine individuals' datasets where the dataset is in a complete format. The second is to insert the existing values into the individuals' datasets where these are incomplete and then examine the missed information. Current research studies prefer the second analytical technique [20].

Different analytic methods are employed for modeling and predicting diabetes, including artificial neural networks, SVM, fuzzy logic, and logistic regression. Researchers have investigated different mathematical models to simulate the behavior and prevalence of diabetes, and have concluded that there is a need to propose mathematical models that can predict future figures. The present research used several keywords to search in the Science Direct database, in order to quantify machine learning models examining the impact of diabetes. The keywords included the following:

- diabetes + "machine learning"
- diabetes + "machine learning" + "prediction"
- diabetes + "machine learning" + "ANN"
- diabetes + "machine learning" + "SVM"
- diabetes + "machine learning" + "fuzzy"
- diabetes + "machine learning" + "logistic regression"

Figure 3.4 depicts the number of published articles in the Science Direct database between 2015 and 2021.

The search criterion "diabetes" + "machine learning" used to determine the total of published articles in 2021 indicates that more than 2,050 articles had been published. Logistic regression was the most used technique by researchers who published about 734 articles, followed by support vector machines with 655 published articles.

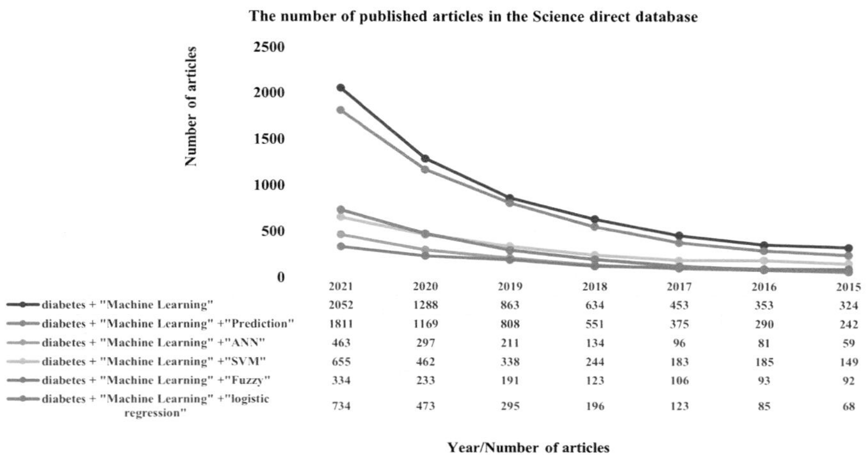


**Figure 3.4 The number of published articles in the Science Direct database.**

## *3.4.1 Artificial Neural Networks*

An artificial neural network (ANN) is a mathematical model of information processing that simulates the functioning of biological nervous systems in the human brain. The critical element of this mathematical model is the formation of the new architecture of the information processing system. A neural model consists of many highly interconnected processing elements (neurons) that cooperate to process data for a specific problem, as shown in Figure 3.5. These models of neural networks can learn from past experiences, store empirical knowledge and make it available for future use. A neural network topology describes the relationship of neurons and how they are related to each other in a unique structure. Each input of the network cells is connected by a weight that determines the power of the input cell on different nodes. These weights are in line with the biological neuron activity model. The activation signal is passed through the activation function (transfer function) to generate the output of each neuron. Each neuron also has a single threshold value used to decide which nodes will give results to the next network cell. Learning in

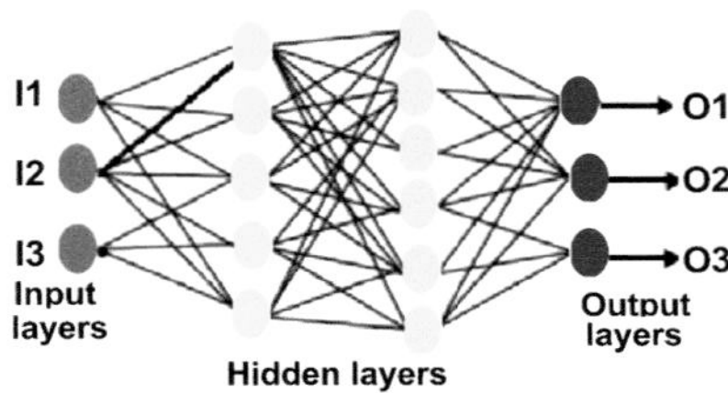


**Figure 3.5 ANN architecture [21].**

biological systems involves modifications to the weight connections between neurons by increasing the proportion of sodium in the cell to be connected to the next cell. It is the same principle by which automated neural networks work, where the value of each input cell is recursively calculated until the weights are adjusted to be the immense value that can exceed the threshold value and send the input to the next cell. The adjustment process continues until the network weights are stable and produce outputs compared with the original data to obtain the best match between them.

In a network with feed-forward structure, signals flow from inputs forward through hidden layers, and ultimately reach the output layers. However, some networks have feedback connections (recurrent) from successive to earlier neurons, which involves complex computation.

The topology can be classified mainly as single layer, multilayer, and self-organizing. A single-layer network is a simple topology of a neural network that has no in-between (hidden) layers. One layer of input nodes directly connects the input layer to the next layer (output layer). A multilayer network is a complex topology of a neural network that has one or more hidden layers. The input layers connect to the output layers not directly but through intermediate layers called hidden layers. The self-organizing topology is a competitive unsupervised machine learning that aims to reduce the higher-dimensional data to a low-dimensional (two-dimensional) structure.

The current node competes with its neighbors to produce a winner node that fits the actual data sets.

### 3.4.2 Support Vector Machine

Support vector machines (SVM) comprise a group of supervised learning approaches used to solve classification or regression problems. SVM was later extended to handle nonlinear models of the generalized Vladimir Vapnik algorithm. The SVM algorithm was developed based on statistical learning theory concepts and the extended Vapnik–Chervonenkis (VC) dimension [22]. SVM uses linear and nonlinear functions to compose multidimensional hyperplane space that separates data into different classes, as shown in Figure 3.6.

The SVM method is deployed in both regression and classification problems, which include continuous numeric and categorical variables. SVM is an iterative training method that produces an optimal hyperplane to minimize an error function.

$$F\left(a,w,b\right) = sign\left(w\ a + b\right) \tag{3.1}$$

Different types of SVM models have been proposed that can be classified into the following groups:

- Type 1 classification SVM is also known as the C-SVM optimization model.

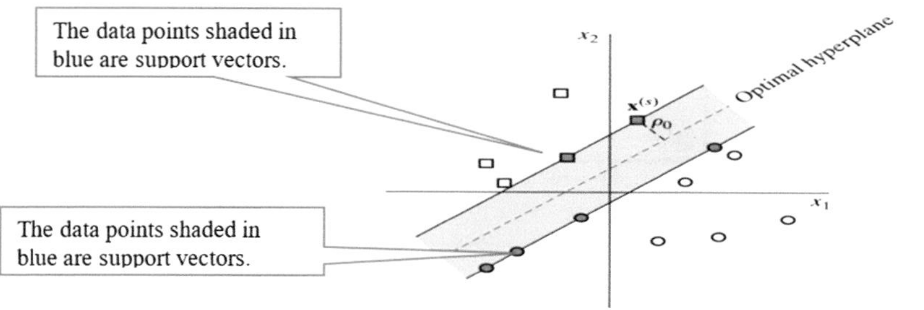


Figure 3.6 **SVM hyperplane space [23].**

- Type 2 classification SVM is also known as the Nu-SVM one-class model.
- Type 1 regression SVM is also known as the epsilon-SVM and achieves the margin of tolerance.
- Type 2 regression SVM is also known as the nu-SVM regression optimization model.

### *3.4.3 Fuzzy Logic*

Fuzzy logic is a knowledge representation based on mathematical principles to examine degrees of membership to mimic human control logic [24]. Fuzzy logic differs from the two-valued Boolean logic in that it is multi-valued. Fuzzy logic generates the degrees of membership of the variable value between 0 (completely false) and 1 (entirely true), as shown in Figure 3.7.

Fuzzy systems are suitable for implementing uncertain or approximate reasoning functions based on fuzzy rules. Fuzzy set methods are appropriate for linguistic

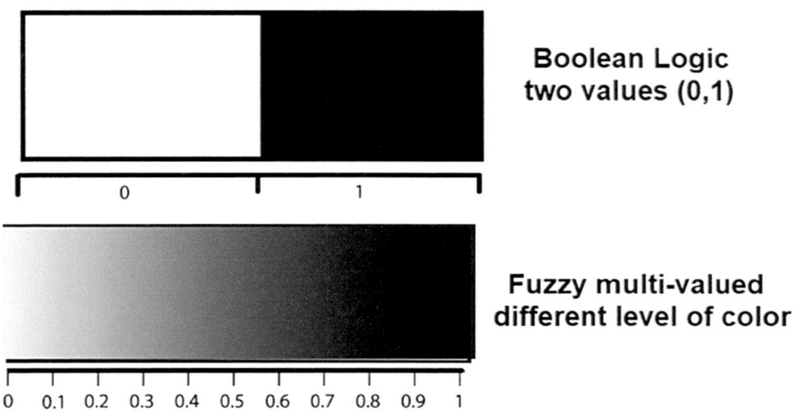


Figure 3.7 **Fuzzy logic multi-valued.**

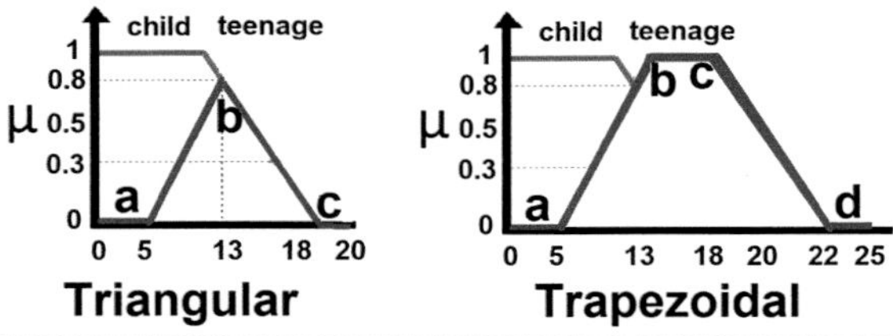


**Figure 3.8 The two-membership function degree computation.**

reasoning modes of nature to humans. The fuzzy set of an input variable's membership function maps a universe of discourse in the interval [0, 1] as defined in Equation (3.2).

$$A = \sum_{i=1}^{n} \left( \frac{\mu_A(x_i)}{x_i} \right) \tag{3.2}$$

where $x$ is a fuzzy set ($A$) member. The fuzzy set membership degree function ($A$) is represented by $\mu_A$. So, $\mu A$: $X \rightarrow [0, 1]$.

The fuzzy membership degree computes the shape of interval determined by the path of variables as shown in Figure 3.8, which includes the following:

**Triangular**

$$f(x,a,b,c) = \begin{cases} \dfrac{x-a}{b-a}; & a < x < b \\ \dfrac{c-x}{c-b}; & b < x < c \\ 0, & \text{otherwise} \end{cases} \tag{3.3}$$

**Trapezoidal**

$$f(x,a,b,c,d) = \begin{cases} \dfrac{x-a}{b-a}; & a < x < b \\ \dfrac{d-x}{d-c}; & c < x < d \\ 1; & b < x < c \\ 0, & \text{otherwise} \end{cases} \tag{3.4}$$

A linguistic variable defines the meaning of a variable that has word-values representing the variable status. It uses semantic concepts to determine more than one value for the variable (a fuzzy set representation).

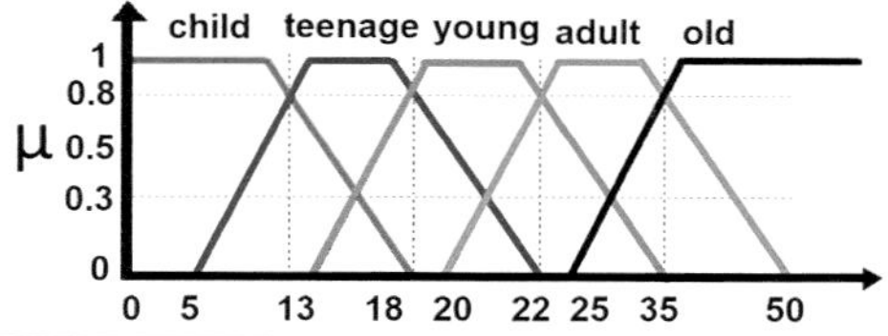


**Figure 3.9 Fuzzy membership function for the variable "age".**

For example, the linguistic variable for the variable age shown in Figure 3.9 could be categorized into the following:

- Child: the age is in the range of [0, 18], written as $0 \leq \text{age} \leq 18$.
- Teenage: the age is in the range of [5, 22], written as $5 \leq \text{age} \leq 22$.
- Young: the age is in the range of [13, 35], written as $13 \leq \text{age} \leq 35$.
- Adult: the age is in the range of [20, 50], written as $20 \leq \text{age} \leq 50$.
- Old: the age is in the range of [25, +∞], written as $\text{age} \geq 25$.

So, now we can evaluate the fuzzy membership function value that occurs in a unique range, such as:

$\mu_{\text{child}}(20)$, which is equal to 0.
$\mu_{\text{child}}(13)$, which is equal to ≈0.8
$\mu_{\text{child}}(15)$, which is equal to ≈0.3
$\mu_{\text{child}}(5)$, which is equal to 1.

However, the joint variables that share two membership function intervals should operate like Join, Intersection, and Complement operations.

**Join**

$$\mu_{A \cup B}(x) = \max\{\mu_A(x), \mu_B(x)\}, \forall x \in X \tag{3.5}$$

**Intersection**

$$\mu_{A \cap B}(x) = \min\{\mu_A(x), \mu_B(x)\}, \forall x \in X \tag{3.6}$$

**Complement**

$$\mu_{\neg A}(x) = 1 - \mu_A(x) \tag{3.7}$$

Figure 3.10 shows the implementation of the joint interval operations.

For example, what is the membership degree of (child (13) AND teenage (13))?

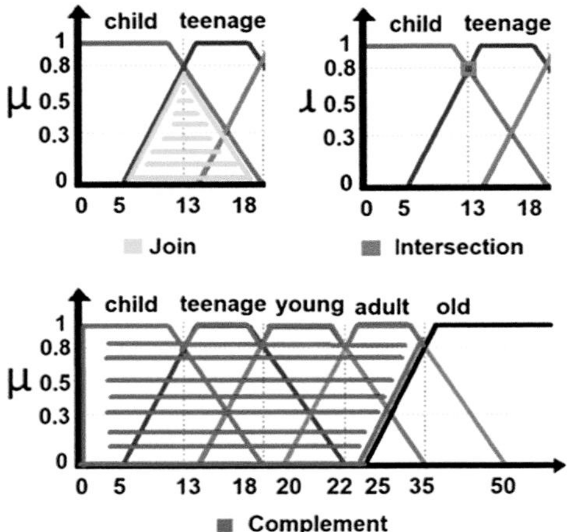


**Figure 3.10 The joint interval operations.**

$\mu_{\text{child}}(13) = 0.8$, $\mu_{\text{teenage}}(21) = 0.8$, and the "AND" is the intersection operation then $\mu_{\text{child}}(10)$ and $\mu_{\text{teenage}}(21) = \min(0.8, 0.8) = 0.8$

## *3.4.4 Logistic Regression*

The purpose of the statistical evaluation of medical data is to express relations among its variables mathematically, for example, to analyze patients affected by diabetes (*Y*) over the years (*X*). Diabetes is the dependent variable to be defined, and the independent variable is over the years. There are three types of regression analyses: linear regression, logistic regression, and cox regression [25].

The linear regression model describes the straight line of the equation:

$$Y = a + b^{*} X, \tag{3.8}$$

where the value of (*a*) is describing y-intersect of the line, and (*b*) is the slope. The linear regression approach is commonly used for modeling univariate time-series applications, used for statistical and predictive analysis. Two methods are used to classify data based on a set of predictors: LR and the linear discriminant analysis method (LDA). LDA analysis can achieve high performance when the prior probability is computed based on the group size [26].

It requires many assumptions, such as multivariate normality and equal variance matrices for all groups. The logistic trend line has a slow increase initially; after that, it will grow to reach a moderate level and then increase slowly [26].

Logistic regression (LR) examines the existence of a nonlinear relationship between the dependent and independent variables [27] as defined in Equation (3.9).

$$Yi = a + b^{*} \log_{10}(Xi) \tag{3.9}$$

where *a* is the intercept (on the y-axis), and *b* is the slope of the regression line.

Logistic regression is deployed in numerous research fields, such as machine learning, medical science, and social sciences. Boyd et al. developed a Trauma and Injury Severity Score that predicts the mortality rate in injured patients [28].

The mathematical definition of the logistic regression function that determines a multiple linear regression model is as follows:

$$\operatorname{logit}(p) = \log\left(\frac{p(y=i)}{1-(p=i)}\right), \text{for } i = 1\ldots n \tag{3.10}$$

which can then be computed as:

$$\operatorname{logit}(p) = \beta_0 + \beta_1.x_n + \beta_2.x_n + \ldots + \beta_p.x_m \tag{3.11}$$

We should consider model fitting in the logistic regression analysis process because adding an independent variable will increase the variance value in the log odds computation. However, adding more variables to the regression model will cause an overfitting problem, which decreases the model's generalization to fit the actual data [29,30].

## 3.5 A Case Study

The case study presented here was utilized in North Al-Batinah, Oman. A well-defined questionnaire was prepared to collect the data needed to examine the impact factors mentioned in Figure 3.2. The collected data (332 samples) were cleaned using a purposive sampling method for selecting 214 diabetes patients' answers. The selected data were then organized and tabulated for robustness using multilinear regression tests (gender-wise), ANOVA, descriptive analysis, etc.

From analysis of the literature it is clear that the type of diabetes affects the medication of diabetes patients. It also impacts the number of times the patient visits the clinic with high blood glucose. Blood glucose status affects the frequency of testing blood glucose at home and visiting the doctor.

We therefore put forward the following hypotheses:

***Hypothesis 1-a.*** *The type of diabetes plays a vital role in the medication type of diabetes patients.*
***Hypothesis 1-b.*** *Types of diabetes play an essential role in the frequency of testing at home.*
***Hypothesis 2-a.*** *The blood glucose status plays an essential role in the frequency of testing at home.*
***Hypothesis 2-b.*** *Testing blood sugar at home plays a vital role in monitoring blood sugar per day.*

***Hypothesis 3-a.*** *The set of tests prescribed by the doctor plays a vital role in visiting a diabetes clinic.*
***Hypothesis 3-b.*** *The Blood glucose status plays an essential role in the frequency of visiting a diabetes clinic.*

## 3.6 Results and Discussion

Table 3.1 presents demographic information on the participants derived from the questionnaire. It shows that age is a significant factor influencing diabetes type.

**Table 3.1 Demographic Information**

| *Characteristics* | *Classification* | *Frequency* | % |
|---|---|---|---|
| Nationality | Omani | 214.0 | 100 |
| Gender | Male | 45.0 | 21.0 |
| | Female | 169.0 | 79.0 |
| Age | Less than 20 years | 15.0 | 7.0 |
| | 20–<40 years | 62.0 | 29.0 |
| | 40–<70 years | 118.0 | 55.1 |
| | 70 years and above | 19.0 | 8.9 |
| Are you overweight? | Yes | 122.0 | 57.0 |
| | No | 64.0 | 29.9 |
| | Don't know | 28.0 | 13.1 |
| Do you smoke? | Never | 171.0 | 79.9 |
| | Sometimes | 25.0 | 11.7 |
| | Always | 18.0 | 8.4 |
| Does anyone in the family have diabetes? | Yes | 124.0 | 57.9 |
| | No | 15.0 | 7.0 |
| | Don't know | 75.0 | 35.1 |

**Table 3.1** *(Continued)* **Demographic Information**

| *Characteristics* | *Classification* | *Frequency* | *%* |
|---|---|---|---|
| What type of diabetes do you have? | Type 1 diabetes (T1 DM) | 31.0 | 14.5 |
| | Type 2 diabetes (T2 DM) | 88.0 | 41.1 |
| | Gestational diabetes (GDM) | 17.0 | 8.0 |
| | Don't know | 78.0 | 36.4 |
| What type of medication do you take? | Tablets | 131.0 | 61.2 |
| | Insulin injection | 17.0 | 8.0 |
| | Tablets and insulin injection | 3.0 | 1.4 |
| | Do diet/lifestyle (e.g., sport) changes only | 43.0 | 20.1 |
| | Do nothing | 20.0 | 9.3 |
| How many times do you visit the diabetes clinic? | 1–4 times a month | 124.0 | 57.9 |
| | More than 4 times a month | 28.0 | 13.1 |
| | 1–4 times a year | 62.0 | 29.0 |
| What kind of tests does your doctor suggest for you? | General | 166.0 | 77.6 |
| | Specific | 8.0 | 3.7 |
| | Both | 40.0 | 18.7 |
| How often you had low/high blood sugar (blood glucose status) | Never | 37.0 | 17.3 |
| | Sometimes | 49.0 | 22.9 |
| | Always | 128.0 | 59.8 |
| Has the doctor advised you on the readings taken at home? | Never | 105.0 | 49.1 |
| | Sometimes | 66.0 | 30.8 |
| | Always | 43.0 | 20.1 |
| How often do you test your blood sugar at home? | Never | 47.0 | 22.0 |
| | Sometimes | 117.0 | 54.6 |
| | Always | 50.0 | 23.4 |

(*Continued*)

**Table 3.1** *(Continued)* **Demographic Information**

| *Characteristics* | *Classification* | *Frequency* | *%* |
|---|---|---|---|
| Do you monitor blood sugar at least once a day | Very important | 131.0 | 61.2 |
| | Important | 70.0 | 32.7 |
| | No idea | 13.0 | 6.1 |
| Do you keep a record of your self-measured readings | Never | 39.0 | 18.2 |
| | Sometimes | 137.0 | 64.1 |
| | Always | 38.0 | 17.7 |
| Recording your readings | On paper | 127.0 | 59.3 |
| | In hospital file | 74.0 | 34.6 |
| | In mobile phone | 13.0 | 6.1 |
| Your reaction to low or high blood sugar | Take medication at home | 27.0 | 12.6 |
| | Go to hospital | 159.0 | 74.3 |
| | Either of the above | 20.0 | 9.4 |
| | Do not react | 8.0 | 3.7 |
| Getting hospital appointments is a costly affair | Yes | 146.0 | 68.2 |
| | No | 37.0 | 17.3 |
| | Don't know | 31.0 | 14.5 |
| You have access to your results | Never | 80.0 | 37.4 |
| | Sometimes | 103.0 | 48.11 |
| | Always | 31.0 | 4.5 |
| Having a smartphone/ tablet | Yes (I use applications) | 141.0 | 65.9 |
| | Yes (use for calling only) | 60.0 | 28.0 |
| | No | 13.0 | 6.1 |
| Using mobile application beneficial to save and give feedback to diabetic patients | Yes | 174.0 | 81.3 |
| | No | 11.0 | 5.1 |
| | Don't know | 29.0 | 13.6 |

### *3.6.1 Multicollinearity Test Results/ Variables*

A multicollinearity test illustrates the degree of relationship (perfect/exact) between the exploratory variables in a regression model. Linear regression supposes there is no perfect/exact relationship among the experimental variables. Therefore, when the assumption is broken, the multicollinearity problem occurs.

Table 3.2 shows the results of the multicollinearity tests.

Table 3.3 presents the independent variables result with a tolerance value > 0.1 and a variance inflation factor value (VIF) < 10, which shows the regression model has no multicollinearity problem. The multilinear regression tests results are presented in Tables 3.4, 3.5, and 3.6.

**Table 3.2 Results of Multicollinearity Test**

| *Model type* | *Tolerance value* | *VIF Value* |
|---|---|---|
| Gender | 0.754 | 1.326 |
| Age | 0.930 | 1.076 |
| Smoking habit | 0.749 | 1.335 |
| Overweight | 0.502 | 1.994 |
| Family history | 0.517 | 1.933 |

**Table 3.3 Results of Multilinear Regression Test (Variables Entered/Removed)**

| *Model* | *Variables entered in the model* | *Variables removed* | *Method* |
|---|---|---|---|
| 1 | Age, gender, smoking habit, overweight, family history | | Enter |

*Note:* Dependent Variable is Diabetes Types; Entered all requested Variables.

**Table 3.4 Multilinear Regression Test Results / Model Summary**

| *Model* | *R* | *R Square* | *Adjusted R Square* | *Std. Error of the Estimate* |
|---|---|---|---|---|
| 1 | 0.747 | 0.557 | 0.547 | 0.752 |

*Note:* Predictors: (constant), age, gender, smoking habit, overweight, family history.

**Table 3.5 Results of Multilinear Regression Test / ANOVA[a]**

| *Model Type* | *Sum of Squares Value* | *df* | *Mean Square* | *F* | *Sig.* |
|---|---|---|---|---|---|
| Regression | 148.118 | 5 | 29.624 | 52.370 | 0.000[b] |
| Residual | 117.658 | 208 | 0.566 | | |
| Total | 265.776 | 213 | | | |

[a] Dependent Variable: Diabetes Types
[b] Predictors: (constant), age, gender, smoking habit, overweight, family history.

**Table 3.6 Results of the Multilinear Regression Test/Coefficients**

| | *Unstandardized Coefficients* | | *Standardized Coefficients* | | |
|---|---|---|---|---|---|
| *Model type* | *B* | *Std. Error* | *Beta* | *t Value* | *Sig. Value* |
| Constant | –1.617 | 0.417 | | –3.873 | 0.000 |
| Gender | 0.304 | 0.145 | 0.111 | 2.090 | 0.038 |
| Age | 0.595 | 0.068 | 0.421 | 8.801 | 0.000 |
| Smoking habit | 0.530 | 0.097 | 0.290 | 5.438 | 0.000 |
| Overweight | 0.295 | 0.102 | 0.189 | 2.900 | 0.004 |
| Family history | 0.560 | 0.076 | 0.471 | 7.340 | 0.000 |

*Note:* Dependent Variable: Diabetes Types

### 3.6.2 Multilinear Regression Test Results / Coefficients

Table 3.6 shows that the coefficients results indicate diabetes is dependent on the independent variables, viz gender, age, overweight, smoking habit, and family history based on the obtained $p$-value less than 0.05.

Thus, we can write the accepted linear regression model as in Equation (3.12):

$$\mathrm{TD} = -1.617 + 0.304\,\mathrm{G} + 0.595\,\mathrm{A} + 0.530\,\mathrm{S} + 0.295\,\mathrm{OW} + 0.560\,\mathrm{FH} \quad (3.12)$$

where TD—Diabetes type, G—Gender, S—Smoking habit, A—Age, OW—Overweight and FH—Family History.

Examining the independent variables coefficients evidence that the age variable has the most significant influence on the diabetes type (0.595), followed by family history (0.560) and smoking habit (0.530). However, the impacts of gender (0.304), and lastly, overweight (0.295) are less.

## 3.7 Conclusions

The results of the proposed approach illustrate that age plays an important role in determining the diabetes type and medication of diabetes patients. It can also be seen that the diabetes type influences the incidence of glucose self-testing at home, with patients visiting the clinic in case of significant variations in the readings. In addition, many of the respondents reported that they do not have access to their medical records. On the other hand, about 66% were already using some applications through their mobile phones.

The main objective is to examine the risk factors that influence the diabetes type and their impact rate. Based on Equation (3.1), the highest impact factor on the types of diabetes is age with a value of 0.595, closely followed by family history (0.560), and smoking habit (0.530). The minor impact factors were gender (0.304) and overweight (0.295).

The literature review analysis concludes that diabetes type is a significant factor influencing the treatment type of diabetes patients. There is a shortage of reliable data related to the actual number of patients with diabetes because it has been obtained from different sources.

The following are some suggestions:

- To issue a monthly bulletin to raise community awareness about diabetes types, their effects on human health and treatment methods, as well as about suitable types of exercise, because many patients do not know the type of diabetes they suffer from or how to treat it.
- To create a database of diabetes patients, their conditions, and the type of medication used to provide advice from specialists and regular follow-up.
- To establish a national, local, or international center to link patients' information and the possibility of follow-up by the doctor and the patient themselves, providing the opportunity to give the necessary advice via phone or email.
- To provide treatment and regular blood sugar level checks in clinics or to distribute self-testing devices for diabetes at a subsidized rate or free to reduce the economic impact on patients.
- To increase awareness campaigns about the effects of obesity and how to reduce it by eating healthy food and increasing daily exercise.
- To follow up on the history of families of diabetic patients and analyze the number and type of diabetes to help reduce the future spread of diabetes in the same family.
- To make family members aware of the need to avoid the negative factors that increase the incidence of disease.

## References


1 WHO. (2021). Global Report. Available online [accessed on 15 September 2021]. https://www.who.int/news-room/fact-sheets/detail/diabetes

2 IDF. (2021). Online source [accessed on 10 October 2021]. https://www.diabetesatlas.org/en/sections/worldwide-toll-of-diabetes.html

3 Statista. (2019). Online source [accessed on 10 October 2021]. https://www.statista.com/statistics/495457/deaths-due-to-diabetes-worldwide-number-by-region/

4 El Naqa, I., and Murphy, M. J. (2015). What is machine learning? In Issam El Naqa, Martin J. Murphy, Ruijiang Li (Eds.), *Machine Learning in Radiation Oncology* (pp. 3–11). Springer, Cham.

5 Lama, L., Wilhelmsson, O., Norlander, E., Gustafsson, L., Lager, A., Tynelius, P., … Östenson, C. G. (2021). Machine learning for prediction of diabetes risk in middle-aged Swedish people. *Heliyon*, 7(7), e07419.

6 Jaiswal, V., Negi, A., and Pal, T. (2021). A review on current advances in machine learning based diabetes prediction. *Primary Care Diabetes*, 15, 435–443.

7 Khanam, J. J., and Foo, S. Y. (2021). A comparison of machine learning algorithms for diabetes prediction. *ICT Express*, 7, 432–439.

8 Khaleel, F. A., and Al-Bakry, A. M. (2021). Diagnosis of diabetes using machine learning algorithms. In *Materials Today: Proceedings*.

9 Kavakiotis, I., Tsave, O., Salifoglou, A., Maglaveras, N., Vlahavas, I., and Chouvarda, I. (2017). Machine learning and data mining methods in diabetes research. *Computational and Structural Biotechnology Journal*, 15, 104–116.

10 Polat, K., and Günes, S. (2007). An expert system approach based on principal component analysis and adaptive neuro-fuzzy inference system to diagnosis of diabetes disease. *Digital Signal Processing*, 17, 702–710. doi: 10.1016/j.dsp.2006.09.005.

11 Manikandan, K. (2019). Diagnosis of diabetes diseases using optimized fuzzy rule set by grey wolf optimization. *Pattern Recognition Letters*, 125, 432–438.

12 Mei, J., Zhao, S., Jin, F., Zhang, L., Liu, H., Li, X., … Xu, M. (2017). Deep diabetologist: Learning to prescribe hypoglycemic medications with recurrent neural networks. *Studies in Health Technology and Informatics*, 245, 1277–1277.

13 Lukmanto, R. B., Nugroho, A., and Akbar, H. (2019). Early detection of diabetes mellitus using feature selection and fuzzy support vector machine. *Procedia Computer Science*, 157, 46–54.

14 Farahmand, B., Dehghani, M., and Vafamand, N. (2019). Fuzzy model-based controller for blood glucose control in type 1 diabetes: An LMI approach. *Biomedical Signal Processing and Control*, 54, 101627.

15 Rahman, M., Islam, D., Mukti, R. J., and Saha, I. (2020). A deep learning approach based on convolutional LSTM for detecting diabetes. *Computational Biology and Chemistry*, 88, 107329.

16 CDC. (2020). National Diabetes Statistics Report. Online source [accessed on 10 October 2021]. https://www.cdc.gov/diabetes/data/statistics-report/index.html

17 Dirar A., and Doupis J. (2017, December 15). Gestational diabetes from A to Z. *World Journal of Diabetes*, 8, 489–511. ISSN 1948-9358 (online).

18 IDF. (2021). Online source [accessed on 10 October 2021]. https://diabetesatlas.org/upload/resources/previous/files/8/IDF_DA_8e-EN-final.pdf

19 Yousif, J. H., Khan, F. R., Zia, K., and Saadi, N. A. (2021). Analytical data review to determine the factors impacting risk of diabetes in North Al-Batinah Region, Oman. *International Journal of Environmental Research and Public Health*, 18(10), 5323.

20 Ibrahim, D. R., Tamimi, A. A., and Abdalla, A. M. (2017, May). Performance analysis of biometric recognition modalities. In *2017 8th International Conference on Information Technology (ICIT)* (pp. 980–984). IEEE.
21 Yousif, J. H., and Fekihal, M. A. (2012). Neural approach for determining mental health problems. *Journal of Computing*, 4(1), 6–11.
22 Vapnik, V., and Izmailov, R. (2020, August). Complete statistical theory of learning: Learning using statistical invariants. In *Conformal and Probabilistic Prediction and Applications* (pp. 4–40). PMLR.
23 Yousif, J. H. (2011). *Information Technology Development*. LAP LAMBERT Academic Publishing, Germany ISBN 9783844316704.
24 Thakkar, H., Shah, V., Yagnik, H., and Shah, M. (2020). Comparative anatomization of data mining and fuzzy logic techniques used in diabetes prognosis. *Clinical eHealth*, 4, 12–23.
25 Schneider, A., Hommel, G., and Blettner, M. (2010). Linear regression analysis: Part 14 of a series on evaluation of scientific publications. *Deutsches Ärzteblatt International*, 107(44), 776.
26 Liong, C. Y., and Foo, S. F. (2013, April). Comparison of linear discriminant analysis and logistic regression for data classification. In *AIP Conference Proceedings* (Vol. 1522, No. 1, pp. 1159–1165). American Institute of Physics.
27 Benoit, K. (2012). Multinomial and ordinal logistic regression. Accessed on 10 December 2017.
28 Boyd, C. R., Tolson, M. A., and Copes, W. S. (1987). Evaluating trauma care: The TRISS method. Trauma score and the injury severity score. *The Journal of Trauma*, 27(4), 370–378.
29 Joshi, R. D., and Dhakal, C. K. (2021). Predicting type 2 diabetes using logistic regression and machine learning approaches. *International Journal of Environmental Research and Public Health*, 18(14), 7346.
30 Tabaei, B. P., and Herman, W. H. (2002). A multivariate logistic regression equation to screen for diabetes: Development and validation. *Diabetes Care*, 25(11), 1999–2003.
31 Nishi, F. K., Khan, M. M., Alsufyani, A., Bourouis, S., Gupta, P., and Saini, D. K. (2022). Electronic Healthcare Data Record Security Using Blockchain and Smart Contract. *Journal of Sensors, 2022.*
32 Sharma, S., Gupta, S., Gupta, D., Juneja, S., Gupta, P., Dhiman, G., and Kautish, S. (2022). Deep learning model for the automatic classification of white blood cells. *Computational Intelligence and Neuroscience, 2022.*
33 Tazin, T., Sarker, S., Gupta, P., Ayaz, F. I., Islam, S., Monirujjaman Khan, M., … Alshazly, H. (2021). A robust and novel approach for brain tumor classification using convolutional neural network. *Computational Intelligence and Neuroscience, 2021.*

*Chapter 4*

# A Highly Reliable Machine Learning Algorithm for Cardiovascular Disease Prediction

Horesh Kumar

*Greater Noida Institute of Technology, Greater Noida, India*

Tarun Jain, Kartik Soni, Amisha Gupta, Rishi Gupta, Arjun Singh and Aditya Sinha

*Manipal University, Jaipur, India*

## Contents

4.1 Introduction ....62
4.2 Literature Review ....62
4.3 Methodology ....63
4.3.1 Dataset ....63
4.3.2 Implementing the Classifiers ....64
4.3.2.1 XGBOOST ....64
4.3.2.2 Random Forest ....64

DOI: 10.1201/9781003322597-4

4.3.2.3 Naïve Bayes ........................................................ 66
4.3.2.4 Majority Voting Ensemble (MVE) ........................................ 69
4.4 Conclusion ........................................................ 71
References ........................................................ 72

## 4.1 Introduction

According to the World Health Organization (WHO), 32% of all deaths worldwide are caused by cardiovascular diseases. Today it is not only the older age groups, but also many young people who are susceptible to serious heart conditions. It is imperative to harness the potential of AI in the field of cardiology, where early detection of heart diseases can save millions of lives worldwide.

For our work to be used in the actual healthcare industry, it needs to be mission critical. Thus, we have placed strong emphasis on having reliable algorithms with high accuracy, such as is yielded by the reliable voting ensemble classifier. Multiple attributes have been taken into account for accurate classification, such as age, gender, chest pain type, resting blood pressure (mm Hg), serum cholesterol, fasting blood sugar level, resting electrocardiographic results, maximum heart rate achieved, exercise-induced angina, depression induced by exercise relative to rest, and slope of peak exercise. These are some of the most important factors in detecting the presence of a cardiac problem.

## 4.2 Literature Review

Rahma Atallah et al. in [1] used a voting ensemble classifier for heart disease prediction and achieved 90% accuracy. Our approach yields higher accuracy. Atharv Nikam et al. in [2] used BMI as an important factor in classification. Devansh Shah et al. in [3] achieved the best results on the same dataset using K-nearest neighbor classifiers. C. Krittanawong et al. in [4] assessed how well ML algorithms predict cardiac diseases. R. Das et al. in [5] obtained 87% accuracy in heart disease prediction using KNN. R. Bharti et al. in [6] used ML as well as DL approaches for heart disease prediction. K.M. Soni et al. in [7] implemented nine ML classifiers for cancer classification, with RNN yielding the highest accuracy level.

Xiao-Yan Gao et al. in [8] used the ensemble method to develop a high accuracy-yielding model. Yang et al. in [9] used the random forest classifier to study cardiovascular disease prediction based on cases in China. Peter W.F. Wilson et al. in [10] used various metrics to predict heart disease risk in middle-aged men. Armin Yazdani et al. in [11] computed strength scores as being important predictors in predicting heart diseases. Vijeta Sharma et al. in [12] also used the UCI repository dataset and applied machine learning techniques. C. Beluah et al. in [13] improved risk prediction accuracy by using ensemble techniques. Dhai Eddine Salahi et al. in

[14] used SVM and KNN with 93% accuracy for cardiovascular disease prediction, after selecting the most relevant features. Some recent work in the fiend of medical image processing are [15–17]

# 4.3 Methodology

## *4.3.1 Dataset*

We obtained a cardiovascular disease detection dataset with nearly 300 cases from UCI's machine learning repository for Switzerland. We trained and tested different machine learning algorithms on the given dataset. Each case (row) had 14 attributes to describe it, i.e., our dataset has 14 attribute columns. Upon proper analysis, these 14 attributes proved to be crucial for the determination of cardiovascular disease detection. Attributes include age, gender, chest pain type, resting blood pressure (mm/Hg), cholesterol level, fasting blood sugar, resting electrocardiograph results, maximum heart rate achieved, exercise-induced angina, etc.

The data split was 20:80 or 30:70 according to the performance of the algorithm. Figure 4.1 represents the basic methodology followed to perform the classification of cardiovascular disease detection.

The target variable had values of '0' and '1', signifying, respectively, that a person is at no risk or might be at risk for cardiovascular disease.

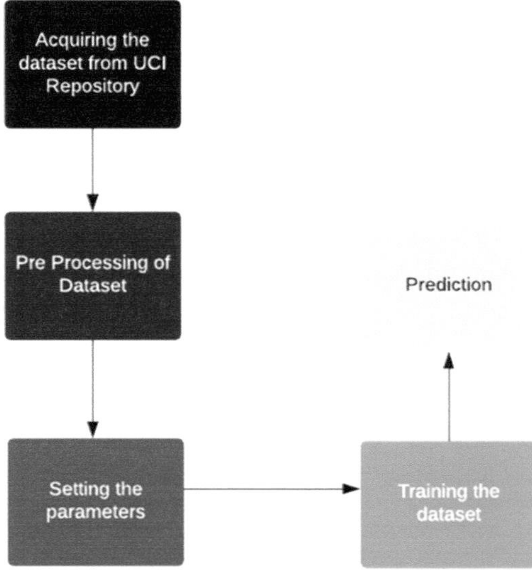


**Figure 4.1 Step-by-step Methodology.**

### 4.3.2 Implementing the Classifiers

The following classifiers have been trained on the training dataset which is further used to check the accuracy of classifiers by prediction on the testing dataset. The majority voting ensemble yielded the highest accuracy among all the high accuracy-yielding classifiers.

#### 4.3.2.1 XGBOOST

XGBoost (XGB) is a gradient boosting, i.e., a supervised machine learning, algorithm. It is known as a gradient boosting algorithm since it attempts to minimize the loss function by using a gradient descent algorithm. With each iteration, it attempts to reduce the loss or errors of previous trees to make the final prediction. Therefore, the XGB classifier is one of the highest accuracy yielding classifiers.[18]

While implementing, a 70:30 split gave the best performance. The parameters of the XGB classifier are indicated in Figure 4.2.

##### 4.3.2.1.1 XGBoost Result Analysis

Figure 4.3 indicates that 11 points in the dataset were misclassified, yielding a final accuracy of 87.91%.

In Figure 4.4, the area under the curve 0.927 indicates high accuracy.

The table in Figure 4.5 scrutinizes the performance of the XGBoost classifier using several evaluation parameters.

As is evident, a wide array of metrics has been used to check the performance of the classifier to ensure a reliable model. This is especially important as our paper addresses a mission-critical domain: if the model is to be put to practical use, it needs to be very reliable in multiple respects.

#### 4.3.2.2 Random Forest

The random forest algorithm consists of multiple trees which are not correlated. For each case (i.e., for each row) an output class prediction is made by the tree and at the end the class with maximum frequency becomes the final output.

```
XGBClassifier(base_score=0.5, booster='gbtree', colsample_bylevel=1,
              colsample_bynode=1, colsample_bytree=1, gamma=0,
              learning_rate=0.1, max_delta_step=0, max_depth=3,
              min_child_weight=1, missing=None, n_estimators=100, n_jobs=1,
              nthread=None, objective='binary:logistic', random_state=0,
              reg_alpha=0, reg_lambda=1, scale_pos_weight=1, seed=None,
              silent=None, subsample=1, verbosity=1)
```

**Figure 4.2 Parameters of XGB Classifier.**

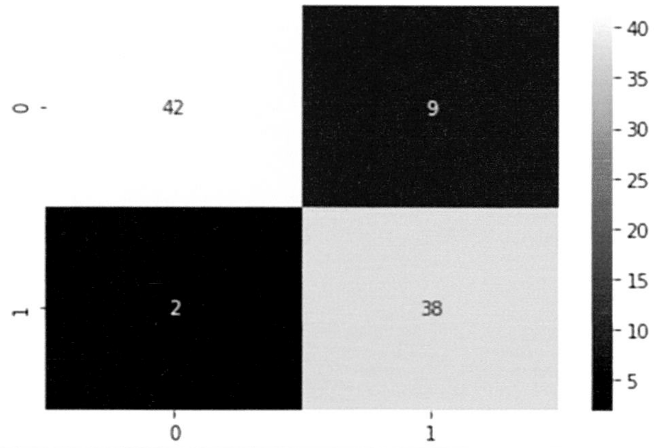


**Figure 4.3 Confusion Matrix of XGBoost Prediction.**

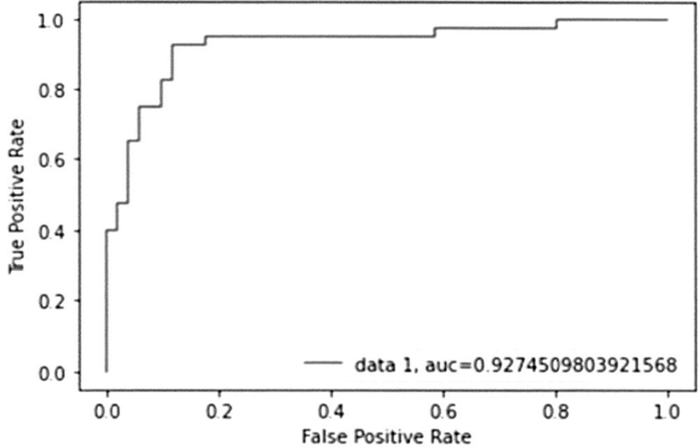


**Figure 4.4 ROC of XGBoost's prediction.**

| Specificity | Sensitivity | Accuracy | Precision | FPR |
|---|---|---|---|---|
| 0.80 | 0.95 | 0.879 | 0.823 | 0.2 |

| FNR | NPV | FDR | F1 score | MCC |
|---|---|---|---|---|
| 0.03 | 0.95 | 0.17 | 0.88 | 0.76 |

**Figure 4.5 Evaluation Parameters of XGBoost.**

```
RandomForestClassifier(bootstrap=True, ccp_alpha=0.0, class_weight=None,
                       criterion='entropy', max_depth=None, max_features='auto',
                       max_leaf_nodes=None, max_samples=None,
                       min_impurity_decrease=0.0, min_impurity_split=None,
                       min_samples_leaf=1, min_samples_split=2,
                       min_weight_fraction_leaf=0.0, n_estimators=10,
                       n_jobs=None, oob_score=False, random_state=0, verbose=0,
                       warm_start=False)
```

**Figure 4.6 Parameters of Random Forest Classifier.**

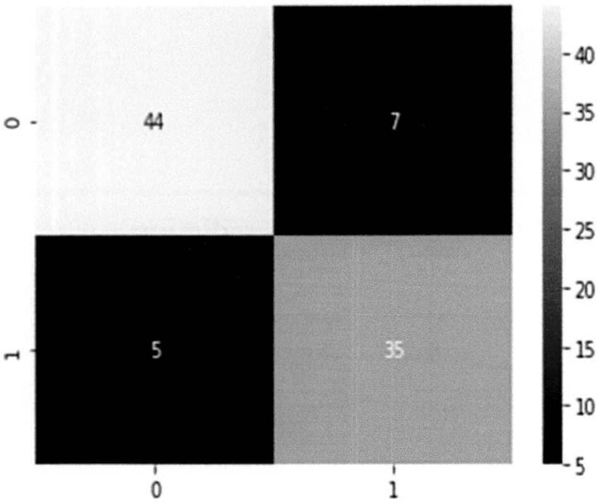


**Figure 4.7 Confusion Matrix of Random Forest Predictions.**

During implementation a 70:30 split resulted in the highest accuracy. The number of estimators used was ten and the criterion chosen was 'entropy'. It was used for information gain. Figure 4.6 indicates the different parameters taken into account by the random forest algorithm for the classification of heart disease prediction.

#### 4.3.2.2.1 Random Forest Result Analysis

Figure 4.7 indicates that 12 points in the dataset were misclassified, yielding a final accuracy of 86.81%.

The area under the curve being 0.933 in ROC (Figure 4.8) indicates a high accuracy level.

Figure 4.9 scrutinizes the performance of Random Forest classifier using various evaluation parameters so as to get a better understanding of algorithm's performance on the dataset [19].

### *4.3.2.3 Naïve Bayes*

The naïve Bayes classifier works on the principle of Bayes' theorem. It predicts the result on the basis of the probability of an entity.

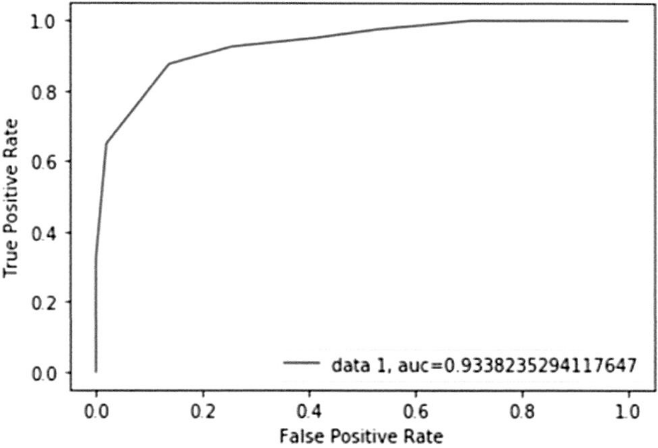


**Figure 4.8 ROC of random forest predictions.**

| Specificity | Sensitivity | Accuracy | Precision | FPR |
|---|---|---|---|---|
| 0.833 | 0.897 | 0.868 | 0.862 | 0.16 |

| FNR | NPV | FDR | F1 score | MCC |
|---|---|---|---|---|
| 0.10 | 0.875 | 0.13 | 0.874 | 0.73 |

**Figure 4.9 Evaluation Parameters of Random Forest.**

In this classifier, an 80:20 split resulted in the maximum accuracy. Gaussian naïve Bayes was used for the implementation because it is a very flexible model which works well on a huge amount of data. It uses the Gaussian naïve Bayes algorithm for classification purposes.

$$P(y) = \frac{1}{\sqrt{\left(2\pi\sigma_y^2\right)}}\left(-\frac{\left(x_i - \mu_y\right)^2}{2\sigma_y^2}\right)$$

The parameters chosen for the naïve Bayes classifier are indicated in Figure 4.10.

$$\text{GaussianNB}(\text{priors} = \text{None}, \text{var\_smoothing} = 1\text{e} - 09)$$

```
GaussianNB(priors=None, var_smoothing=1e-09)
```

**Figure 4.10 Parameters of Naïve Bayes Classifier.**

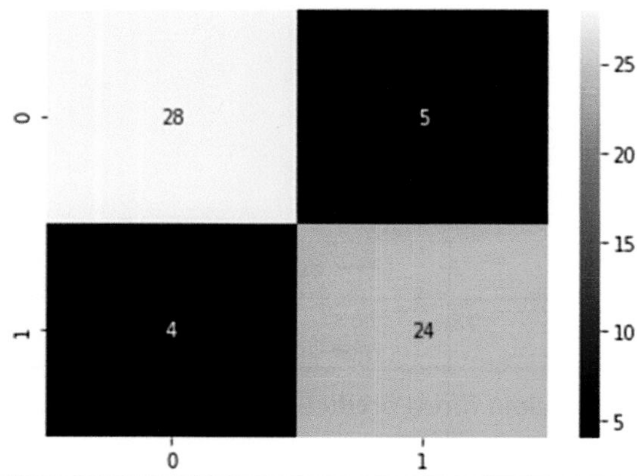


**Figure 4.11 Confusion Matrix of Naïve Bayes Predictions.**

#### 4.3.2.3.1 Naïve Bayes Result Analysis

Figure 4.11 indicates through the confusion matrix of naïve Bayes prediction that only nine points were misclassified in the dataset, yielding a high accuracy of 85.24% (Figure 4.12).

Figure 4.13 scrutinizes the performance of Naïve Bayes classifier using various evaluation parameters. The high AUC of 0.93 in Figure 4.14 indicates high accuracy and an efficient prediction.

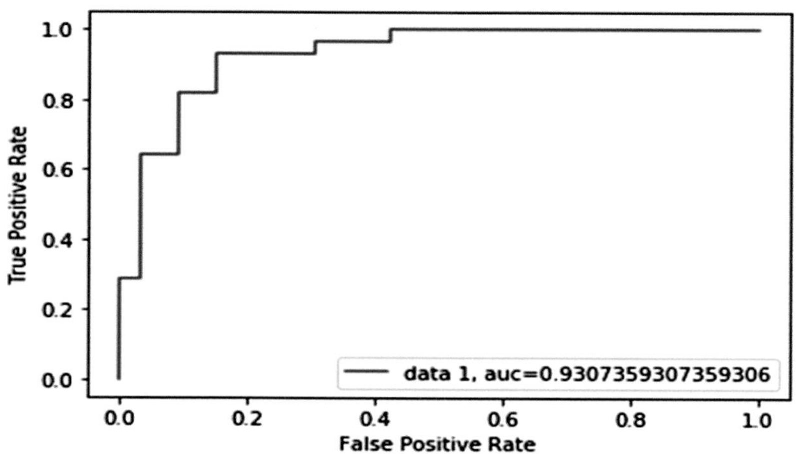


**Figure 4.12 ROC of Naïve Bayes Predictions.**

| Specificity | Sensitivity | Accuracy | Precision | FPR |
|---|---|---|---|---|
| 0.827 | 0.875 | 0.852 | 0.848 | 0.17 |

| FNR | NPV | FDR | F1 score | MCC |
|---|---|---|---|---|
| 0.125 | 0.857 | 0.15 | 0.854 | 0.70 |

**Figure 4.13 Evaluation Parameters of Naïve Bayes.**

### *4.3.2.4 Majority Voting Ensemble (MVE)*

The majority voting ensemble classifier works on the principle of majority voting, i.e., it makes prediction by taking the average of the results of multiple classifiers. Therefore, it results in very high accuracy compared to all the other classifiers.

Majority voting prediction involves two techniques, hard voting and soft voting.

- *Hard Voting* ensemble outputs the class with the maximum number of votes from all the classifiers.
- *Soft Voting* ensemble outputs on the basis of probability. It sums the probabilities of all the class labels and finally outputs the class label with maximum probability.

In the implementation of the majority voting ensemble for classification of cardiovascular diseases, a total of five classifiers were used:

1. Logistic regression classifier
2. Support vector classifier
3. Decision tree classifier
4. Random forest classifier
5. K-neighbor classifier

The different parameters taken into account for the above classifiers are as specified in Figure 4.14.

```
estimator = []
estimator.append(('LR',
                  LogisticRegression(solver ='lbfgs',
                                     multi_class ='multinomial',
                                     max_iter = 200)))
estimator.append(('SVC', SVC(gamma ='auto', probability = True)))
estimator.append(('DTC', DecisionTreeClassifier(criterion="entropy", random_state=0)))
estimator.append(('RFC', RandomForestClassifier(n_estimators=10, criterion="entropy", random_state=0)))
estimator.append(('KNC',KNeighborsClassifier(n_neighbors=5,metric='minkowski',p=2)))
```

**Figure 4.14 Parameters for Different Classifiers Considered.**

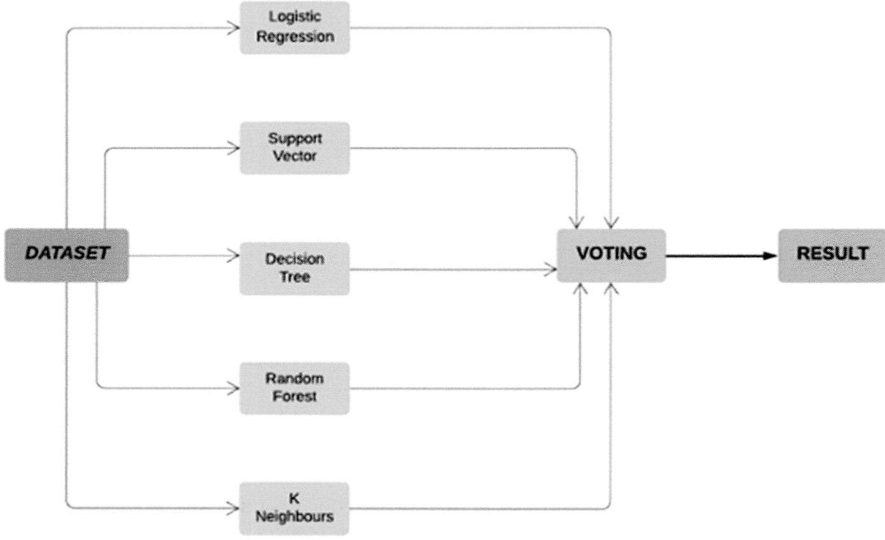


**Figure 4.15 Working of Majority Voting Ensemble.**

Figure 4.15 demonstrates the working of the majority voting ensemble, in which the dataset is fed to a number of classifiers, following which the class with maximum number of votes is selected as the final result class on the basis of voting.

#### 4.3.2.4.1 Majority Voting Ensemble Result Analysis

Figure 4.16 indicates through the confusion matrix of naïve Bayes prediction that only 12 points were misclassified out of 1891 points in the dataset, yielding a high accuracy of 99.35%.

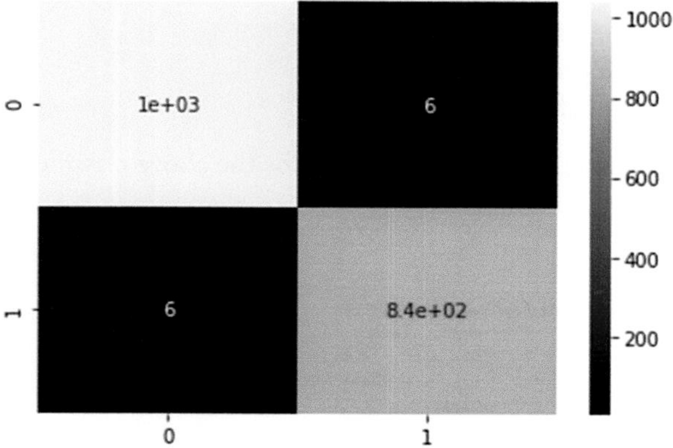


**Figure 4.16 Confusion matrix of MVE's predictions. A figure showing parameters of confusion matrix and their values obtained in MVE's predictions.**

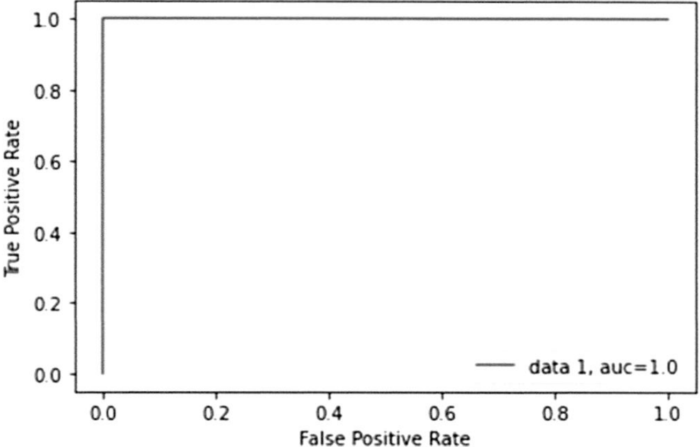


**Figure 4.17 ROC curve of MVE Predictions.**

| Specificity | Sensitivity | Accuracy | Precision | FPR |
|---|---|---|---|---|
| 0.99 | 0.992 | 0.993 | 0.994 | 0.007 |

| FNR | NPV | FDR | F1 score | MCC |
|---|---|---|---|---|
| 0.007 | 0.99 | 0.005 | 1.18 | 0.98 |

**Figure 4.18 Naïve Bayes evaluation parameters.**

The extremely high AUC of 1.0 in Figure 4.17 indicates very high accuracy and an efficient prediction.

Figure 4.18 takes into account all the important evaluation parameters required to evaluate the performance of majority voting ensemble.

## 4.4 Conclusion

We implemented multiple classifiers for the heart disease prediction dataset in order to compare the accuracies provided by different classifiers and further designed a high-accuracy majority voting classifier which resulted in 99.3% accuracy. It is important to have an extremely high-accuracy classifier for the prediction of cardiovascular disease so as to determine whether the disease is in a benign or malignant state.

## References


1 R. Atallah and A. Al-Mousa, Heart Disease Detection Using Machine Learning Majority Voting Ensemble Method, *2019 2nd International Conference on New Trends in Computing Sciences (ICTCS)*, 2019. doi:10.1109/ictcs.2019.8923053.

2 A. Nikam, S. Bhandari, A. Mhaske and S. Mantri, Cardiovascular Disease Prediction Using Machine Learning Models, *2020 IEEE Pune Section International Conference (PuneCon)*, 2020. doi:10.1109/punecon50868.2020.9362367.

3 D. Shah, S. Patel and S. Bharti, Heart disease prediction using machine learning techniques, *SN Computer Science*, vol. 1, no. 6, 2020. doi:10.1007/s42979-020-00365-y.

4 C. Krittanawong et al., Machine learning prediction in cardiovascular diseases: A meta-analysis, *Scientific Reports*, vol. 10, no. 1, 2020. doi:10.1038/s41598-020-72685-1.

5 R. Das, I. Turkoglu and A. Sengur, Effective diagnosis of heart disease through neural networks ensembles, *Expert Systems with Applications*, vol. 36, no. 4, pp. 7675–7680, 2009. doi:10.1016/j.eswa.2008.09.013.

6 R. Bharti, A. Khamparia, M. Shabaz, G. Dhiman, S. Pande and P. Singh, Prediction of heart disease using a combination of machine learning and deep learning, *Computational Intelligence and Neuroscience*, vol. 2021, pp. 1–11, 2021.

7 K. Soni, A. Gupta and T. Jain, Supervised Machine Learning Approaches for Breast Cancer Classification and a high performance Recurrent Neural Network, *2021 Third International Conference on Inventive Research in Computing Applications (ICIRCA)*, 2021.

8 X. Gao, A. Amin Ali, H. Shaban Hassan and E. Anwar, "Improving the accuracy for analyzing heart diseases prediction based on the ensemble method", *Complexity*, vol. 2021, pp. 1–10, 2021.

9 L. Yang, H. Wu, X. Jin, P. Zheng, S. Hu, X. Xu, W. Yu and J. Yan, Study of cardiovascular disease prediction model based on random forest in eastern China, *Scientific Reports*, vol. 10, no. 1, p. 5245, 2020.

10 P. Wilson, R. D'Agostino, D. Levy, A. Belanger, H. Silbershatz and W. Kannel, Prediction of coronary heart disease using risk factor categories, *Circulation*, vol. 97, no. 18, pp. 1837–1847, 1998.

11 A. Yazdani, K. Varathan, Y. Chiam, A. Malik and W. Wan Ahmad, "A novel approach for heart disease prediction using strength scores with significant predictors", *BMC Medical Informatics and Decision Making*, vol. 21, no. 1, p. 194, 2021.

12 V. Sharma, S. Yadav and M. Gupta, Heart Disease Prediction using Machine Learning Techniques, *2020 2nd International Conference on Advances in Computing, Communication Control and Networking (ICACCCN)*, 2020.

13 C. Latha and S. Jeeva, Improving the accuracy of prediction of heart disease risk based on ensemble classification techniques, *Informatics in Medicine Unlocked*, vol. 16, p. 100203, 2019.

14 D. Salhi, A. Tari and M. Kechadi, Using machine learning for heart disease prediction. In *Advances in Computing Systems and Applications*, pp. 70–81, 2021.

15 Nishi, F. K., Khan, M. M., Alsufyani, A., Bourouis, S., Gupta, P., & Saini, D. K. Electronic Healthcare Data Record Security Using Blockchain and Smart Contract. *Journal of Sensors*, *2022*, 2022.

16 Sharma, S., Gupta, S., Gupta, D., Juneja, S., Gupta, P., Dhiman, G., & Kautish, S. Deep learning model for the automatic classification of white blood cells. *Computational Intelligence and Neuroscience*, *2022*, 2022.

17 Tazin, T., Sarker, S., Gupta, P., Ayaz, F. I., Islam, S., Monirujjaman Khan, M., … Alshazly, H. A robust and novel approach for brain tumor classification using convolutional neural network. *Computational Intelligence and Neuroscience, 2021*, 2021.

18 K. M. Soni, A. Gupta and T. Jain, Supervised Machine Learning Approaches for Breast Cancer Classification and a High Performance Recurrent Neural Network, *2021 Third International Conference on Inventive Research in Computing Applications (ICIRCA)*, 2021, pp. 1–7, doi:10.1109/ICIRCA51532.2021.9544630.

19 T. Jain, A. Jain, P. S. Hada, H. Kumar, V. K. Verma and A. Patni, Machine Learning Techniques for Prediction of Mental Health, *2021 Third International Conference on Inventive Research in Computing Applications (ICIRCA)*, 2021, pp. 1606–1613, doi:10.1109/ICIRCA51532.2021.9545061.

# Chapter 5

# Machine Learning Algorithms for Industry Using Image Sensing

Aakash Dhall and Hemant K Upadhyay
*BM Institute of Engineering and Technology Sonepat, India*

Sapna Juneja and Abhinav Juneja
*KIET Group of Institutions, Delhi NCR, India*

## Contents

5.1 Introduction ....76
5.2 What is Manufacturing Artificial Intelligence? ....77
5.3 Defining the Industrial Internet of Things ....77
5.4 IoT History ....78
5.5 IIoT Architectures ....78
5.6 Applications of IIoT ....79
    5.6.1 Smart Manufacturing ....80
5.7 Securing the Internet of Things ....81
    5.7.1 Safety ....82
    5.7.2 Security ....83
    5.7.3 Privacy ....84
5.8 Challenges and Opportunities ....85
5.9 Future of IIoT ....86
5.10 Communication 5G and Beyond ....88

DOI: 10.1201/9781003322597-5

5.11 How Did AI Develop in Production? ..........88
5.11.1 AI in Manufacturing Current State ..........89
5.11.2 What is AI's Future in Production? ..........90
5.12 Process and Factory Floors that are Flexible and Configurable ..........92
5.13 Manufacturing and AI: Applications and Benefits ..........92
5.14 Impact of COVID-19 on Industrial Internet of Things ..........94
5.15 Conclusion ..........95
References ..........95

## 5.1 Introduction

The IoT is a networking of such items as computers, apparatuses, cars, home applications, houses, and similar objects that are equipped with mechatronics and networking communication to capture and share information. Schneider et al. [3] state "The IoT enables items for sensing and operating over present networks, allowing in directly linked blend of the environment in software structure and increased productivity and accuracy."

The very first industrial revolution improved productivity through the use of hydroelectric power, improved steam power, and the development of machine tools; the second revolution introduced electricity and mass manufacturing through assembly lines; the third revolution advanced automation through electronics and information technology; and the fourth industrial revolution is now under way (see Figure 5.1). CPS (cyber-physical systems) is a new field involving engineered

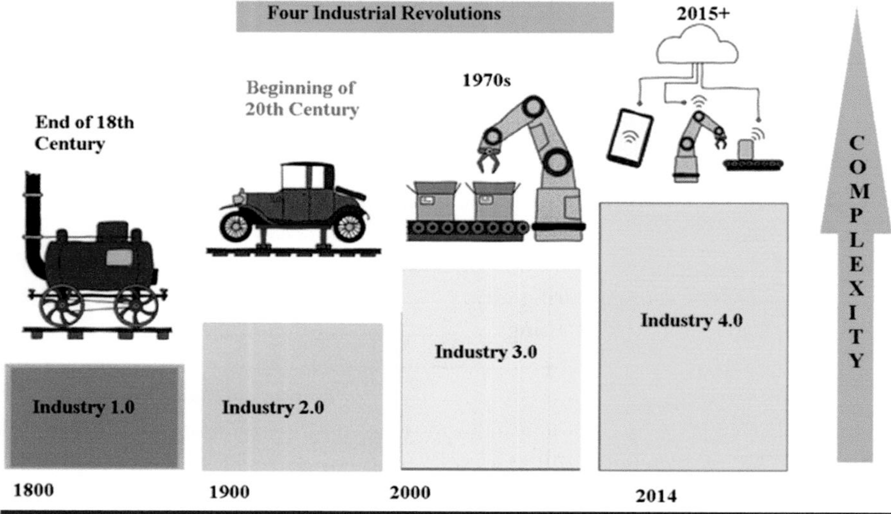


Figure 5.1 Four Industrial Revolutions.

computing and communication systems that interact with their surroundings. The IIoT is speeding up the advance of industrial growth and changing economies, ushering in a new age of growth and competitiveness.

The purpose of this chapter is to introduce the reader to the general idea of the IIoT, its design, implementation and uses, and the challenges and opportunities it poses.

According to Sapna Juneja et al. [27], the self-contained factory remains a provocative vision, commonly seen in speculative fiction. It is almost autonomous and operates entirely through neural network systems that control robot production lines. But the way neural networks are used in production in the realistic preparation horizon is immersive.

The practical design of AI in the automotive industry is more like a series of applications for lightweight, isolated systems managing production processes. They are more or less independent and are increasingly wise and even human in their reactions to external events – events ranging from a system outage, a tool wearing out to a fire or natural disaster.

## 5.2 What is Manufacturing Artificial Intelligence?

Historians monitor man's advances from Stone Age to Bronze Age, Iron Age, etc., based on human knowledge of the natural world, resources, instruments and technology. Evolutionary progression is measured. Humanity is now in the Information Age, or Silicon Age. In this electronic period, people have the potential to do tasks that were inconceivable a few years ago utilizing machines, and use unprecedented power in the natural environment.

With the progress of computer technology people can now do tasks that historically were difficult, and AI encourages determined people to do better. In the production sector, they can design and make parts and products using AI. According to Hwaiyu Geng et al. [22], AI in production is a machinery intelligence that performs human tasks automatically – responding internally and externally to events, including anticipation of events.

H. Ding et al. [17] suggest that most self-sufficient and "intelligent, industrial robots don't need much monitoring. AI and engineering make them more intelligent, safer and more powerful.

## 5.3 Defining the Industrial Internet of Things

The Industrial Internet of Things (IIoT) is a network that connects devices and services to a web-based system. It transforms vast data into powerful new knowledge and information by using tools to apply deep analytics. The IoT has been expanded into manufacturing industries where its applications are called the Industrial Internet of Things (IIoT). IIoT allows businesses and companies to improve performance and reliability by concentrating on machine-to-machine connectivity, machine learning, and big data.

Jeschke et al. [5] explain that based on use and customer base, IoT can be divided into three categories:

Consumer IoT comprises linked components like technology-based smart vehicles, mobile sets, time instruments, laptops and linked devices.

Commercial IoT involves products such as inventory management, system trackers and medical equipment.

Industrial IoT covers electrical connectors, wastewater systems, flow gauges, monitors for pipelines, production robots, and similar industry-based items.

We have come into the era of newer change as the whole planet these days maximizes our most important physical assets' efficiency. We are faced with unbelievable creativity on the Internet by accelerating the connection between objects and people and other objects – applications of IIoT pledge to give our lives tremendous importance.

## 5.4 IoT History

To fully understand the IoT concept, we first need to understand how it has evolved. Newer software may modify the industrial structure rapidly in today's technology-riven era. However, though the IIoT is now global, linking unlimited computers, resources, and sets worldwide – this is an overnight sensation. In the last few decades, technical steps large and small – ranging from significant breakthroughs in machine architecture to small steps – have contributed to IIoT in its present form.

In 1968, Dick Morley started to develop the IIoT as one of the most important success stories in production history. That year, Morley and a group of geek friends invented the PLC which would eventually become irreplaceable in factories with automated assembly lines and industrial robots.

## 5.5 IIoT Architectures

Hugh Boyes at el [6] explained, the choice of architecture is very important significant issue businesses deal when choosing in case of Industrial Internet of Things. Since Industrial Internet of Things idea is on the basis of a networking connection device, the IIoT architecture is very essential part. Industrial Internet of Things sets have been generally a modular staged digital technology architecture. There are different IIoT specifications in various industries. An aeroplane, for example, is very different from a simple gasket production process in the data output of the discharge and landing. Therefore, the choice of exemplary IIoT architecture is important because IIoT involves data transmission.

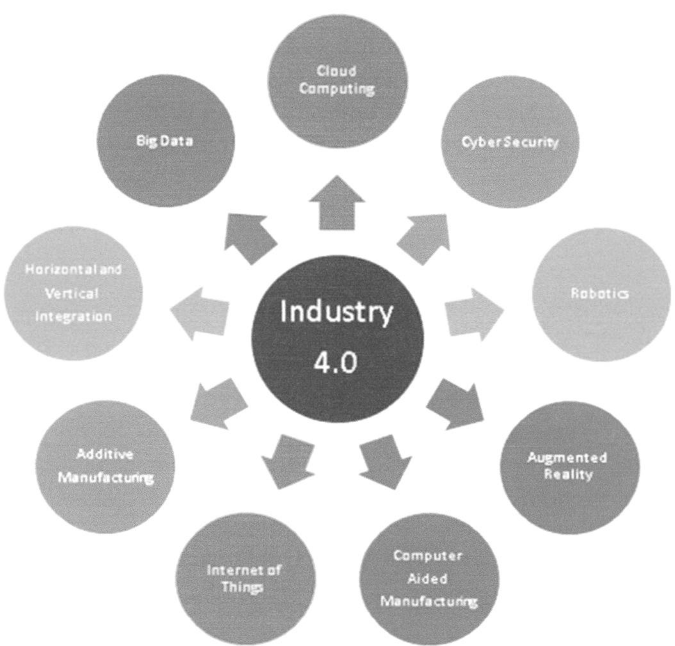


**Figure 5.2 Industry Connectivity.**

A well-founded business strategy and the overall operating framework are driving successful digital transformation implementations. The design of the IoT (IIoT) Industrial systems enforces new software/system architecture decision sets as shown in Figure 5.2.

## 5.6 Applications of IIoT

Tyler Ainsworth et al. [8] explained, The Industrial Internet of Things would boost production and will allow much greater data collection and much rapid accessibility and much effectively. Numerous firms began implementing IIoT by leveraging their factories with intelligent connected devices. The IIoT drives huge requirement in a wide range of vertical industry for more information collection and connectivity. The IIoT for businesses worldwide is going to demand of the hour soon.

Ting Zheng et al. [18] explained, The way business is done is more and more competitive. Consumers love smart house, smart automobiles, smart infrastructure, clever appliances, and IIoT generates knowledge. Companies discover newer commercial possibilities from the additional cutting edges that can be arranged through AI into clear and comprehensible ideas.

Abhinav Juneja et al. [29] explained, The development of value in IoT is based on the capacity of decision making based on data in real-time. Data collection and subsequent processes are needed. Data collection uses include billions of smart and semi-smart connected matters. The transfer of data involves several layers of connectivity and relies on linking distributed IoT equipment to decision-making systems. More computing power and memory are needed to analyze data – primarily for making decisions in real-time. As digital content and the content produced by machines increase, data storage needs are also increasing.

### 5.6.1 Smart Manufacturing

Q. Qi et al. [4] explained, A vision of future production goods in the production process finding their path. In intelligent factories, devices and goods interact cooperatively, the Internet of Things interconnects driving raw materials and machinery. There are already factories in the future with network machines and products; however, these previously autonomous devices would be linked to a full grid. The sensors, communication technologies and cyber-physical systems link all devices, machines and materials (CPS). They converse with one another and collaborate to influence one another. The logic of Cyber-physical systems underpins Industry 4.0.

Smart manufacturing enables management of any organization to appropriately capture and evaluate the information to take wise execution of plans and maximize efficiency. The key to smart manufacturing is the database; that is accountable for "what to do", "when to do it." This is a dynamic disruptive set of efforts along the ability to recreate manufacturing's present era landscaping. Progressive wear is popular in industrial production equipment. As a result, maintenance methodologies and monitoring mechanism are required.

Production processes are ideal operations for remote monitoring technologies because they must track potentially inaccessible areas while maintaining near-continuous output. G. Laput et al. explained [12], Uses of sensors in the industrial applications are growing because of substantial cost decrement in sensors, developments in sensor engineering and the emergence of advanced modern uses those may be utilized to derive, discover information from data.

- Chu Anh My et al. explained [16], For years, IIoT has harnessed sensor data, machine-to-machine (M2M) communication, and automation innovations in industrial settings by integrating machine learning and big data technology.
- The driving theory behind the IIoT is that intelligent machines are better than humans at collecting and transmitting data accurately and reliably.
- The driving theory behind the IIoT is that intelligent machines are better than humans at collecting and transmitting data accurately and reliably. This data will help businesses detect inefficiencies and issues earlier, saving time and resources and promoting business intelligence efforts.

- In particular, IIoT has tremendous potential in manufacturing for quality management, fair and green practices, supply chain traceability, and overall supply chain performance.

IoT networking systems installed in the factory communicate database from sensing equipments and machineries to the Cloud. This database is integrated with the contextual data and further distributed to the stakeholders. Industrial Internet of Things facilitates this flow of data by using wired and wireless networking, allowing for remote monitoring and management of processes and the ability to adjust production plans rapidly as required. This significantly enhances manufacturing results by minimizing wastage, increasing the speed of the production and increasing product quality.

Smart manufacturing necessitates vertical as well as horizontal database combining with the organization. Vertical digitization can involve production, sourcing, distribution processes and efficiency. Data integration with vendors, consumers, and vital stakeholders can be part of horizontal digitalization. Integrating includes updating and the procedures before you are satisfied.

The IoT is the world's digital nervous system. Total IoT implementation concerns with alive bodies those sees, hears, and feels its surroundings. If the data obtained from a part like finger indicates that something is too cold, this data must be transmitted rapidly to our brain so that our hand may be withdrawn. Cameras, microphones, as well as sensory organs, can monitor anything from temperature to pressure change.

The most obvious symptom of mechanical failure is audio. The majority of faults in this domain are caused by the motor pumps' action, which induces frictional disturbances. Microphones listens for indicators of wear – variations in system noises – so that repairs can be planned until it gets broken and becomes the reason for downtime.

Downtime is probably the worst thing which may happen to a production plant. Instead of analyzing the waveform of time Vs series directly, audio based signals are converted into the spectrograms. The definition of a "auxel," which is similar to pixels in images, was used to describe the intensity value at a particular time Vs frequency spot.

An important IIoT projects in the semiconductor industry is the use of acoustic sensing devices on wafer processing machineries to capture signals like wafers are brushed. We may distinguish irregular sounds and recognize potentially hazardous tool environments by matching background sound signatures from wafer's auditory signals to sound patterns found during brushing.

## 5.7 Securing the Internet of Things

Most people are aware of the onslaught of web based gadgets which are supposed to be a part of human lives within the upcoming decade. This linkage will result in unprecedented efficiency, innovative commercial models, and effectiveness previously unimaginable. This would provide appealing objectives for newer generation of crime minded people and other factors trying for break through virtual back doors which did not exist.

Unsecured IoT devices have become a legitimate reason, considering that IoT devices would be used in more than 25% of cyberattacks. Putting measures in place would protect citizens thus allowing this process to take place. Gartner expects that 26 billion new computers will be connected to the Internet by 2025, excluding PCs, tablets, and smartphones. It is important to protect all of these systems, which are quickly becoming integral parts of human lives. These devices use to be small and focused on a single goal like to do: reliable data collection or its linking to the Internet. That signifies that extra security hardware of that scale is still in its infancy.

IoT threats may be generally divided into three categories: protection, security, and data privacy.

### 5.7.1 Safety

E. Vasilomanolakis et al. [23] explained, The Internet of Things (IoT) has gifted us the ever-growing digitalized risks along with cyber security, generating a slew of newer vulnerabilities such as serious threats for general security, physical damage, and devastating planned attacks on widely shared general infrastructure. We know about an petroleum pipeline in Turkey that was hacked, resulting in an blast and thousands of liters of spilled oil, the cyber attackers bypassed the current safety plan, shutting down the alarming devices, cutting off the communicating connections, and pressurizing the line with crude oil. A local water supply organization suffered a breach, that compromised consumer info. There is a chance that linked apparatus could fail and injure the public.

Furthermore, if hackers get access to related machines and cause it to act in undetectable methods for a period of time, which can become reason for apparatus to produce faulty apparatus. This probability also jeopardizes life. Your protection programmers are inextricably connected in industrial development. Plenty of customers use IIoT to access manufacturing resources virtually, provide wireless connectivity to pump stations to maximize asset efficiency and reduce overall cost. However, improved communication could enhance safety risks that is to be managed by improved business risk management.

Users' raised expectations for these legacy systems to operate consistently and without interruption. That is particularly valid for critical establishments.

The crucial criterion for system collectivity is that it has protection. It has considerable advantages for connecting all automobiles and related infrastructure to the Internet of Things; but have huge danger. We may reduce the likelihood of potential cyber-attacking as cars are interconnected. As opposed to the possibility of someone managing of the car from the remote and safety is compromised.

The development of an combined device networking to link automobile systems along through the Internet of Things for real time communication and interaction with the environment and assurance for much protection for everyone engaged is the next technological move which may provide much safety for the automobile.

### 5.7.2 Security

Securing industrial Internet of Things devices is necessary to preserve data combining and to secure against attacking that can jeopardize system reliability. Since structures can transmit vast quantities of sensitive information over the web and the end-users can monitor devices easily, the protection of "stuff" will permeate each layer of the possible solution.

Vital issue with the growing number of Internet of Things devices is the enhanced complication needed for their safe operation. The enhance complication generates safety problems that are much more challenging than the complex challenges individuals encounter when protecting a unit. We focus few negative issues caused by intelligent systems and collected devices, and discuss the problems connected to safety, privacy, and utility are inextricably linked, and factors those focus all the four at the same time are required. Individual system safety and security requirements based on current technologies are required. Similarly, future implementations of such systems must be driven by technology which defines for the individuals for appropriately handling collecting devices.

To secure its embedded products, the industry requires the equivalence of a flu shot. Until attacks can occur, all future nodes inside the linked castle must be immunized. This is only possible along security features integrated into the memory system. This protects the computing system on the networking and at almost points before the networking, with the conception with the supply chain.

Good memory protection would not remove the need for good code sign and measuring activities. Better security is often built on multiple levels of protection. However, the objective is to make the calculating device as much resilient for attacking by shielding the memory and machine logic.

We know that the future is a hybrid of types of computing. The initial database may be processed on-site and modified database will be submitted to the Cloud for review, and the on-site applications may allow regular feedback on the system health to focus possible scope for betterment.

Although threats may still occur in the Internet of Things, as these may do in other technological endeavors, there is thin probability to enhance the protection of Internet of Things surroundings by utilizing safety techniques as encryption of database, safe user authenticating tools, resilient codes which respond predictably.

Security must be built into IoT systems as the basis, with stringent validity checks, authentication, data verification, and encryption of all data. At the application level, software development organizations must improve their ability to write code that is stable, resilient, and trustworthy, through improved code development standards, training, threat detection, and testing. When systems communicate with one another, it is essential to provide an agreed-upon interoperability specification that is both secure and accurate. Without a solid bottom-to-top structure, each system added to the IoT would introduce new threats. We require a stable Internet of Things with safety protection, that is a difficult next to impossible trade-off.

### 5.7.3 Privacy

Privacy concern is difficult to comprehend and ensure in a global scenario while smart devices do collection, transmit, and monetize data. The radically different privacy vulnerabilities can pose an even greater threat to the IoT's performance. Data collection by Internet of Things devices is gradually raising the warning that Internet of Things users may become attentive for processing of collected data by Internet of Things devices. This type of devices are put on the Internet for ease, causing a major public nuisance at best, a real intrusion on privacy in some cases.

Important in person details such as the location and activity. Such situation creates questions about the confidentiality of personal data. Several embedded connection devices may be reviewed remotely before going live on the Internet to ensure that they have not been compromised and the real brains and nervous systems of each linked computer as well as the safeguarded code that runs on them are considered.

The definition of "trusted" or "measured" boot is one of the Trusted Computing Community's core players and several others in the security industry. The theory is that a virtual system is at the very heart of the programme and checked.

The code will test themselves and subsequently measure other modules of code before passing power to them at the system boot's earliest step. As each calculation following is considered right and trusted, the device progresses safely through the boot phase and ultimately becomes a trustworthy linked device.

The industry's code protection response is code protection calculation before it is implemented to respond to a question already raised. The thing is that it looks very much like being sick and checking with the throat swab or blood test the cause of your illness. While it's good to know that you're still ill and there's medication to better your situation, you may not help but might have avoided the scourge.

We described few impacts of the modifications in a discussion on usage structures and the protection. We assume that the transition rate is changing, and the challenge and volatility are strong enough to prioritize expenditure in research to offset future problems. Potential advantages for human life, the national priorities, and the economy are enough to guarantee significant investment in innovation in the most advantageous technologies.

For data brokers, data markets' regulatory requirements are lacking; these are the organizations who provide the data from different sources. While knowledge appears to be the IoT money, the openness remains, who has availability of the database and this is utilized to design goods and market to marketers. Clear guidance on preservation, usage and data protection, including metadata, are required.

## 5.8 Challenges and Opportunities

Chetna Chauhan et al. [20] explained, The Internet of Things is applied to almost forms of companies along with businesses and offers a variety of advantages. The adoption of IIoT raises some of the most urgent problems and questions. The problems are: Vulnerabilities to the authentication system (privacy, sabotage, service denial): hacking profile targets still leaves this risk in mind.

For instance, sabotage and service denial may have much more drastic implications than a private concession. Changing the disinfectant mix ratio in a water treatment plant or stopping the nuclear power plant's cooling system may pose an immediate hazard to the whole region.

Connectivity: IoT's potential problem slink too many computers, defying the very nature of existing communications models and underlying technology. We now focus on the server/client model for authentication, authorization and connection of various nodes in a network.

Issues of regulation and law: This covers primarily medical instruments, banking, insurance, equipment for infrastructures, manufacturing equipment and particularly equipment relating to pharmaceuticals and food. Today, this means compliance with legislation like CFR 21 section 11, HIPAA, 95/46/EC and GAMP 5, etc. This raises the time and costs involved to sell these goods.

Network Determinism: This is critical for almost all IoT fields, including control applications, defence, production, transport, general infrastructure and medical devices. Usually, the use of the Cloud needs about 200 milliseconds or longer.

This is ideal for most applications, but not for safety applications or other applications requiring quick, almost immediate response. A safety management device signal that was issued 5s later could be too late.

Jan Stentoft et al. [21] explained about, the absence of the universal architecture and standardization of IoT would minimize its usefulness and raise end users' costs through continual fragmentation. Currently there are Google Brillo and Weave, AllJoyn and Higgins, to name just a handful, in addition to the brands listed above. Any of these goods are specifically targeted. Any of the reasons for the fragmentation are concerns about security and privacy (privacy through obscure behaviour, fear of not being invented), market domination, attempts to escape concerns about intellectual property rights for rivals, and the current lack of strong leadership this field. Scalability: This isn't much of a concern at present however, as the number of devices in use grows, it will mainly become a problem in connections with generic market cloud. The bandwidth and time taken to validate transfers would be increased.

Restrictions of the sensors available: Fundamental sensor types are now very performing, such as temperature, illumination, move, sound, colour, radar, the laser scanner, echography and X-ray. Moreover, in addition to developments in microelectronics in solid-state sensors, bare sensors will no longer be a problem in future. In busy, chaotic and diverse conditions, the challenge would be to increase prejudice. The use of algorithms close to fleeting logic promises to make this less a problem in the future.

Off-grid electricity sources: dense and sustainable: While most networking problems could be resolved via Ethernet, WIFI, 3G and Bluetooth, by accommodating the form factors of different users, battery life limitations remain. Most smartphones still need to be charged daily and most sensors still need routine battery modification or grid link. If power can be wirelessly transmitted from a distance to such equipment or power sources that last for at least a year can be incorporated into the sensors, it will change.

## 5.9 Future of IIoT

Thommie Burström et al. [10] explained, The future of Industrial Internet of Things may be unlimited. The growth of Internet of Things may make the future plant come true shortly. Industrial internet progress is accelerated by increasing network resilience, advanced artificial intelligence, the ability to launch and ensure hypermarket applications. A thrilling flood of future IoT technologies will be generated by intuitive interactivity between people and machines. Human 4.0 enables people to communicate with each other and equipment in real-time over great distances and to have sensory input close to what they have locally. This will allow new ways to learn, surgeon and cure remotely. Our three dimensional audio as well as Haptic experiences and the key interface for the real life the following platform after smartphone apps will become. To build future IoTs, close synergies between IoT platforms and network networks are needed.

The Ignition IIoT solution strengthens communication, performance, scalability, saving time and expense for the industry. The processes and staff on the floor should be united with those on the business stage. It will also allow companies to make their system the best without technical and economic constraints. For these and other purposes, Ignition provides the perfect forum to carry IIoT's power into your company.

To achieve the upper hand of these powers, the implementation of an IIoT approach in the industry becomes invaluable. These adapters can learn from large-scale IIoT technologies that easily solve today's market needs and satisfy potential demands. As such ventures broaden and these changing demands need solutions offered by vendors with the right mixture of innovations, domain expertise and an environment of collaboration to fill the gaps. The skill of IIoT providers is obvious further. Successful Industrial Internet of Things installations in production and operating procedures may begin to span the company's hierarchy to allow coordinated operating with Industrial Internet of Things touch points from a CXO to frontline employee.

Myriad world powers transform companies "digital" faster to deter disruption, make them more productive and leverage new opportunities. This digital revolution entails various items with various industries. It is becoming more scalable and versatile in production and organizational efficiencies.

In comparison to manufacturing networks, the industrial Internet of things would fundamentally transform the future. We can already see the pattern coming to life from wrist watches to smart appliances for the multiple participants. If the Industrial IOT project achieves its full potential, many will have the chance to improve their jobs and living levels, as the full potential of this vision leads to innumerable possibilities for value growth. When new "revolutions" are in place, this is still the case.

Industrial IoT's full capacity would contribute to smart power grids, intelligent health care, smart transportation, intelligent diagnostics, etc. The handling, packaging, delivery of products and maintenance of supply chains may be made automatic up to some extent in the coming decade. In near future, analysts say that IIoT would further increase output volumes and become the motor behind different inventions. This allows the production of ecosystems powered by intelligent systems with independent configuration, monitoring and healing on its own. Consider the technology of the "Terminator" fashion. Rather, this technique would enhance our operating efficiency and drive product development at an unparalleled pace.

While a series of adoption problems will also need to be solved, statistical data indicates that 50 billion connected devices will be available worldwide by 2025. It would be a shame to stay unused to strengthen manufacturing processes in such a large network. Remember that IoT is not about the invention of intelligent products. Instead of reactionary interference, it would contribute to a higher degree of productivity and prediction – today's a major challenge industry is striving for. Figure 5.3 shows the future of world with IoT and industry.

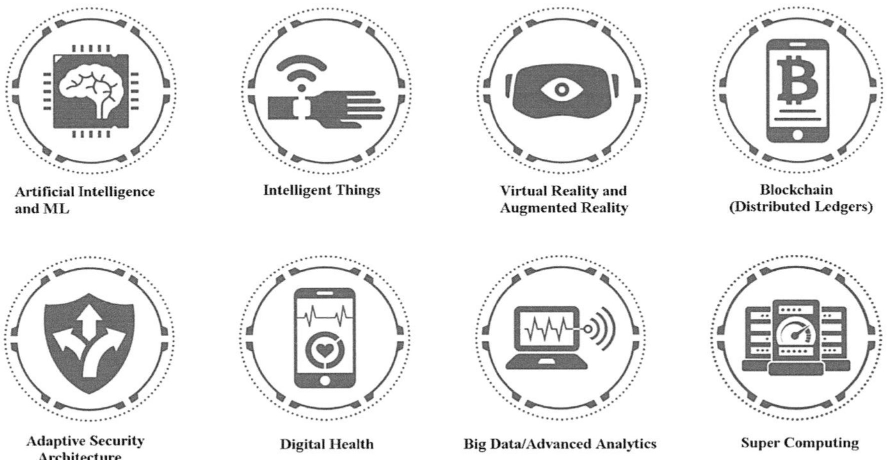


**Figure 5.3 Future of IIoT.**

## 5.10 Communication 5G and Beyond

S. Mumtaz et al. [24] explained, 3GPP is the standardization of telecommunications from seven corporate guidelines to an individual paper. The 5G vision was planned and studied from the 3GPP platform. Contact is the foundation for open networking in the concept of 5G communications to infuse the automobile industry into industry 4.0. The guiding requirement for 5G is low latency, trustworthiness, connectivity, data transfer speed and high-precision positioning. The requirement mentioned above for autonomous flexibility requires high levels of automation in the automotive industry. The promise of providing real-time networking, a low-cost approach, adaptable industries and redundancy in hard-wired products would allow the automobile industry, Industry 4.0, to improve and grow 5G communication. Many sensors can be remote from the factory floor in automation, but these sensors must reactivate, be stable and run in real-time. 5G can accelerate these. It's fundamental component of its proposed performance is the potential to link thousands of smartphones with the large 5G bandwidth. The bandwidth can be contrasted with a multi-lane road and the sensors thus reflect the 5G wide potential compared to an intelligent vehicle. It reminds us that the focus for returning critics on the network should be due to the need for dedicated network software for mobile devices, computers and sensors. Safety for 5G in the factory or sensor/appliances is the main concern. Any business must protect itself against these possibilities through IIoT networks with increasing cybercrime. Sapna Juneja et al. [28] explained, Futuristic Cyber Twin Architecture for 6G Technology to support Internet of Everything Automotive machines perform accurately, many operate remotely, and many are interactive robots. 5G and 6G communications can improve industrial automation, and superior security is required in this connectivity network.

## 5.11 How Did AI Develop in Production?

Today, most AI manufacturers concern with calculation instruments, nondestructive testing (NDT) and other methods. AI supports product design, but manufacturing is also in the early stages of AI adoption. Tools of machines remain very obtuse. However, the news is that shop instruments remain the topic of old machines, either with mechanical or minimal digital interface, for most manufacturers worldwide.

New manufacturing systems have screens – human-computer interfaces and electronic sensors for input on availability of raw materials, device state, power usage and several other variables. On television or the machine, you will see what you are doing. As are the possibilities for the way AI is used in the automotive sector, the way forward is simple.

Serkan Ayvaz et al. [26] explained, the nearest situations require real-time control of machining and monitoring of status inputs such as equipment use. This form of application is referred to as "predictive maintenance." This is an obvious opportunity for AI: algorithms that use endless data streams from sensors, identify meaningful trends and use analytics to anticipate problems and alert maintenance teams to repair them before their occurrence. Sensors inside the system will detect the event. It may be a sound sensor that listens to the belts or gears' wear-out or a sensor that tracks wear. This knowledge is related to an empirical model that can estimate how long life remains in this instrument.

Additive production is a significant method on the store floor and has led to the addition to the systems of several different types of sensors, tracking new material and packaging technology conditions that have only been broadly implemented within the past 10 years.

### 5.11.1 AI in Manufacturing Current State

Guanghui Zhou et al. [1], explained With the help of a digital simulation, AI makes even more detailed design of production processes and diagnostics and solutions for problems when manufacturing defects occur. An exact visual copy of the actual component, the machine tool or the part you make is a digital twin. It's far more than a model of CAD. It represents exactly how and how the component is portrayed digitally when, for instance, a defect occurs. (This is the reason they fail) all pieces have flaws. AI is needed in the design and maintenance of production processes for the implementation of the digital twin.

Akshay G. Khanzode et al. [19] explained, The use of AI and the financial resources to support these technologies have greatly benefited large companies. However, some of the more innovative applications, such as contract designers and suppliers supplying high-tech sectors such as aviation, is financed by small to medium-sized companies (SMEs).

Frank Lynch et al. [13] explained, By introducing quickly modern equipment or innovations, often small companies attempt to take on larger rivals. The resources provided are differentiating in industrial fields, but in some situations, without the prerequisite expertise, they incorporate new tools and processes. That can be valid in terms of architecture or development; it is also difficult to break into additive production. In this case, small and medium-sized firms may have greater AI benefits than big companies: The use of intelligent systems that can provide guidance and help set up and operationalize a small start-up could help create a disturbing market position.

In essence, engineering knowledge from the end of the process should be incorporated into a development process. In other words, onboard AI tools can be supplied with the know-how to manage their implementation, acceptance, sensors analysis for operating and maintenance problem detection. (These analyses may involve so-called unattended models, trained to find input patterns from sensors rather than known problems, through scanning for unusual or "false" aspects to be examined.)

Understanding each part's impact on each part is essential because human beings can automate and then use AI design to allow the software design to function closer to the physical object.

### 5.11.2 What is AI's Future in Production?

Tao, F et al. [2], explained This situation means that an end-to-end work method to sell to a manufacturer is easily packaged. It may contain anything from software to physical equipment at the plant, the machines' digital twin, the ordering mechanism that shares data with the factory's supply chain processes, and the analysis for process monitoring and data collection as inputs pass through the system. In turn, creating structures for "factory in a box."

**Factory in a Box**
Laurence McHauser et al. [25] explained, as a producer, this method will allow you to examine the part you have done today, comparing it to the part you did yesterday, verifying that quality testing is carried out, and analyzing the NDT made for each phase. The input allows you to understand precisely what parameters you used to create those sections and then see where faults exist from the sensor data.
The operation's ultimate goal is to put components onto one end, and the pieces are extracted. People are required only to manage the installations where robotics will ultimately do most of the job. However, people also plan and decide on the new conception, supervise the production process, and serve other line functions. The device allows you to consider the real implications of your actions.

**Autonomous AI Machine Learning**
Patrik Zajec et al. [15] explained, AI's biggest asset is the capacity to learn from its own experience without human intervention. These systems can quickly detect large trends in data volumes beyond human analysts' ability. However, human specialists in manufacturing today also drive AI applications and encode their experience from previous programmers. Human experts carry their opinions on what happened, what went wrong, what went right.

Autonomous AI is eventually building on this body of professional experience so that a new employee can learn from operational input in additive manufacture by analyzing and refining the onboard sensor data for preventative maintenance. This is a breakthrough in technologies such as self-reflecting devices – the device adapts to improve efficiency when replacing used parts as wear-out resources.

**Optimization of factory architecture and configuration**
AI applications do not restrict themselves to the production process. Think of it from a strategy point of view. Multiple factors influence the facility architecture, from operator protection to process flow quality. It can cause the facility to be

reconfigured to accommodate several short-term tasks or procedures that are always evolving.

Sometimes improvements may contribute to room and content problems that are unexpected and may cause performance or security concerns. However, these conflicts can be monitored and calculated by sensors and AI to play in factory layout optimization.

**Real-time AI research catch data sensors**

A significant move is the use of NDT after the component is made when implementing modern techniques, about which there is much confusion as additive fabrication. Nondestructive testing can be very costly, particularly when incorporating CT scanners for capital equipment (used to analyze manufactured parts' structural integrity). Computer sensors may attach to models made of a wide collection of data learned from manufacturing for particular components. Once data is available, a machine learning model can be built using sensor information – to compare, for example, with a defect in the CT scan. The sensor data indicate components that may be faulty by the analysis model without needing the component to be scanned by CT. Instead of regularly screening all parts once they leave the line, only certain parts will be screened.

The operation will also control the use of the equipment by citizens. Production engineers assume that the device is equipped to control the machinery. An additional step may be taken or a step missed for human examination. Sensors can reliably collect AI measurement knowledge.

AI also contributes to adjusting production methods and tools to a variety of environmental factors. Take humidity, for instance. Additive manufacturing equipment engineers have discovered that such devices do not operate in certain countries as planned. Humidity sensors have been used in warehouses to track temperatures and to locate counterintuitive artefacts often. In one situation, moisture caused problems in what was meant to be a moisture-controlled environment.

Developing effective AI models requires the efficient use of sensor data. Such models must be educated to learn what the data shows, affect them, find the causes, and what they can do. Machine learning algorithms today will use sensor data to prevent a problem and warn a human problem solver.

Piero Formica et al. [14] explained, In the end, AI systems will anticipate problems and respond to them in real-time. The role of AI models is soon to create proactive means of resolving challenges and improving production processes.

**Design**

Wu, D., Terpenny et al. [26] explained, AI plays a significant role in the design, where a design engineer sets out a list of project specifications, and then design software produces numerous iterations. This AI Prototype understands how the material properties vary depending on how human characteristics and geometry are affected in the process.

AI based Design is a suitable technique of optimization. Many conventional optimization strategies consider wider alternatives to section optimization. AI design algorithms may be much more precise, based on individual traits, and use material testing to understand the function's mechanical characteristics. While plans are idealized, production methods occur in the real world; conditions cannot be consistent. This degree of comprehension requires an efficient design algorithm.

The AI design will create the optimum design and software requirements for several tooling facilities. This means that smaller geographically scattered installations can provide a wider variety of components. Such facilities could be close to where they are needed; one day and the next, aerospace components could be made for other vital goods, thereby saving delivery and storage costs. For example, in the automobile industry, this is becoming an important term.

## 5.12 Process and Factory Floors that are Flexible and Configurable

Con Cronin et al. [7] explained, AI can also be used to optimize production systems and the flexibility and reconfiguration of such processes. Current demand will decide the factory floor's configuration and create a mechanism that is still possible for potential requests. Those versions can then be compared and compared. This research would also decide if fewer great additives, or many smaller devices, may be less expensive and, if demand is weak, redirected to other ventures. Study of "What-if" is a popular AI app.

Both shop floor layout and sequencing processes will be optimized using the model. For instance, thermal treatment can be performed directly from the 3D printer on an additive component. The substance can be pre-tempered or re-tempered and require a particular heat cycle. Engineers may use different examples to decide what facilities the plant could have – subcontracting portions of the operation to another local business might make more sense.

These AI implementations could alter the business case focused on a single captive technique or working with many items or programs. Lastly, the factory will become more robust. In aeronautics, a decreasing sector, its production activities can also be adapted by producing medical components.

## 5.13 Manufacturing and AI: Applications and Benefits

Yi-Chun Chen at el [9] explained, Both fields of production are AI architecture, process development, wear reduction and energy consumption optimization. That has already started.

The robots are becoming smarter and more interconnected, with each other and with the supply chain. Materials in portions of the sensors tracking any interaction on the chain will preferably be included. People manage the mechanism, but they don't act in the world. This frees critical production capital and workers from routine, programmed jobs to concentrate on innovation, creating innovative designing and processing components.

There has been opposition to AI implementation, as in any structural reform. There will be very costly and limited expertise and expertise needed for AI; many producers do not have these facilities on site. To warrant an investment to develop something different or upgrade a procedure, they require extensive evidence and risk-free from upscaling a plant. They consider themselves as effective in advanced skills.

This will make businesses more attractive to the idea of "factory in a box." More companies, especially SMEs, will confidently follow an end-to-end packaging method using sensors and analytics to enhance the software's tooling. It also makes decisions less costly by incorporating digital twin power, in which engineers can test a new development process as a simulation.

Predictive management is another key field for AI manufacturing. In this way, engineers will outfit factory machines with pre-trained AI models incorporating their combined experience. Based on computer input, the models can learn on-site new trends of causes and effects to avoid problems.

In quality inspection, there is also a function for the AI, which generates much data to make machine learning suitable. Consider the manufacture of additives: One construction produces as many terabytes of data on how the process produces the component, the conditions on-site and any problems found during construction. This amount of data is beyond study, but now it is feasible for AI systems. What works with additive tools can be conveniently used to produce, cast, inject, and other production processes across a wide variety.

Complementary technology such as VR and AR are introduced, AI solutions minimize the design time and simplify assembly line processes. VR/AR systems were already designed for line staff to visualize the production process, provide visual direction to enhance their work speed and accuracy. The operator should have AR glasses that illustrate how to install the components in project charts. You have rotated this clamp enough, and you did not rotate it enough or pulling the button. The device will control the job and deliver prompts.

Larger businesses and small and medium-sized enterprises have distinct fields of AI implementation emphasis. SMEs aim to manufacture a huge variety of components, and larger firms also assemble certain components from other countries. There are exceptions; car manufacturers do many chassis spot soldering but buy and assemble other pieces, such as rooms and plastics.

A trend for the components is evolving using smart materials and components and integrated sensors to track their condition, friction, torque, etc. This is a particularly provocative concept for automobile manufacture, as those considerations are more important than how long the vehicle is powered; more maintenance is needed if it is driven through many slats every day.

Intelligent modules will inform you they are at or are due to be tested at the end of their lives. The components themselves will check on AI systems from time to time to report normal status instead of checking these points externally until situations are sideways, where the component begins to need treatment. This method reduces the amount of data transport within the system, and the analytical processing efficiency can drag on a large scale.

In additional processing, AI's largest, most urgent potential to add value is. The main targets of additive processes are their products, which are both cheaper and smaller. In the future, as humans evolve and grow AI, the entire manufacturing value chain is likely to become significant.

## 5.14 Impact of COVID-19 on Industrial Internet of Things

No one expected the COVID-19 outbreak to wreak havoc on the global economy and their personal businesses. Governments, healthcare authorities, and corporate leaders are focusing on protecting lives and controlling the pandemic as the coronavirus continues to spread. Simultaneously, they aim to reduce the humanitarian toll by safeguarding the livelihoods of millions of people who are currently furloughed, jobless, or facing job loss. Industrial IoT (IIoT), may assist businesses on their journey. It has proven its usefulness on several occasions in recent years.

Hemant Upadhyay et al. [31] explained, many industries, including education, have seen major changes as things move online, resulting in new disorders among students and teachers, including sitting postures and the impacts of studying online.

Hemant Upadhyay et al. [32] also discussed the, social isolation barriers amid COVID-19 that can affect the whole humanity in general and how to prevent form those. Off-the-shelf. The use of IIoT technologies enables the continuation of operations with fewer people on-site. A tier-one supplier in the Bangalore, for example, is utilizing a manufacturing-execution system (MES) to improve production and boost transparency. When it comes to machine breakdowns, for example, IVIs can assist in identifying issues such as damaged components or oil leaking that could disrupt production. Over videoconference, one method allows teams to see the tool results and debate potential causes of inaccuracy.

With off-the-shelf IIoT solutions, industrial organizations can make a major effect on labour tracking in as little as a few weeks. If employees test positive for the coronavirus, employers might utilize location data from wearable devices to warn coworkers with whom they had been in close contact. Vision-based control systems can help identify diseased or contagious individuals, maintain physical separation, and guarantee that sick employees stay at home. Amazon, for example, analyses footage from on-site video cameras using machine-learning algorithms to ensure that staff keep safe distances from one another throughout shifts. For the same goals, several businesses combine low-tech methods with vision-based control systems. These preconfigured solutions generally include an IIoT kit (sensors, edge transmitters) and an IIoT platform (data platform, dashboards, interfaces).

## 5.15 Conclusion

The IIoT will change our way of life, working and playing. The IIoT has a bright and optimistic future. The IoT affects every facet of our lives from cartridge communication to portable body sensing devices and domestic equipment. We are "authoring" our lives across networks that alter and grow continuously depending on our world and other systems' feedback. Self-sufficient IoT vehicles make it safer for cars to prevent collisions. With wearable that track cardiac problems and strokes before they happen, it will make our lives easier.

As the technological developments and customers' wish to combine electronics such as smart phones with household machinery led to a nearly infinite IoT future. Wi-Fi allowed people and machinery to be connected in air, on the water and on the ground. Huge amount of data flow from one device to the other, engineering protection would have to evolve as rapidly as networking to satisfy demands. In the field of robotics and knowledge sharing, governments will certainly face difficult choices to compete with the private organizations.

The ethical solution to the Fourth Industrial Revolution must bear in mind with both technological firms and governments. Safety and privacy are the first challenges facing the Industrial IoT. If several of the protection and security problems which affect the IIoT cannot be alleviated, we cannot fully fulfill our capacity. IoT and the convergence revolution mean huge information to facilitate real-time actions and boost income, competitiveness and performance. The opportunities are thrilling, the efficiency is increasing, and the future is connected to incredible stuff. The IoT of 2025 has a long way to go. However, one thing for sure, it will be incredible.

## References

[1] Guanghui Zhou, Chao Zhang, Zhi Li, Kai Ding, & Chuang Wang, "Knowledge-driven digital twin manufacturing cell towards intelligent manufacturing," *International Journal of Production Research*, 58 (4), 1034–1051, 2020, doi: 10.1080/00207543.2019.1607978.

[2] F. Tao, J. Cheng, Q. Qi et al., "Digital twin-driven product design, manufacturing and service with big data," *Int J Adv Manuf Technol*, 94, 3563–3576, 2018, doi: 10.1007/s00170-017-0233-1

[3] S. Schneider, "The Industrial Internet of Things (IIoT)". In Geng H. (ed.), *Internet of Things and Data Analytics Handbook*, Hoboken, NJ, 2017, John Wiley & Sons, Inc.

[4] Q. Qi & F. Tao, "Digital twin and big data towards smart manufacturing and industry 4.0: 360 degree comparison," *IEEE Access*, 6, 3585–3593, 2018, doi: 10.1109/ACCESS.2018.2793265.
[5] S. Jeschke, C. Brecher, T. Meisen, D. Ozdemir, & T. Eschert, "Industrial internet of things and cyber manufacturing systems". In *Industrial Internet of Things*, Cham, 2017, Springer, pp. 3–19.
[6] Hugh Boyes, Bil Hallaq, Joe Cunningham, & Tim Watson, "The Industrial Internet of Things (IIoT): An analysis framework," *Computers in Industry*, 101, 1–12, 2018, ISSN 0166-3615, doi: 10.1016/j.compind.2018.04.015.
[7] Con Cronin, Andrew Conway, & Joseph Walsh, "Flexible manufacturing systems using IIoT in the automotive sector," *Procedia Manufacturing*, 38, 1652–1659, 2019, ISSN 2351-9789, doi: 10.1016/j.promfg.2020.01.119.
[8] T. Ainsworth, J. Brake, P. Gonzalez, D. Toma, & A. F. Browne, "A comprehensive survey of industry 4.0, IIoT and areas of implementation," *SoutheastCon*, 2021, 1–6, 2021, doi: 10.1109/SoutheastCon45413.2021.9401860.
[9] Y. Chen, B. He, S. Lin, J. Soeseno, D. Tan, T. Chen, & W. Chen, "Demystifying data and AI for manufacturing: Case studies from a major computer maker," *APSIPA Transactions on Signal and Information Processing*, 10, E4, 2021, doi:10.1017/ATSIP.2021.3.
[10] Thommie Burström, Vinit Parida, Tom Lahti, & Joakim Wincent, "AI-enabled business-model innovation and transformation in industrial ecosystems: A framework, model and outline for further research," *Journal of Business Research*, 127, 85–95, 2021, ISSN 0148-2963, doi: 10.1016/j.jbusres.2021.01.016.
[11] G. Laput, Y. Zhang, & C. Harrison, "Synthetic sensors: Towards general-purpose sensing," *CHI'17-Proceedings of the 2017 CHI Conference on Human Factors in Computing Systems*, May 2017, pp. 3986–3999, doi: 10.1145/3025453.3025773.
[12] Frank Lynch, Charles Marshall, Dennis O'Connor, & Mike Kiskiel II, "AI in manufacturing at digital," *AI Magazine*, 7 (5), 53, 1986, doi: 10.1609/aimag.v7i5.565.
[13] Piero Formica, "Human manufacturing and the challenges of AI," *Industry and Higher Education*, 35 (3), 147–149, June 2021. doi: 10.1177/09504222211000279.
[14] Patrik Zajec, Jože M. Rožanec, Inna Novalija, Blaž Fortuna, Dunja Mladenić, & Klemen Kenda, "Towards active learning based smart assistant for manufacturing," 2021. https://arxiv.org/abs/2103.16177
[15] Chu Anh My, "The role of big data analytics and AI in smart manufacturing: An overview". In Kumar R., Quang N.H., Kumar Solanki V., Cardona M., Pattnaik P.K. (eds.), *Research in Intelligent and Computing in Engineering. Advances in Intelligent Systems and Computing*, vol. 1254. Singapore, 2021, Springer. doi: 10.1007/978-981-15-7527-3_87.
[16] H. Ding, R. X. Gao, A. J. Isaksson, R. G. Landers, T. Parisini, & Y. Yuan, "State of AI-based monitoring in smart manufacturing and introduction to focused section," In *IEEE/ASME Transactions on Mechatronics*, vol. 25, no. 5, pp. 2143–2154, Oct. 2020, doi: 10.1109/TMECH.2020.3022983.
[17] Ting Zheng, Marco Ardolino, Andrea Bacchetti, & Marco Perona, "The applications of Industry 4.0 technologies in manufacturing context: A systematic literature review," *International Journal of Production Research*, 59 (6), 1922–1954, 2021, doi: 10.1080/00207543.2020.1824085.
[18] Akshay G. Khanzode, P.R.S. Sarma, Sachin Kumar Mangla, & Hong Jun Yuan, "Modeling the Industry 4.0 adoption for sustainable production in micro, small & medium enterprises," *Journal of Cleaner Production*, 279, 123489, January 2021. doi: 10.1016/j.jclepro.2020.123489.

[19] Chetna Chauhan, Amol Singh, & Suni lluthra, "Barriers to industry 4.0 adoption and its performance implications: An empirical investigation of emerging economy," *Journal of Cleaner Production*, 285, 124809, February 2021, doi: 10.1016/j.jclepro.2020.124809.

[20] Jan Stentoft, Kent Adsbøll Wickstrøm, Kristian Philipsen, & Anders Haug, "Drivers and barriers for Industry 4.0 readiness and practice: Empirical evidence from small and medium-sized manufacturers," *Production Planning & Control*, 2020, doi: 10.1080/09537287.2020.1768318.

[21] Hwaiyu Geng, "The Industrial Internet of Things (IIoT)," In *Internet of Things and Data Analytics Handbook*, Hobokenn NJ, 2017, Wiley, pp. 41–81, doi: 10.1002/9781119173601.ch3.

[22] E. Vasilomanolakis, J. Daubert, M. Luthra, V. Gazis, A. Wiesmaier, & P. Kikiras, "On the security and privacy of Internet of Things architectures and systems," *2015 International Workshop on Secure Internet of Things (SIoT)*, 2015, pp. 49–57, doi: 10.1109/SIOT.2015.9.

[23] S. Mumtaz, A. Bo, A. Al-Dulaimi, & K. Tsang, "Guest editorial 5G and beyond mobile technologies and applications for industrial IoT (IIoT)," *In IEEE Transactions on Industrial Informatics*, vol. 14, no. 6, pp. 2588–2591, June 2018, doi: 10.1109/TII.2018.2823311.

[24] Laurence McHauser, Christoph Schmitz, & Markus Hammer, "Model-Factory-In-A-Box: A portable solution that brings the complexity of a real factory and all the benefits of experiential-learning environments directly to learners in industry," *Procedia Manufacturing*, 45, 246–252, 2020, ISSN 2351-9789, doi: 10.1016/j.promfg.2020.04.102.

[25] Serkan Ayvaz, & Koray Alpay, "Predictive maintenance system for production lines in manufacturing: A machine learning approach using IoT data in real-time," *Expert Systems with Applications*, 173, 114598, 2021, ISSN 0957-4174, doi: 10.1016/j.eswa.2021.114598.

[26] D. Wu, J. Terpenny, & D. Schaefer, "Digital design and manufacturing on the cloud: A review of software and services – RETRACTED," *Artificial Intelligence for Engineering Design, Analysis and Manufacturing*, *31* (1), 104–118, 2017. doi: 10.1017/S0890060416000305.

[27] Sapna Juneja, Abhinav Juneja, Gaurav Dhiman, Sanchit Behl, & Sandeep Kautish, "An approach to thoracic syndrome classification with convolutional neural network," *Computational and Mathematical Methods in Medicine*, 2021, 3900254, 2021, doi: 10.1155/2021/3900254.

[28] Sapna Juneja, Mamta Gahlan, Gaurav Dhiman, & Sandeep Kautish, "Futuristic cyber twin architecture for 6G technology to support internet of everything," *Scientific Programming*, 2021, 2021, doi: 10.1155/2021/9101782.

[29] Abhinav Juneja, Sapna Bajaj, & Rohit Anand, "Improvising green computing using multi criteria decision making," *Journal of Advanced Research in Dynamical and Control Systems*, 12 (03), 1161–1165, March 2020, doi: 10.5373/JARDCS/V12SP3/20201362.

[30] Hemant Upadhyay, Sapna Juneja, Abhinav Juneja, Gaurav Dhiman, & Sandeep Kautish, "Evaluation of ergonomic related Disorders in online education using Fuzzy AHP," *Computational Intelligence and Neuroscience*, 2021, 221497, 2021, doi: 10.1155/2021/2214971.

[31] Hemant Upadhyay, Sapna Juneja, Sunil Maggu, Grima Dhingra, & Abhinav Juneja, "Multi criteria analysis of social isolation barriers amid Covid 19 using Fuzzy AHP," *World Journal of Engineering*, 2021, doi: 10.1108/wje-04-2021-0195.

# Chapter 6

# Solutions Using Machine Learning for COVID-19

Muhammad Shafi, Kashif Zia and Jabar H. Yousif
*Sohar University, Sohar, Oman*

## Contents

6.1 Introduction ........ 100
6.2 Application of ML and AI Methods to COVID-19 ........ 100
6.2.1 Screening and Diagnosis ........ 101
6.2.1.1 Using the Patient's Symptoms and Routine Tests ........ 101
6.2.1.2 Using Chest X-rays and CT Images ........ 102
6.2.2 Population Monitoring ........ 103
6.2.2.1 Monitoring Patients ........ 103
6.2.2.2 Contact Tracing ........ 104
6.2.2.3 Avoiding Physical Contact ........ 105
6.2.3 Models for Prediction and Forecasting of the Disease ........ 105
6.2.3.1 An Example Model Predicting the Spread of COVID-19 ........ 109
6.2.4 Models of Vaccinations ........ 112
6.2.4.1 An Example Model of Global Vaccination Drive ........ 113
6.3 Conclusion ........ 117
References ........ 117

DOI: 10.1201/9781003322597-6

## 6.1 Introduction

COVID-19 is the latest outbreak of a pandemic at a global scale. Like other such incidents in the history of humanity, the pandemic started as a localized epidemic in Wuhan, China in December, 2019. According to Lippi and Plebani, COVID-19 is a respirational and zoonotic disease, caused by a virus of the *coronaviridae* family [1]. The virus strain is severe acute respiratory syndrome coronavirus 2 (SARS-CoV-2), resulting in fever, coughing, breathing difficulties, fatigue, and myalgia. It may develop into pneumonia of high intensity. COVID-19 acquired an unprecedented momentum after mid-2020, and this has continued even after almost a year and a half. By 5 October 2021, COVID-19 had infected 234,553,539 people and claimed 4,796,222 lives [2].

Nevertheless, there are signs that it may turn into a normal flu by the spring of 2022 [3]. A series of global-scale interventions were required to arrive at a position where we feel hopeful about getting back to normalcy. During the last two years, the global community as a whole has devised, tested and implemented policies and technologies to overcome the challenge focusing on the following areas: (i) rapid diagnosis, (ii) screening patients (for seriousness categorization), (iii) accurate and efficient clinical trials, (iv) imposing social-distancing measures, (v) imposing vaccination measures, (vi) risk assessment, and (vii) contact tracing. In many of these areas, machine learning (ML) and artificial intelligence (AI) have played pivotal roles.

This chapter focuses on ML and AI technologies that have been employed to deal with various challenges during the last two years. First, we elaborate on how ML and AI is relevant for COVID-19. Next, we discuss models and technologies used so far, with their purpose and the extent of their success. Sufficient details of each set of ML and AI methods employed are given, along with the dataset used (if any). Finally, we examine the pros and cons of the methods used, providing an informed perspective that can be considered if a similar pandemic arises in the future.

## 6.2 Application of ML and AI Methods to COVID-19

The relationship of healthcare with AI dates back to 1976 when the first expert diagnosis support system, MYCIN, was developed [4]. This evolution has continued for decades, bringing us to diagnosis (decision support) systems that are particularly designed for infectious diseases [5–7]. Overall, ML and AI applications had already cemented their footprint in various health-related fields before COVID-19. These include prognostics [8], health informatics [9, 10], medical imaging [11], diagnosis [12, 13] and more.

It was natural to exploit and further enhance this knowledge as the devastation of COVID-19 began. In many of these medical practices, further research was conducted specifically to deal with the outbreak. However, some new aspects specific to COVID-19 were also considered. These areas are explored in the following sections.

### 6.2.1 Screening and Diagnosis

Early detection of a disease, particularly an infectious one, is critically important to reduce the spread from infected patients to other susceptible contacts. ML and AI can be used to achieve early diagnosis and screening. Lalmuanawma et al. [14] have documented four systems that are particularly designed for COVID-19 screening. The authors in [15] have proposed a deep convolutional network for COVID-19 diagnosis that is based on scanning CT images. They reported a high level of accuracy and specificity compared to existing systems. Similarly, authors in [16] have also used a convolutional neural network for the classification of CT images. They also measured the accuracy of the screening based on two sets of classifiers, i.e., binary and multi classes.

In addition to CT scans and X-ray images, patient screening can also be performed based on related features. Authors in [17] have proposed a model of predicting the potential threat of COVID-19 to a patient based on four features: age, GSH, CD3 ratio and total protein. A learning mechanism based on support vector machine (SVM) was adopted. They found this model extremely useful as they were able to identify the more acute cases with almost 100% success. Another indirect way of screening for COVID-19 is proposed by Wu et al. [18]. They used patient blood samples for screening purposes. The features of blood used were bilirubin total, creatine kinase isoenzyme, GLU, creatinine, kalium, lactate dehydrogenase, platelet distribution width, calcium, basophil, total protein, and magnesium. They then employed a random forest algorithm for prediction with an overall accuracy of 95.95% and 96.97% specificity, respectively.

Real-time reverse transcription polymerase chain reaction (RT-PCR) is the most effective and widely used tool for diagnosis of COVID-19. However, there are some challenges with RT-PCR test such as high cost, supply shortages, a sizable false negative rate, and the fact that it is time-consuming. Therefore, researchers are seeking alternate mechanisms for the diagnosis of COVID-19 without RT-PCR test. These attempts can be broadly classified into two groups.

#### 6.2.1.1 Using the Patient's Symptoms and Routine Tests

Most studies in the literature try to predict COVID-19 using normal blood tests and patients' symptoms. Most such schemes utilize classification algorithms with binary class as the output. The data is pre-processed before feeding it into a classification scheme.

[19] utilizes 151 published studies of machine learning techniques for the diagnosis of COVID-19 using routine tests and patients' symptoms. They demonstrated a relationship between being a male and higher levels of lymphocytes and neutrophils. They used the XGBoost model for the diagnosis of COVID-19 with a claimed sensitivity of 92.5% and specificity of 97.9%. Similarly, undetected COVID-19 is diagnosed from collected data from hemodialysis patients, due to kidney failure,

using machine learning algorithms [20]. [21] utilizes machine learning to predict COVID-19 positivity using patient symptoms. The symptoms are collected from patients using a question-and-answer session. Some studies use ensemble models instead of relying on a single machine learning algorithm. For example, [22] combines four machine learning algorithms for diagnosis of COVID-19 using processed patient data: random forest, SVM, decision trees, and logistic regression. Similarly, [23] combines K-nearest neighbors (KNN), artificial neural networks (ANN), and naïve Bayes for COVID-19 diagnosis.

In [24], a voice signal is obtained containing a patient's cough. This signal is then pre-processed and fed into an end-to-end portable machine learning system for COVID-19 diagnosis. A similar system is proposed by [25] for the diagnosis of COVID-19 using cough and breath data from patients.

#### *6.2.1.2 Using Chest X-rays and CT Images*

Chest X-rays and CT scans provide vital information about COVID-19 patients. These images contain visual information which can be utilized to diagnose COVID-19 patients. Numerous studies have been conducted in the literature that utilize these images for the diagnosis of the disease. Deep neural networks particularly convolutional neural networks (CNN) and their variants have proven to be very effective. Unlike traditional machine learning schemes where features are extracted from the original data then fed to a classifier, these methods work in an end-to-end style and there is no need for explicit feature extraction from the images. The original images are fed into a CNN and the features extraction task is carried out implicitly by the earlier layers of the networks. Figure 6.1 shows a typical CNN architecture that could be utilized for COVID-19 detection from X-rays or CT scan images. Most deep neural network architectures behave like a black box. However, an analysis of trained deep networks shows that the early layers usually extract low-level features such as lines, edges, etc., while the later layers perform high-level tasks such as classification and recognition. In Figure 6.1, ReLU has been used as the activation function for early layers while Softmax activation has been used in the final layer to do the classification task. Usually, these deep convolutional network architectures are very deep (with several layers) and therefore require a huge amount of training data, high processing power and long training time. A possible solution to this issue is to use off-the-shelf pre-trained networks which are already trained for thousands of images. Fine tuning is carried out, usually in the initial and final layers, to tune these networks according to the training data. This phenomenon is called transfer learning. Some researchers have utilized this transfer learning mechanism for COVID-19 diagnosis from CT and X-ray images. The following are some notable studies on the use of machine learning for COVID-19 diagnosis from X-ray and CT images.

A large dataset comprising 1065 cases was used to train a deep neural network for COVID-19 detection [27]. [28] employed a self-supervised learning mechanism

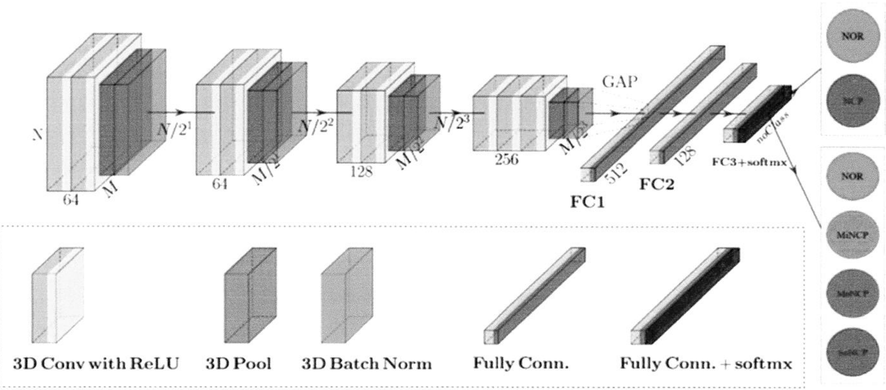


**Figure 6.1 A typical CNN architecture for COVID-19 detection in CT scan images, adopted from [26].**

for a convolutional neural network to detect COVID-19 in CT scan images.[29] incorporated deep neural networks for the detection, localization and quantification of COVID-19 in chest images. As stated earlier, some researchers have utilized pre-trained neural network architectures instead of building new networks from scratch. [30] uses the transfer learning paradigm and some well-known pre-trained deep neural networks such as ResNet18, ResNet50, Squeeznet, and RseNet101. Similarly, [31] utilizes the VGG16, ResNet-50, Xception and Inception-v3 pre-trained networks for COVID-19 diagnosis in chest images. Some recent work in the fiend of medical image processing are [32–34]

## 6.2.2 Population Monitoring

Population monitoring relates to monitoring patients and managing non-patients in such a way that the probability of the spread of the decrease is reduced. We categorize related work into three areas: monitoring patients, contact tracing, and mechanisms for reducing physical contact.

### 6.2.2.1 Monitoring Patients

Among the key challenges in handling COVID-19 are monitoring patients in terms of predicting recovery and mortality, monitoring symptoms, and predicting severity.

*Predicting recovery and mortality.* It has been observed that health care facilities became overloaded during the COVID-19 pandemic and there is a need to prioritize patients for intensive care (ICU) beds. [35] have proposed a machine learning scheme to predict the mortality of patients more than 10 days in advance with more than 90% accuracy. Similarly, [36] proposed a machine learning-based system to predict ICU transfer within 24 hours. [37] utilized data from 117,000 patients to predict the mortality of COVID-19 patients. [38] suggested an ensemble machine learning model by combining five classifiers including KNN, logistic regression, SVM, gradient boosting, and random forest to predict mortality in confirmed COVID-19 patients.

*Predicting Severity.* Some patients deteriorate over time and they die after their symptoms become severe. Researchers have tied to predict the severity ahead of time using various machine learning methods. For example, [39] predicts the severity of COVID-19-positive patients using multivariate logistic regression. [40] combines self-supervised and supervised learning in a graph neural network to predict the severity of COVID-19 patients. Most of these mechanisms use blood test and voice signal data for prediction of severity.

*Monitoring Symptoms.* Researchers have also tried to incorporate artificial intelligence for symptom monitoring of COVID-19 patients, helping to the necessary action to be taken if the symptoms get worse. [41] proposes COVID-19 symptom monitoring systems using different sensors such as camera, microphone, temperature, and color sensors. [42] predicts the need for ICU admission for a particular patient by combining natural language processing, machine learning, and classic epidemiological methods to process the health record of a COVID-19 patient.

#### 6.2.2.2 Contact Tracing

As COVID-19 is an infectious disease and it spreads due to close contacts, contact tracing is crucial for identifying potentially infected people who have been in close contact with an infected person. Most governments launched digital contact-tracing applications to identify potential infected people and break the chain of infection. Contact-tracing applications can be broadly classified into centralized and decentralized architectures. In centralized architecture, the users' data are stored on a central server. The server uses the data for contact matching, risk analysis and sending notifications. In decentralized systems, the mobile phone itself stores the data of close contacts and performs contact matching and notification. Figure 6.2 shows typical centralized and decentralized contact-tracing architectures.

Table 6.1 lists communication technologies used in contact-tracing applications.

The US National Institute of Standards and Technology arranged a month-long event that was focused on the use of artificial intelligence for improving Bluetooth-based contact-tracing applications. The event was mainly focused on analyzing data collected from Bluetooth to accurately estimate the distance between various devices using artificial intelligence and data analysis techniques. The data collected in the digital contact-tracing applications (which is stored on a centralized server or in individual smartphones) is then parsed using various artificial intelligence algorithms to trace close contacts, risks and other predictions.

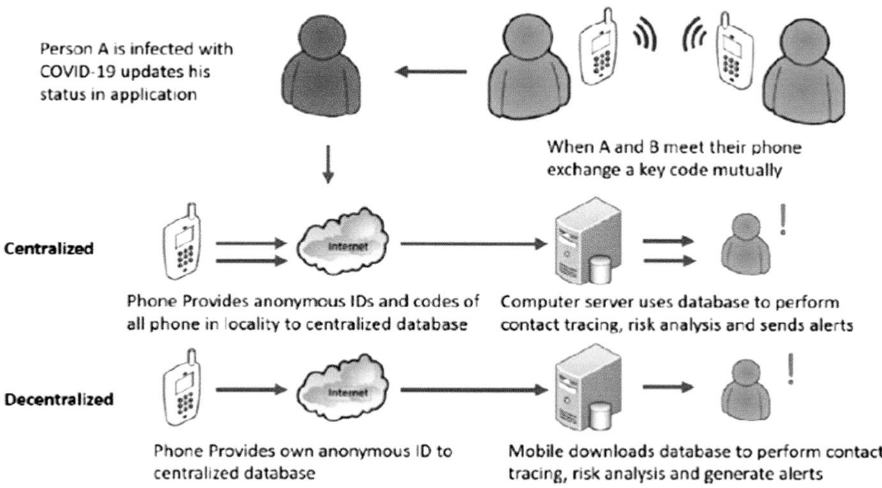


**Figure 6.2 Centralized vs. Decentralized Contact-Tracing Architectures, adopted from [43].**

According to Hellewell et al. [44], isolation of confirmed cases and tracing their contacts has been used in controlling infectious diseases and is also used in the current COVID-19 outbreak. To achieve control using this strategy, however, depends on the characteristics of both virus and response. They assessed the isolation and contact-tracing technique for controlling the transmission of disease from COVID-19 cases imported to the UK from China. They tested their model for various scenarios and concluded that in most of the scenarios, a highly effective tracing and isolation technique was sufficient to control the outbreak in three months. They learnt that where there were long delays in isolation in those cases where the symptoms were detected late, an increase in disease transmission was observed.

#### 6.2.2.3 Avoiding Physical Contact

Facial recognition systems have been widely employed for tracking workers' attendance during the COVID-19 pandemic. This contactless scheme has greatly reduced the probability of physical contacts and thus contributed to controlling the spread of the disease. Some countries such as China used drones for disinfection spray. Robots and drones were also utilized for the delivery of food, medicines and other items to avoid physical contact.

### 6.2.3 Models for Prediction and Forecasting of the Disease

Forecasting the spread of the virus is important for effective policy making and is usually dealt with by modeling and simulation.

**Table 6.1 Communication Technologies Used in Contact-Tracing Applications**

| *Name* | *Description* |
|---|---|
| WiFi | WiFi is one of the most effective communication technologies for contact tracing in indoor environment such as shopping malls, community centers, cinema theaters, etc. As compared to other technologies, WiFi is cheap and has greater accuracy for localization and tracing of close contacts. |
| Bluetooth | Bluetooth is perhaps the most widely used technology for contact tracing. Available in almost all modern smartphones and with no associated cost other than the smartphone battery consumption, Bluetooth is a popular choice for contact-tracing applications. Whenever two Bluetooth devices come into sufficiently close proximity, both devices store the information of this collision which can be further used for identifying potentially infected individuals. |
| Global Positioning System | GPS has been effectively used in curbing COVID-19 disease. As almost all smartphones are equipped with GPS these days, their location can be used to identify people who have come into close contact with a person testing positive. Similarly, GPS has also played a crucial role in contactless shopping and online delivery to implement social distancing and reduce the probability of COVID-19 spread. |
| Zigbee | Zigbee is a communication technology used for low-power and low-cost communication networks. Zigbee devices can communicate up to a distance of 20m which makes it an effective choice for modern COVID-19 contact-tracing applications. The close proximity of two mobiles can be predicated using the Zigbee technology which can further be used for contact tracing and notification. |
| QR Codes | Some countries have used QR codes for COVID-19 contact tracing. QR codes are installed in different locations especially inside buildings and individuals are encouraged or required to scan those codes whenever they pass through that point. This collected data is further processed for finding close contacts, matching, risk analysis and sending notifications to potentially infected COVID-19 patients. |

**Table 6.2 Contact-tracing applications, adopted from [43].**

| *App Name* | *Country* | *Tech* |
|---|---|---|
| Aarogya Setu | India | Bluetooth, Location |
| Beat Covid Gibraltar | Gibraltar | TBD |
| BeAware | Bahrain | Bluetooth, Location |
| Belgium's app | Belgium | Bluetooth, Google/Apple |
| Chinese health code system | China | Location, Data mining |
| COCOA | Japan | Google/Apple |
| Corona-Warn-App | Germany | Bluetooth, Google/Apple |
| COVID Alert | Canada | Bluetooth, Google/Apple |
| CovidRadar | Mexico | Bluetooth |
| COVIDSafe | Australia | Bluetooth |
| CovTracer | Cyprus | Location,GPS |
| E7mi | Tunisia | Bluetooth |
| Ehteraz | Qatar | Bluetooth, Location |
| eRouska | Czech | Bluetooth |
| Estonia's App | Estonia | Bluetooth, DP-3T, Google/Apple |
| GH COVID-19 Tracker | Ghana | Location |
| HaMagen | Israel | Location |
| Hayat Eve Sığar | Turkey | Bluetooth, Location |
| HSE Covid-19 App | Ireland | Bluetooth, Google/Apple |
| Immuni | Italy | Bluetooth, Google/Apple |
| Ketju | Finland | Bluetooth, DP-3T |
| Mask.ir | Iran | Location |
| Mor Chana | Thailand | Location, Bluetooth |
| MyTrace | Malaysia | Bluetooth, Google/Apple |
| NHS COVID-19 App | United Kingdom | Bluetooth, Google/Apple |

(*Continued*)

**Table 6.2** *(Continued)* **Contact-tracing applications, adopted from [43].**

| *App Name* | *Country* | *Tech* |
|---|---|---|
| Northern Ireland's app | Northern Ireland | Bluetooth, Google/Apple |
| NZ COVID Tracer | New Zealand | QR codes |
| PeduliLindungi | Indonesia | TBD |
| ProteGO | Poland | Bluetooth |
| Rakning C-19 | Iceland | Location |
| Shlonik | Kuwait | Location |
| Smittestop | Denmark | Bluetooth, Google/Apple |
| Smittestopp | Norway | Bluetooth, Location |
| StaySafe | Philippines | Bluetooth |
| StopKorona | North Macedonia | Bluetooth |
| Stopp Corona | Austria | Bluetooth, Google/Apple |
| Swiss contact-tracing App | Switzerland | Bluetooth, DP-3T, Google/Apple |
| Tawakkalna | Saudi Arabia | TBD |
| Trace together | Singapore | Bluetooth, Blue Trace |
| TraceCovid | United Arab Emirates | Bluetooth |
| ViruSafe | Bulgaria | Location |
| VirusRadar | Hungary | Bluetooth |

The modeling of infectious diseases has been of interest to scientists for quite a long time. It started with modeling the dynamics of the spread of viruses/diseases at the system level, also known as state-transition systems. The oldest ones are SI (susceptible infectious) and SIR (susceptible-infectious-recovered) models [45]. In both, a rate termed $\beta$ is used to let a population of agents transit from susceptible to infected state. However, in the SIR models, we also have a recovery rate, $\mu$, which is used to let the agent transit from infectious state to a recovered state permanently. Later, for epidemics like COVID-19, the SIR model was extended to SEIR [46], with a new state exposed, sometimes also called the latent state. The respective rate is denoted by $\varepsilon$.

Typically for COVID-19, the closest representative model in the category is the one proposed for the H1N1 epidemic [47]. As in H1N1, in COVID-19, we have two types of infectious individuals, those who show symptoms (Symp) and those who do not show symptoms (ASymp). An exposed individual can transit to state infectious Symp with rate $\varepsilon$ or to a state infectious ASymp with rate $1-\varepsilon$.

In addition to modeling the spread of the disease to predict its long-term dynamics, models have also been used for short-term predictions. In [48], the authors proposed a model that could predict new cases of COVID-19 for the next six days. Instead of using a state-based system, they used a statistical measure of support vector regression. Further, a pure AI technique of long-short-term-memory (LSTM) deep learning was used to predict when the pandemic would end at the global level [49]. Unfortunately, the end date of June 2020 did not turn out to be true, indicating both the complexity of the phenomenon and the limitations of a model.

#### 6.2.3.1 An Example Model Predicting the Spread of COVID-19

We now present one of our recent model studies on the spread of COVID-19 [50]. In this model, we have used the model from [47] as the base model. We incorporated a new state for COVID-19, namely isolated or quarantined. The isolated state represents the possibility of transferring an infectious individual with symptoms to isolation with a rate $\alpha$. The logic of using $\alpha$ is that the model is able to map the preparedness of a country for the pandemic. All three states – infectious Symp, infectious ASymp, and isolated – transit to recovered state with same rate $\mu$. Also, a transition from infectious ASymp to infectious Symp is made possible with a rate $\rho$. The final model is shown in Figure 6.1. The model is implemented in GLEAMviz [51], the global epidemic and mobility model. GLEAMviz is a simulator which uses real-world data from population and mobility networks (both airways and commuting) on the server side. It integrates these data with the model developed by a user on the client side.

The simulation not only captures the model dynamic of the spread of the virus, but also takes care of population and mobility data. The model is calibrated based on epidemic data and events as they happened. The simulation results are quite disturbing, indicating that, during a process of stringent social distancing and testing strategies, a small perturbation can lead to quite undesirable outcomes. The simulation results, although consistent in their expected outcomes across changing parameter values, also indicate a substantial mismatch with real numbers. An analysis of the reasons for this mismatch is also performed. Within these contradictions, a comparative analysis of the COVID-19 outbreak between two geographically close but demographically very different countries is performed (Figure 6.3).

The model is based on two concepts.

1. *Carriership and Mobility*. A carrier of the virus is a person who is infected by the virus. He/she may or may not show symptoms. Due to this an isolated/quarantined person is also considered as a carrier, but being isolated make him not able to transmit further. The model captures the mobility of

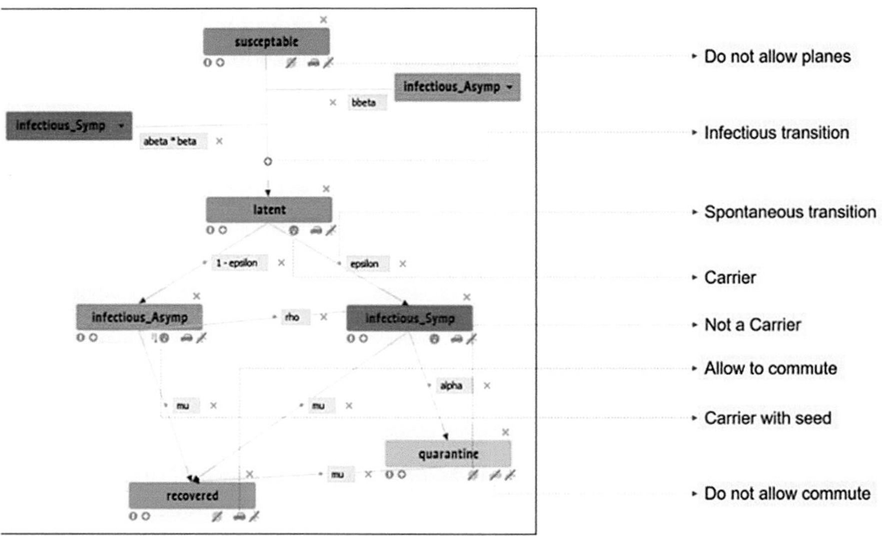


**Figure 6.3 The COVID-19 system dynamics model.**

the population based on situational evidence. For example, considering all air traffic is suspended, no compartment allows air travel, whereas all individuals who are not quarantined are allowed to commute locally. The commuting restrictions are further modified by using different transition variables.

2. *Transition Rates*. The detail of transition rate between the compartments (states) is given below.
   - beta (β): rate of exposure to the virus, where bbeta is for asymptotic infectors, and abeta is for symptotic infectors.
   - epsilon (ε): rate of exposed to infectious state, where epsilon is used for positive infection and 1 – epsilon is used for negative infection. Also, the value of epsilon is reciprocal to the exposed period, which is equal to 5.2 days in our model.
   - rho (ρ): rate of asymptotic infection to symptotic infection. The value of rho is reciprocal to the symptoms appearing period, which is equal to 2.3 days in our model.
   - mu (μ): rate of infectious or isolated to recovered, where this value is reciprocal to the infection period (30 days).
   - alpha (α): rate of symptotic infectious to isolated state.

Next, we categorized different situations and mimicked them by tuning transition rates and timings. For predictions, three categories were considered: case 1 (extremely bad), case 2 (extremely good), and case 3 (intermediate or neutral).

Case 1 is what can be perceived as complete inaction by the authorities. Case 2 represents extremely strict action. And case 3 represents an optimistic view due to (i) weather intervention (case 1a), and (ii) successful extended lockdown (case 3a). For all these cases, we did a simulation of one year and compared two countries, Oman and Pakistan.

## CASE 1

For Oman, the results suggested that the outbreak would be rapid and extreme, reaching 0.2 million cases (nearly 4% of the population) per day after 45 days of the outbreak, and then it would start dropping rapidly. When accumulated, it was noted that 80% of the population would be affected. For Pakistan, the results suggest that the outbreak would be rapid and extreme, reaching 4 million cases (nearly 2% of the population) per day after 75 days of the outbreak, and then it would start dropping. When accumulated, it was noted that 80% of the population would be affected.

## CASE 2

The results are shown in Figure 6.4. Nevertheless, both case 1 and case 2 are unrealistic, so we focus on case 3.

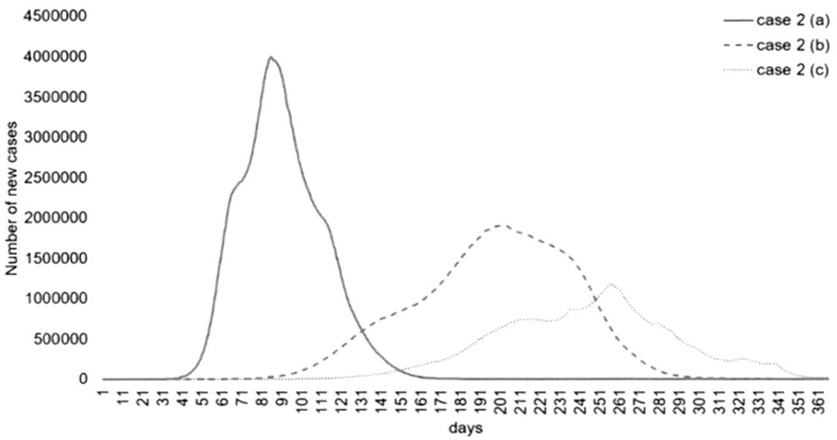


**Figure 6.4 Infections with symptoms (case 2).**

**CASE 3 FOR CASE 3, WE CREATED SOME EXCEPTIONS.**

- At the start of the simulation, we introduced a few patients with symptoms and the same number of patients without symptoms, at the three cities identified for both countries.
- The following exceptions were applied (based on real events): after the first three weeks, real isolation activity was realized, first in small cities and after a further three weeks, all across the country, by setting alpha = 0.95, and abeta = 0.05.
- A complete lockdown was implemented after one month by setting bbeta = 0.05. But then the lockdown was partially relaxed after two weeks by setting the values of abeta and bbeta to 0.1 for the rest of the simulation time.

Further, we introduced bulk cases (patients traveling and entering the country). Initially many of these cases went undetected. These people were integrated with their families and all of them were infected without any symptoms. Hence, the results of this case (case 3) can be considered as the nearest to reality according to the current actions of the authorities. The results of case 3 are given in Figure 6.5.

## 6.2.4 Models of Vaccinations

Right from the start, the world knew the only cure for COVID-19 is vaccination. Work to develop a vaccine started early [52]. It resulted in success. However, the

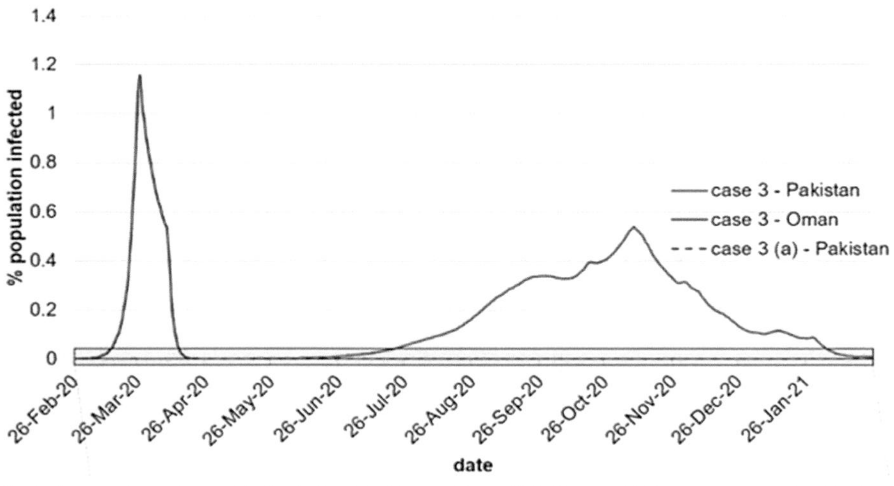


**Figure 6.5 Infections with symptoms (case 3).**

problem of how the vaccine should be distributed remained unsolved and apparently delayed the eradication of the virus.

#### 6.2.4.1 An Example Model of Global Vaccination Drive

In [53] we proposed an agent-based model to evaluate the impact of COVID-19 vaccination distribution disparities on the eradication of the virus. The model proposed is simple yet novel, in the sense that it captures the spatial transmission-induced activity through which we are able to relate the transmission model to the mutated variations of the virus.

Some important "what if" questions have been asked in terms of number of deaths, time required and percentage of population needing to be vaccinated before the pandemic is eradicated. The simulation results have revealed that it is necessary to maintain a global (rather than regional or country-oriented) vaccination drive in case of a new pandemic or continual efforts against COVID-19.

The problems of vaccination distribution/use disparity have been highlighted before [54, 55]. A few agent-based models concerning vaccination efficiency have already been proposed. Authors in [56] have proposed vaccination strategies with a delayed second dose. They have compared different vaccination products and provided a projected number of infections, serious cases and deaths. Authors in [57] proposed a mathematical model to estimate the impact on mortality and total infections of completely lifting COVID-19 restrictions. A qualitative study on who should be prioritized for COVID-19 vaccination is given in [58]. Another focused attempt is a simulation study to estimate future infection rates among children with vaccination [59].

Closer to our model is [60], in which the authors emphasize accelerating the vaccination drive to mitigate high transmissibility resulting in more deadly variants. However, the model proposed is population based, without spatial (regional/country-wise) variations. Another similar model is presented by the authors in [61]. But the system dynamic model again does not cater for spatial considerations and mobility. Another sound piece of research is published in [62], in which the authors combine real data with an agent-based model to estimate the impact of lockdown and vaccination against COVID-19. But this model concerns a single country and does not take non-availability of vaccine as an option. Therefore, a simplistic model of virus transmission is used, consisting of minimal states of susceptible, vaccinated, infected and recovered. A moving agent in one of these states is tightly bound to the underlying space, where the space is divided into regions to evaluate the region-based vs. global vaccination drive. Additionally, the virus gets mutated, where the extent of mutation is directly related to spatial activity representing the transmissions. And the inactivity is directly proportional to the mutated variant at a given location.

In summary, the results of the simulation suggest that it is necessary to maintain a global (rather than regional or country-oriented) vaccination drive in case of a new pandemic or continual efforts against COVID-19. It results in a lesser number of deaths, time and quantity of vaccination required.

We evaluated four cases as shown in Table 6.3.

Since in the simulation, the vaccination happens from day 1, the vaccination_rate equal to 0% means that the transmission of virus happens along with the vaccination drive. Obviously, this did not happen in the case of COVID-19. Hence, 0% vaccination_rate depicts a futuristic (ideal) situation in which vaccination is available before the virus outbreak happens. A vaccination_rate of 20% is about 20% population already vaccinated when the transmission starts. This can be equated to (probably) the end of the second global wave of COVID-19, when active cases were quite low and a substantial population was vaccinated. Therefore, the former represents an *ideal* and the latter a *real* scenario (but an intermediate one).

Since the vaccination drive (as we have seen in the case of COVID-19) was/has been country centered, the (mostly) developed countries vaccinated their own population first, followed by provision of the vaccine to other countries. We call this scenario *self-centered*, and it is implemented in the simulation by introduction of regional blocks (blocks? = true). Therefore, some blocks have more vaccines in comparison to others. An alternate strategy would have been a globally balanced vaccination drive irrespective of country of manufacturing. Thus, that would have been a *global* drive, in which all the blocks would have been the same (hence, block? = false).

In fact, there are 12 regional blocks, as shown in Figure 6.6. Although a clear differentiation is enough for modeling purposes, the blocks/regions are sorted from left to right and from bottom to top, in terms of availability of vaccine. So for example, region 1 is the worst, followed by region 2, 3, and so on. The last column of Table 6.3 summarizes the scenarios in terms of the above two dimensions.

So the idea is to measure the performance of the vaccination drive in all four scenarios and do a comparative analysis. The simulations are an average of a sufficient number of runs. The results are compared based on the following outcomes. The results shown in Figure 6.6 represent the number of agents in different states

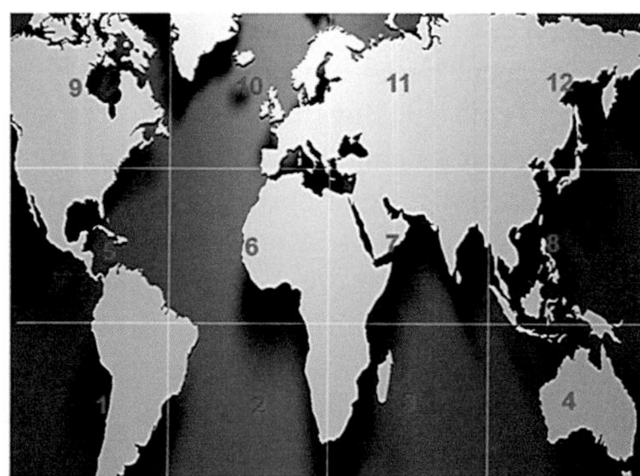


**Figure 6.6 World arranged in vaccination blocks.**

**Table 6.3 Simulation Cases**

| Case | Blocked? | Vaccination_rate | Scenario |
|---|---|---|---|
| Case1 | False | 0 | Global ideal |
| Case2 | False | 20 | Global real |
| Case3 | True | 0 | Self-centered ideal |
| Case4 | True | 20 | Self-centered real |

after the simulation ends (there are no more infected agents in the population). The graph in Figure 6.7 shows the number of people who have died and the time when the simulation ends, with a particular focus on the blocks situation.

Closure occurring early is absolutely beneficial as the world is tired of restrictions and is seeking normal social and economic activity. At the timescale of the simulation, it is evident in the graph shown in Figure 6.6 that the worst-case time is for case 4. We gain at least 20% in case 2. When comparing case 3 with case 1, the gain is 10%. So the global vaccination drive is also beneficial in terms of time needed to eradicate the pandemic. The timing dynamics aspect is visually shown in Figure 6.8 where we compare case 3 with case 1 in terms of time taken to vaccinate 20% of the population. In the sample run, it took 110 iterations to do it in case 3 as compared to 45 iterations in case 1.

Finally, we have the results of how much of the population needs to be vaccinated in each case in Figure 6.9. Obviously, if the vaccine is invented late (case 2 and 4), it will require more, almost 85% of the population. And there is no difference between these two cases. However, the time to achieve this number is less in case 4. While the time to achieve the required percentage between cases representing availability of vaccine right from the start is not much different between cases 3

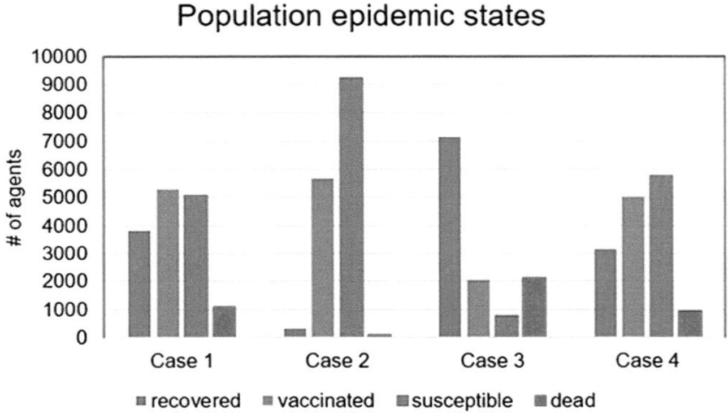


**Figure 6.7 Epidemic states at the end of the simulation.**

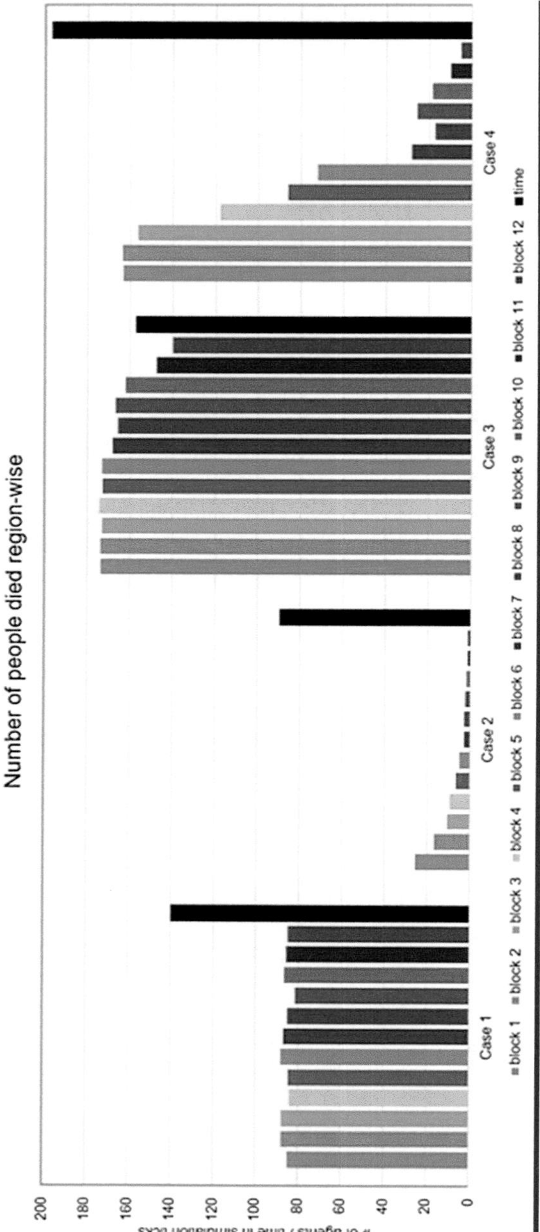


**Figure 6.8 Epidemic states at the end of the simulation (block-wise situation).**

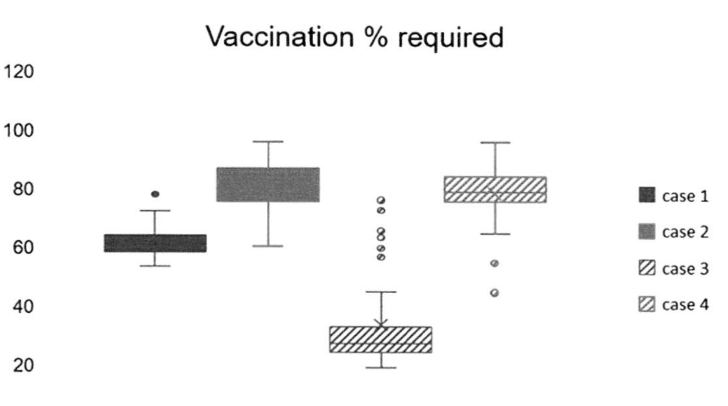


**Figure 6.9 Vaccination percentage required for four cases.**

and 1, the percentage required decreases to almost 30% in case 3, compared to more than 60% in case 1.

## 6.3 Conclusion

Machine learning has played a vital role in combating the COVID-19 pandemic. This chapter has highlighted the applications of machine learning in tackling the pandemic. Various tools, techniques, and methods have been explained that have been utilized for COVID-19. The role of machine learning can be broadly classified into screening and diagnosis, patient monitoring and contact tracing, and prediction and forecasting. All these aspects have been covered in detail with demonstration examples in this chapter. Some challenges are also highlighted. Sufficient detail of each set of ML and AI methods employed is given along with the dataset used (if any). The current research suggests that, as in many other fields, the role of machine learning will be crucial in predicting and dealing with any future pandemics.

## References

[1] Lippi, G., and Plebani, M. (2020). Laboratory abnormalities in patients with COVID-2019 infection. *Clinical Chemistry and Laboratory Medicine (CCLM)*, 58(7), 1131–1134.

[2] WHO: World Health Organization (2021). Coronavirus disease (COVID-2019) situation reports. https://www.who.int/emergencies/diseases/novel-coronavirus-2019/situation-reports/ (accessed 5 October 2021).

[3] Charumilind, S., Craven, M., Lamb, J., Sabow, A., and Wilson, M. (2021). When will the covid-19 pandemic end? an update. McKinsey & Company.

[4] Shortliffe, E. (Ed.). (2012). *Computer-based medical consultations: MYCIN* (Vol. 2). Elsevier.
[5] Agrebi, S., & Larbi, A. (2020). Use of artificial intelligence in infectious diseases. In *Artificial intelligence in precision health* (pp. 415–438). Academic Press.
[6] Peiffer-Smadja, N., Rawson, T. M., Ahmad, R., Buchard, A., Georgiou, P., Lescure, F. X., … Holmes, A. H. (2020). Machine learning for clinical decision support in infectious diseases: a narrative review of current applications. *Clinical Microbiology and Infection*, 26(5), 584–595.
[7] Toğaçar, M., Ergen, B., and Cömert, Z. (2020). COVID-19 detection using deep learning models to exploit Social Mimic Optimization and structured chest X-ray images using fuzzy color and stacking approaches. *Computers in Biology and Medicine*, 121, 103805.
[8] Colubri, A., Hartley, M. A., Siakor, M., Wolfman, V., Felix, A., Sesay, T., … Sabeti, P. C. (2019). Machine-learning prognostic models from the 2014–16 Ebola outbreak: data-harmonization challenges, validation strategies, and mHealth applications. *EClinicalMedicine*, 11, 54–64.
[9] Choi, S., Lee, J., Kang, M. G., Min, H., Chang, Y. S., and Yoon, S. (2017). Large-scale machine learning of media outlets for understanding public reactions to nation-wide viral infection outbreaks. *Methods*, 129, 50–59.
[10] Nápoles, G., Grau, I., Bello, R., and Grau, R. (2014). Two-steps learning of Fuzzy Cognitive Maps for prediction and knowledge discovery on the HIV-1 drug resistance. *Expert Systems with Applications*, 41(3), 821–830.
[11] Chockanathan, U., DSouza, A. M., Abidin, A. Z., Schifitto, G., and Wismüller, A. (2019). Automated diagnosis of HIV-associated neurocognitive disorders using large-scale Granger causality analysis of resting-state functional MRI. *Computers in Biology and Medicine*, 106, 24–30.
[12] Vaka, A. R., Soni, B., and Reddy, S. (2020). Breast cancer detection by leveraging Machine Learning. *ICT Express*, 6(4), 320–324.
[13] Saxena, S., & Gyanchandani, M. (2020). Machine learning methods for computer-aided breast cancer diagnosis using histopathology: a narrative review. *Journal of Medical Imaging and Radiation Sciences*, 51(1), 182–193.
[14] Lalmuanawma, S., Hussain, J., and Chhakchhuak, L. (2020). Applications of machine learning and artificial intelligence for Covid-19 (SARS-CoV-2) pandemic: A review. *Chaos, Solitons & Fractals*, 139, 110059.
[15] Ardakani, A. A., Kanafi, A. R., Acharya, U. R., Khadem, N., and Mohammadi, A. (2020). Application of deep learning technique to manage COVID-19 in routine clinical practice using CT images: Results of 10 convolutional neural networks. *Computers in Biology and Medicine*, 121, 103795.
[16] Ozturk, T., Talo, M., Yildirim, E. A., Baloglu, U. B., Yildirim, O., and Acharya, U. R. (2020). Automated detection of COVID-19 cases using deep neural networks with X-ray images. *Computers in Biology and Medicine*, 121, 103792.
[17] Sun, L., Song, F., Shi, N., Liu, F., Li, S., Li, P., … Shi, Y. (2020). Combination of four clinical indicators predicts the severe/critical symptom of patients infected COVID-19. *Journal of Clinical Virology*, 128, 104431.
[18] Wu, J., Zhang, P., Zhang, L., Meng, W., Li, J., Tong, C., … Li, S. (2020). Rapid and accurate identification of COVID-19 infection through machine learning based on clinical available blood test results. MedRxiv.

[19] Li, W. T., Ma, J., Shende, N., Castaneda, G., Chakladar, J., Tsai, J. C., … Ongkeko, W. M. (2020). Using machine learning of clinical data to diagnose COVID-19: a systematic review and meta-analysis. *BMC Medical Informatics and Decision Making*, 20(1), 1–13.

[20] Monaghan, C., Larkin, J. W., Chaudhuri, S., Han, H., Jiao, Y., Bermudez, K. M., … Maddux, F. W. (2020). Artificial intelligence for covid-19 risk classification in kidney disease: Can technology unmask an unseen disease? *MedRxiv*.

[21] Zoabi, Y., and Shomron, N. (2020). COVID-19 diagnosis prediction by symptoms of tested individuals: a machine learning approach. *MedRxiv*.

[22] Nan, S. N., Ya, Y., Ling, T. L., Nv, G. H., Ying, P. H., and Bin, J. (2020). A prediction model based on machine learning for diagnosing the early COVID-19 patients. *MedRxiv*.

[23] El Boujnouni, M. (2020). *A study and identification of COVID-19 viruses using N-grams with Naïve Bayes, K-nearest neighbors, artificial neural networks, decision tree and support vector machine*. Research Square.

[24] Belkacem, A. N., Ouhbi, S., Lakas, A., Benkhelifa, E., and Chen, C. (2021). End-to-End AI-Based Point-of-Care Diagnosis System for Classifying Respiratory Illnesses and Early Detection of COVID-19: A Theoretical Framework. *Frontiers in Medicine*, 8, 372.

[25] Brown, C., Chauhan, J., Grammenos, A., Han, J., Hasthanasombat, A., Spathis, D., … Mascolo, C. (2020). Exploring automatic diagnosis of COVID-19 from crowd-sourced respiratory sound data. arXiv preprint arXiv:2006.05919.

[26] Hasan, M., Jawad, M., Hasan, K. N. I., Partha, S. B., Masba, M., Al, M., and Saha, S. (2021). COVID-19 identification from volumetric chest CT scans using a progressively resized 3D-CNN incorporating segmentation, augmentation, and class-rebalancing. arXiv preprint arXiv:2102.06169.

[27] Wang, S., Kang, B., Ma, J., Zeng, X., Xiao, M., Guo, J., … Xu, B. (2021). A deep learning algorithm using CT images to screen for Corona Virus Disease (COVID-19). *European Radiology*, 2, 1–9.

[28] Abbas, A., Abdelsamea, M. M., and Gaber, M. M. (2021). 4S-DT: Self-Supervised Super Sample Decomposition for Transfer Learning With Application to COVID-19 Detection. *IEEE Transactions on Neural Networks and Learning Systems, 32*(7), 2798–2808.

[29] Zhang, H. T., Zhang, J. S., Zhang, H. H., Nan, Y. D., Zhao, Y., Fu, E. Q., … Zhang, T. (2020). Automated detection and quantification of COVID-19 pneumonia: CT imaging analysis by a deep learning-based software. *European Journal of Nuclear Medicine and Molecular Imaging*, 47(11), 2525–2532.

[30] Ahuja, S., Panigrahi, B. K., Dey, N., Rajinikanth, V., and Gandhi, T. K. (2021). Deep transfer learning-based automated detection of COVID-19 from lung CT scan slices. *Applied Intelligence*, 51(1), 571–585.

[31] Ko, H., Chung, H., Kang, W. S., Kim, K. W., Shin, Y., Kang, S. J., … Lee, J. (2020). COVID-19 pneumonia diagnosis using a simple 2D deep learning framework with a single chest CT image: model development and validation. *Journal of Medical Internet Research*, 22(6), e19569.

[32] Nishi, F. K., Khan, M. M., Alsufyani, A., Bourouis, S., Gupta, P., and Saini, D. K. (2022). Electronic Healthcare Data Record Security Using Blockchain and Smart Contract. *Journal of Sensors, 2022.*

[33] Sharma, S., Gupta, S., Gupta, D., Juneja, S., Gupta, P., Dhiman, G., and Kautish, S. (2022). Deep learning model for the automatic classification of white blood cells. *Computational Intelligence and Neuroscience, 2022.*

[34] Tazin, T., Sarker, S., Gupta, P., Ayaz, F. I., Islam, S., Monirujjaman Khan, M., … Alshazly, H. (2021). A robust and novel approach for brain tumor classification using convolutional neural network. *Computational Intelligence and Neuroscience, 2021.*

[35] Yan, L., Zhang, H. T., Goncalves, J., Xiao, Y., Wang, M., Guo, Y., … Yuan, Y. (2020). An interpretable mortality prediction model for COVID-19 patients. *Nature Machine Intelligence*, 2(5), 283–288.

[36] Cheng, F. Y., Joshi, H., Tandon, P., Freeman, R., Reich, D. L., Mazumdar, M., … Kia, A. (2020). Using machine learning to predict ICU transfer in hospitalized COVID-19 patients. *Journal of Clinical Medicine*, 9(6), 1668.

[37] Pourhomayoun, M., and Shakibi, M. (2020). Predicting mortality risk in patients with COVID-19 using artificial intelligence to help medical decision-making. *MedRxiv.*

[38] Das, A., Mishra, S., and Gopalan, S. S. (2020). Predicting community mortality risk due to CoVID-19 using machine learning and development of a prediction tool. *MedRxiv.*

[39] Yao, Z., Zheng, X., Zheng, Z., Wu, K., and Zheng, J. (2021). Construction and validation of a machine learning-based nomogram: A tool to predict the risk of getting severe coronavirus disease 2019 (COVID-19). *Immunity, Inflammation and Disease*, 9(2), 595–607.

[40] Sehanobish, A., Ravindra, N. G., & van Dijk, D. (2020). Gaining insight into SARS-CoV-2 infection and COVID-19 severity using self-supervised edge features and Graph Neural Networks. arXiv preprint arXiv:2006.12971.

[41] Maghded, H. S., Ghafoor, K. Z., Sadiq, A. S., Curran, K., Rawat, D. B., and Rabie, K. (2020, August). A novel AI-enabled framework to diagnose coronavirus COVID-19 using smartphone embedded sensors: design study. In *2020 IEEE 21st International Conference on Information Reuse and Integration for Data Science (IRI)* (pp. 180–187). IEEE.

[42] Izquierdo, J. L., Ancochea, J., and Soriano, J. B. (2020). *Clinical Characteristics and Prognostic Factors for ICU Admission of Patients with COVID-19 Using Machine Learning and Natural Language Processing medRxiv* (2020).

[43] Shahroz, M., Ahmad, F., Younis, M. S., Ahmad, N., Boulos, M. N. K., Vinuesa, R., and Qadir, J. (2021). COVID-19 Digital Contact Tracing Applications and Techniques: A Review Post Initial Deployments. *Transportation Engineering*, 100072.

[44] Hellewell, J., Abbott, S., Gimma, A., Bosse, N. I., Jarvis, C. I., Russell, T. W., … Eggo, R. M. (2020). Feasibility of controlling COVID-19 outbreaks by isolation of cases and contacts. *The Lancet Global Health*, 8(4), e488–e496.

[45] Brauer, F., Castillo-Chavez, C., and Castillo-Chavez, C. (2012). *Mathematical Models in Population Biology and Epidemiology* (Vol. 2, p. 508). New York: Springer.

[46] Perez, L., and Dragicevic, S. (2009). An agent-based approach for modeling dynamics of contagious disease spread. *International Journal of Health Geographics*, 8(1), 1–17.

[47] Balcan, D., Hu, H., Gonçalves, B., Bajardi, P., Poletto, C., Ramasco, J. J., … Vespignani, A. (2009). Seasonal transmission potential and activity peaks of the new influenza A (H1N1): a Monte Carlo likelihood analysis based on human mobility. *BMC Medicine*, 7(1), 1–12.

[48] Ribeiro, M. H. D. M., da Silva, R. G., Mariani, V. C., and dos Santos Coelho, L. (2020). Short-term forecasting COVID-19 cumulative confirmed cases: Perspectives for Brazil. *Chaos, Solitons & Fractals*, 135, 109853.

[49] Chimmula, V. K. R., and Zhang, L. (2020). Time series forecasting of COVID-19 transmission in Canada using LSTM networks. *Chaos, Solitons & Frac*tals, 135, 109864.
[50] Zia, K., Farooq, U., and Shafi, M. (2021). COVID-19 Outbreak: Model-Driven Impact Analysis Comparing Oman and Pakistan. *Applied Computing Journal*, 38–54.
[51] Van den Broeck, W., Gioannini, C., Gonçalves, B., Quaggiotto, M., Colizza, V., & Vespignani, A. (2011). The GLEAMviz computational tool, a publicly available software to explore realistic epidemic spreading scenarios at the global scale. *BMC Infectious Diseases*, 11(1), 1–14.
[52] Callaway, E. (2020). Coronavirus: Labs Worldwide Scramble to Analyse Samples. *Nature*, 578(16), 127–146.
[53] Zia, K. (2021). Why a Globally Fair COVID-19 Vaccination? An Analysis based on Agent-Based Simulation. *MedRxiv*.
[54] Iyanda, A., Boakye, K., and Lu, Y. (2021). Covid-19: Evidenced health disparity. *Encyclopedia*, 1(3), 744–763.
[55] Liu, Y., Salwi, S., and Drolet, B. C. (2020). Multivalue ethical framework for fair global allocation of a COVID-19 vaccine. *Journal of Medical Ethics*, 46(8), 499–501.
[56] S. M. Moghadas, T. N. Vilches, K. Zhang, S. Nourbakhsh, P. Sah, M. C. Fitzpatrick, A. P. Galvani, Evaluation of covid-19 vaccination strategies with a delayed second dose, *PLoS Biology* 19 (4) (2021) e3001211.
[57] L. Matrajt, H. Janes, J. T. Schiffer, D. Dimitrov, Quantifying the impact of lifting community nonpharmaceutical interventions for covid-19 during vaccination rollout in the united states, in: *Open forum infectious diseases*, Vol. 8, Oxford University Press US, 2021, p. ofab341.
[58] F. M. Russell, B. Greenwood, Who should be prioritised for covid-19 vaccination?, *Human Vaccines & Immunotherapeutics* 17 (5) (2021) 1317–1321.
[59] S. M. Moghadas, M. C. Fitzpatrick, A. Shoukat, K. Zhang, A. P. Galvani, Simulated identification of silent covid-19 infections among children and estimated future infection rates with vaccination, *JAMA Network Open* 4 (4) (2021) e217097.
[60] P. Sah, T. N. Vilches, S. M. Moghadas, M. C. Fitzpatrick, B. H. Singer, P. J. Hotez, A. P. Galvani, Accelerated vaccine rollout is imperative to mitigate highly transmissible covid-19 variants, *EClinicalMedicine* 35 (2021) 100865.
[61] T. N. Vilches, F. A. Rubio, R. F. Perroni, G. B. de Almeida, C. P. Ferreira, and C. M. C. B. Fortaleza, Vaccination efforts in brazil: scenarios and perspectives under a mathematical modelling approach, *MedRxiv*.
[62] J. Thompson, and S. Wattam, Estimating the impact of interventions against covid-19: from lockdown to vaccination, *MedRxiv*.

## Chapter 7

# Big Data Analytics in Healthcare Data Processing

Tanveer Ahmed
*Bennett University, Greater Noida, India*

Rishav Singh
*NIT Delhi, Delhi, India*

Ritika Singh
*CSIR CSIO, Chandigarh, India*

## Contents

7.1 Introduction ........ 124
7.2 Big Data ........ 126
7.2.1 Big Data Analytics in Healthcare ........ 126
7.2.1.1 Big Data Characteristics in Healthcare: The 5 Vs ........ 127
7.2.1.2 Demand for Big Data Analytics in Healthcare ........ 128
7.2.1.3 Big Data Analytics Platforms and Tools in Healthcare ........ 129
7.3 Big Data Analytics and Artificial Intelligence ........ 129
7.3.1 Artificial Intelligence and its Uses in Healthcare ........ 131

DOI: 10.1201/9781003322597-7

7.4 Big Data Analytics and Deep Learning ....132
7.4.1 Convolutional Neural Networks (CNN) ....132
7.4.2 Recurrent Neural Networks (RNN) ....133
7.4.3 Long Short-Term Memory (LSTM) ....133
7.5 Different Machine Learning Techniques Used in Healthcare ....133
7.6 Advantages of Big Data in Healthcare ....133
7.7 Application of Big Data Analytics in Healthcare ....136
7.7.1 Healthcare Monitoring ....136
7.7.2 Healthcare Risk Prediction ....136
7.7.3 Behavioral Monitoring ....136
7.7.4 Treatment of Cancer and Genomics ....136
7.7.5 Detect and Prevent Fraud ....136
7.7.6 Hospital Network ....137
7.7.7 Clinical Decision Support System ....137
7.7.8 Clinical Trials and Drug Development ....137
7.7.9 Telediagnosis and Image Informatics ....137
7.7.10 Healthcare Knowledge System ....137
7.8 Challenges and Recommendations ....137
7.8.1 Obtaining and Cleaning Huge Amounts of Health Data from Different Sources ....138
7.8.2 Maintaining the Storage and Quality of Large Amounts of Health Data ....138
7.8.3 Big Health Data Can Be Scaled Up or Down Depending on Need ....139
7.8.4 Using Big Health Data to Make Faster and Better Decisions ....139
7.9 Future Direction in Healthcare for Big Data ....140
7.9.1 Issues in the Collection of Health Data ....140
7.9.2 Data Governance ....140
7.9.3 The Importance of Recent Technologies ....140
7.9.4 Investigating the Success of Big Data Analytics ....140
7.10 Conclusion ....141
References ....141

## 7.1 Introduction

Big data analytics covers a wide spectrum of techniques ranging from classification to regression, outlier detection, exception handling and several others. Although it is a part of the standard data-preprocessing paradigm, the scale at which the models that perform these tasks are applied is breathtaking. Recent developments in artificial intelligence have also really elevated the performance and development of methods to a whole new level. Naturally, big data analytics has attracted a wide variety of applications in a plethora of fields. One such field is healthcare. Big data analytics in this domain covers amalgamation of and development of large datasets and huge models to cover several aspects of patient care. The field is complemented by the advent of personalized and predictive models that use the idea of electronic healthcare records to continuously monitor and delivery timely medical care to a patient. This is generally accomplished by complementing the delivery mechanism with the internet of things. In this context, the internet of things (IoT) is a community of gadgets and other objects attached to the human body that are equipped with electronics, software programs, sensors, and network connectivity to accumulate and share facts [3].

Throughout 2020, health-related IoT accounts for 40% of all IoT-related activity, a US$117 billion enterprise [4], and clinical informatics, combining treatment and data technology that is transforming healthcare as we understand it, lowering charges, reducing inefficiencies, and saving lives. The combination of IoT with healthcare requires careful handling, as it produces massive amounts of previously unseen data. Big data analytics enables users to observe and analyze large datasets consisting of millions of electronic health records, helping to identify previously unseen patterns and developing previously undiscovered data mining techniques. Precision medicine [5] is an idea that will become increasingly popular in the coming years. Starting from genomics, it has moved towards omics systems, providing multiscale statistics for evaluation and interpretation [6]. The Collaborative Cancer Cloud project, which keeps confidential scientific facts that can be utilized for research into most cancers, was introduced by Intel and Oregon Health Science College in 2015. Intel aims to make the federated cloud community available to different universities, including those that specialize in the treatment of Parkinson's disease via the medical internet of things (mIoT).

Data available for such applications is highly unstructured. To make matters worse, the complexity and highly technical nature of the data makes iit highly challenging for standard machine learning methods to be straightforwardly applied to a cloud platform. Such data would therefore require hand-crafted and manually engineered features to be useful at all. This is challenging, especially considering the diverse nature of the problem. According to the McKinsey Global Institute, efficient processing of big data would reduce global medical expenditure by around 8%. It would therefore be highly beneficial to engineer techniques to discover previously undiscovered patterns and use them to find effective solutions to healthcare problems. This article is focused on analyzing the application of big data analytics to healthcare. More specifically, in this article, we aim to analyze and study various techniques that could help guide future research in the field. Through analysis of work in this field, we have also identified a few challenges that demand immediate attention. We discuss recent work in the field of healthcare and highlight important points to which research should direct its focus.

## 7.2 Big Data

The term 'big data' means the collection of huge data sets that pose a challenge for system designers. It is one of the tools and methods that a firm can use to generate, store, and exploit massive amounts of data. On a daily basis, every one of us generates a vast amount of data at an unparalleled rate from a variety of sources: from cameras, mobile phones, associated applications and several others [7]. A great deal of computer power, analytical skills, and knowledge is needed to get anything useful out of such a massive amount of data.

Figure 7.1 illustrates the general framework of big data analytics. The amount generated at the big data source is primarily raw, and must be processed or converted, at which time there are a number of options. The unprocessed data are used by service-oriented architectures which combine with web services (middleware) [1, 8] such as data pre-processing, call and retrieve. Following that, the data are stored on a big data platform such as Hadoop, Pig, and so on. Finally, data are prepared for processing.

The merits of several distributed designs with diverse areas, tool choices, and analytics models for healthcare are discussed in the following sections.

### *7.2.1 Big Data Analytics in Healthcare*

Figure 7.2 summarizes the usage of big data analytics in healthcare. Data can be gathered from a variety of sources, including medical imaging, electronic health records (EHR), and other sources [9]. Big data is currently developing new data analysis tools that incorporate machine learning models in relation to various sources. In the context of contact tracing, big data is contact information obtained from a variety of sources that can be used to track down everyone who has been in close proximity to a COVID-positive person.

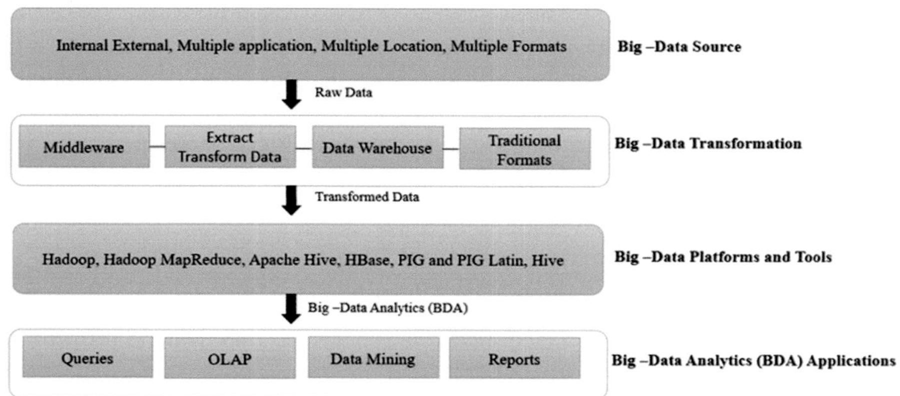


**Figure 7.1 Layered Architecture of Big Data Analytics (BDA).**

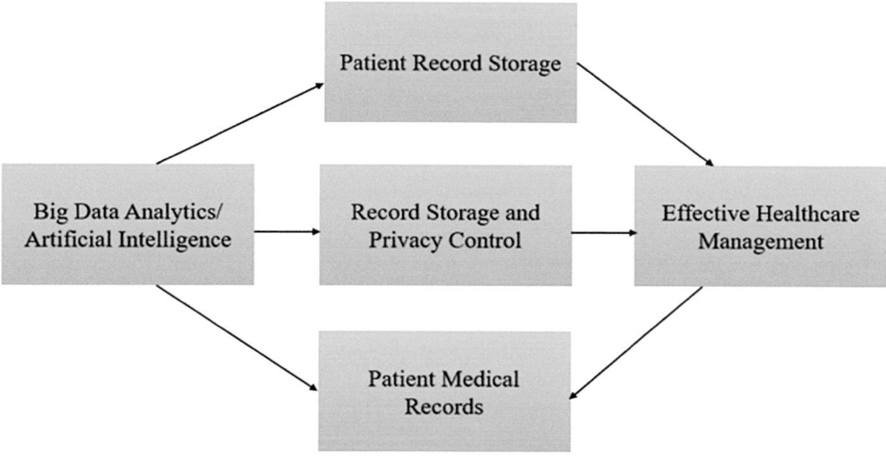


**Figure 7.2 Use of Big Data Services for Analyzing Patient Records.**

#### *7.2.1.1 Big Data Characteristics in Healthcare: The 5 Vs*

The qualities of large data that we have discussed apply to a variety of issues in the health domain, including the present coronavirus pandemic. Figure 7.3 shows the overall structure of the 5Vs of healthcare big data.

*Volume*: Large amounts of data that must be managed, analyzed with the help of traditional databases and data processing architecture are referred to as "big data" [1]. These data are calculated in exabytes [9]. The volume of data generated by modern IT and the healthcare system has been growing, owing to decreasing storage and processing costs, as well as a need to extract valuable

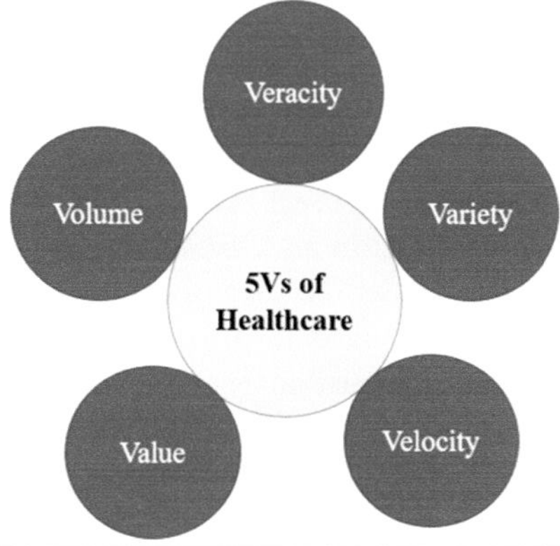


**Figure 7.3 The 5 Vs of Healthcare in Big Data.**

insights from data in order to improve business processes and consumer services [10].

*Veracity:* Data veracity refers to the degree of certainty that a data interpretation is consistent [11]. Varied data sources have different levels of data reliability and dependability [12]. Unsupervised machine learning algorithms, on the other hand, are used in healthcare for automated machines to make decisions based on data which may be deceptive or useless [10].The purpose of healthcare analytics is to obtain useful information that can be used to make better decisions and provide better patient care.

*Variety*: We have different type of data in society, whether structured or unstructured (e.g., email, call center transcripts, blogs and social media posts, radiograph films, audio, video files, and machine data such as log files from websites, servers, and mobile system apps) [13, 14]. Clinical data (patient record data) is an example of structured data that requires specific equipment to collect, store, and evaluate. Only 5%–10% of all healthcare data is structured.

*Velocity:* Velocity refers to how quickly data is created, processed, and updated, as well as how quickly an information consumer requires outcomes from a processing system [15]. The fundamental explanation for the exponential expansion of data is velocity, which denotes the rate at which this type of data is collected [1]. Owing to the way structured or unstructured data is acquired, further, the speed with which this data is generated necessitates quick decisions.

*Value:* The term "value" refers to how the user will receive or benefit from the study findings. It is the ability to take any form of raw data and transform it into valuable information that forms the most significant feature of big data analysis. Its premise is identical to that of healthcare information

#### *7.2.1.2 Demand for Big Data Analytics in Healthcare*

*Providing patient-centered services*: To give patients faster relief by providing effective medication to counteract any effects of a disease at the early stages. Further, big data can also minimize drug doses to reduce side-effects. This helps patients save money by lowering readmission rates [16].

*Treatment procedures should be improved*: Personalized patient care involves monitoring the effects of medication and, based on the findings, changing drug dosages to provide better relief. To give proactive treatment to patients, vital signs are monitored. Analyzing data provided by patients who have already had the same symptoms can assist doctors in prescribing effective medications to new patients [16].

*Monitoring the hospital's quality*: Checking to see if the hospitals are set up in accordance with the Indian Medical Council's guidelines. This routine inspection aids the government in taking appropriate action against hospitals that are disqualified.

*Predicting viral infections before they spread*: Using live analysis, predict viral diseases before they spread. This can be determined by looking through the social logs of patients infected with a disease in a specific place. This aids healthcare workers in advising victims and taking the required precautions.

### 7.2.1.3 Big Data Analytics Platforms and Tools in Healthcare

*Hadoop:* Hadoop common platforms have different frameworks such as MapReduce, Apache, HDFS and Hadoop Common. It also refers to a set of common utilities which assist all different Hadoop framework modules.

*Hadoop MapReduce*: Hadoop MapReduce has two main frameworks, Map and Reduce, which handles structured and unstructured data [17–20]. This is also the main factor in Hadoop, which handles the large amount of data processed in parallel when used in a distributed computing environment.

*Hadoop Distributed File System (HDFS):* Unstructured data is processed using this file system. HDFS is a popular data storage system that divides each file into fixed-size blocks and distributes them across several servers (nodes). HDFS uses NameNode (master node) and Data-Node (slave node) [21, 22].

*Apache Hive*: Hive by Apache Hive is a data warehouse architecture for querying and analyzing large amounts of Hadoop HDFS data. It is a Hadoop ETL tool (extract, transform, and load). Hive is a Hadoop-based data warehouse that uses a declarative language is known as Hive query language (HiveQL) which allow SQL programmers to easily analyze data [23].

*HBase*: is based on the Distributed File System (DFS) from Hadoop (HDFS). Apache Hbase is a multidimensional distributed database system that is part of the Hadoop ecosystem. It can store a larger amount of data from terabyte (TB) to petabyte (PB) level [24].

*PIG and PIG Latin*: PIG is designed to work with a wide range of organized and unorganized data. It has two primary modules: the PIG Latin programming language the PIG Latin runtime version [25].

*Hive:* is a Hadoop framework for runtime which combines SQL. It can run Hive Query Language (HQL) queries, which are equivalent to SQL queries.

## 7.3 Big Data Analytics and Artificial Intelligence

The structure of big data analytics is presented in Figure 7.4. The ever-increasing complexity of computational systems and the increasing demand to understand the complex system has paved the way for big data analytics and has provided various excellent opportunities for its applications in a variety of fields. The ever-increasing demand to make computers smart has driven the world to achieve great success, and correspondingly, research has tried to push the boundaries beyond the existing potential of big data. In this regard, healthcare has become data driven.

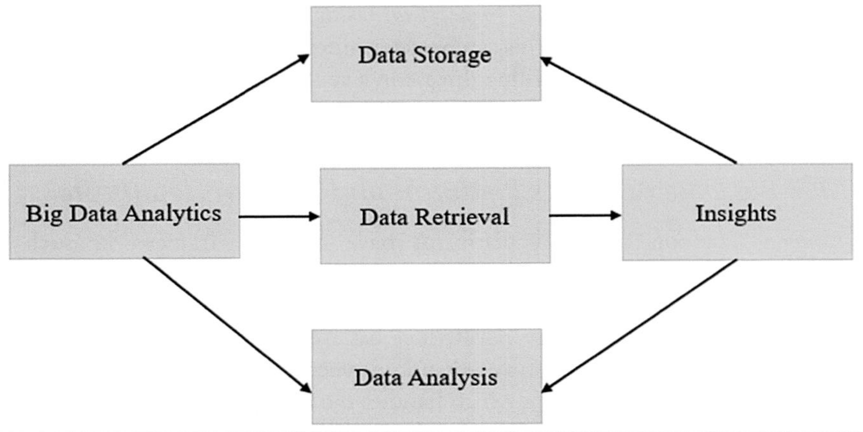


**Figure 7.4 Overall Structure of Big Data Analytics.**

This statement is evidenced by the fact that the way data is now generated from patients to medical practitioners, the way information and instructions are shared among the conglomerate of hospitals or health care institutions has become crucial for decision making. With increased digitization, whether it is test report generation, insurance, or usage of medical equipment, etc., everything is now driven by data. Naturally, with the increase in the amount of data there has been a multifold increase in the information hidden in this complex maze of data. It is imperative that the usage of advanced analytics and machine learning also increase with it.

We have seen that big data analytics has become one of the important tools for uncovering hidden pattens in the huge volumes of data available to a medical practitioner. This idea involves discovery, interpretation, and communication of new and actionable insights from the huge volume of data in a plethora of domains for timely and efficient decision making. Big data analytics is altogether a continuously evolving methodology that involves using various algorithms from a wide variety of fields, e.g., data mining, artificial intelligence, machine learning, mathematics, cloud computing, and HPC, to address the issue of huge volumes of data. It has traditionally been applied to multiple fields such finance [26] and biomedicine [27, 28], among others. With recent advances in cloud computing technologies, the field has taken a new turn and the capabilities of the paradigm have been increased multiple times. As with any data-driven field there are challenges, including privacy, integration [29], security, and disparity among multiple sources of data. Even governance and anonymization of data is a problem these days.

AI as a branch is geared towards the advance, development and application of human-like intelligence in lifeless machines. The goal of the paradigm is to induce knowledge-driven reasoning and enable a machine to make decisions based on a human-like reasoning process. The field has shown potential and there is a huge amount of work dedicated to the study of such methodologies. This field involves the use of multiple algorithms from mathematics and statistics. With recent developments in the field of deep learning, the paradigm has also taken multiple strides forward. Today, researchers are able to address issues that were unpredictable to solve just a few years back.

Healthcare was identified as one of the interesting areas of application of this paradigm. As mentioned in the previous paragraph, there are a lot of useful insights available in the raw data. It would be very useful for any system designer to apply automated algorithms and use those insights for the betterment of the system.

## 7.3.1 Artificial Intelligence and its Uses in Healthcare

It has been suggested that artificial intelligence will revolutionize practically every aspect of healthcare. AI can assist physicians in making more informed clinical decisions and improving patient outcomes. The broad categories of AI applications in healthcare are summarized in Figure 7.5. In this section, we summarize the benefits that AI can bring in various biomedical tasks. It is important to note that using AI-based techniques also forms an important part of big data analytics (BDA). The most important advantages are:

- Checking for abnormalities and recommending medical action.
- Predicting the onset of new diseases.
- Accurate and efficient diagnosis.
- A good outcome for the patient.
- Improving the experience of doctors and surgeons.
- Improving the quality of medical care.
- **Improving pathological** outcome.

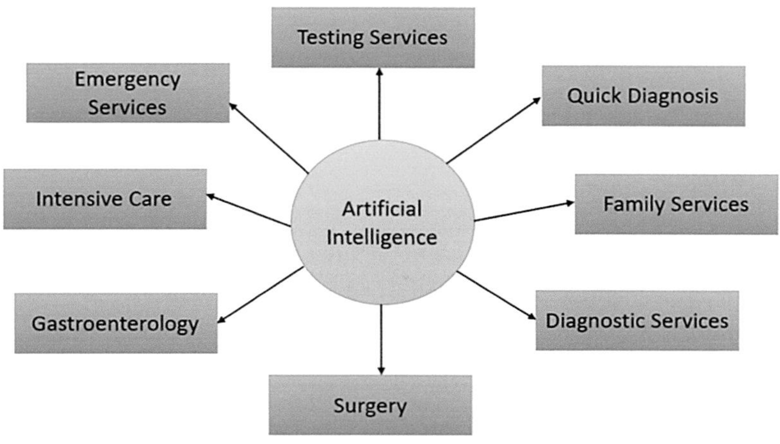


**Figure 7.5 Use of AI in healthcare services.**

- Maintaining a clinical record.
- Providing the patient with outstanding service.
- **Providing support to** doctors and patients.
- Proper instruction for medical students.
- Enhancing hospital security.
- Helpful in the treatment of complex and novel conditions.
- Balancing patient blood/glucose levels.
- Patient monitoring.

## 7.4 Big Data Analytics and Deep Learning

Deep learning models have a variety of applications such as genomics sequencing structure [30], image detection, and structure of drugs. For visual tracking [31] and object detection, deep learning has also been employed in medical picture analysis. Deep learning is making tremendous progress in detecting unstructured and complex structures in high-dimensional data, allowing it to better predict the activity of potential therapeutic drugs [32] and the effects of non-coding DNA mutations on gene expression and disease [33] (Table 7.1).

### *7.4.1 Convolutional Neural Networks (CNN)*

CNNs emerged as a result of the development of deep network topologies. CNNs outperform traditional networks. Following AlexNet's excellent performance on the ImageNet dataset in 2012, many additional deep designs have been developed in recent years. A collection of filters is applied to each layer of the CNN in order to extract and learn the data's relevant attributes. Early CNNs, such as AlexNet and VGG16, were sequential networks where the output was pushed from one layer to the other. There are also models that use CNNs as a basis model for feature

**Table 7.1 Deep Learning Algorithms**

| *Deep Learning Algorithms* | *Application* |
|---|---|
| CNN | When it comes to picture classification and detection, radiology imaging can be used to detect COVID-19 early on [34]. |
| RNN | For predicting the health of patients in the future [35] |
| LSTM | Diagnoses patients in a pediatric intensive care unit based on clinical measurements [36], predicts future medical outcomes [37], and discovers new drugs [38, 39]. |

extractions, such as object detection models, SSD [40], YOLO [41], segmentation models, SegNet [42] and Unet [43], and generative models, GAN [44]. CNNs are also widely employed in the biomedical field for a variety of applications, including disease classification [45], detection [46], and segmentation [47].

### 7.4.2 Recurrent Neural Networks (RNN)

Recurrent neural network is another well-known type of deep learning that works with sequence data and is commonly used in applications like financial time-series, speech recognition, music production, natural language processing (NLP), and language translation, to name a few. Traditional RNNs suffer from the gradient vanishing problem and are unable to sustain long-term dependency when utilized in NLP applications. More complex sequence models, such as long short-term memory (LSTM) [48] and GRUs (gated recurrent units) [49] have evolved to solve the limitations of traditional RNNs.

### 7.4.3 Long Short-Term Memory (LSTM)

Long short-term memory (LSTM) networks [50] are one of the types of recurrent neural network that can retain patterns selectively across time. They represent a better choice for modeling data. Owing to their advantages, they are often employed to find underlying hidden dynamics in human behavior. The LSTM cell's memory is stored and transformed from input to output in the cell state. An LSTM cell is made up of the forget, output, input, and update gates. The forget gate determines what to forget from previous memory units, the input gate determines what to take into the neuron, the update gate refreshes the cell, and the output gate, as its name implies, generates new long-term memory.

## 7.5 Different Machine Learning Techniques Used in Healthcare

Most of the techniques (summarized in Table 7.2) are described in the literature [51, 52].

## 7.6 Advantages of Big Data in Healthcare

By efficiently using the ideas of BDA, healthcare workers and industrial organizations are expected to gain significant benefits by analyzing and discovering patterns that were previously unknown to the world. Potential benefits include, for example, early detection of disease that can then be treated and effectively managed using automated drug delivery systems. Finding relevant cuts in the healthcare budget

**Table 7.2 Different Techniques Used in Healthcare**

| *Techniques* | *Healthcare Applications* |
|---|---|
| Genetic Algorithm (GA) | Data dependencies, bandwidth consumption, computational resources. |
| Firefly Swarm Optimization (FSO) | Protein complex identification, brain tissue segmentation, multilayer color image thresholding, heart disease prediction. |
| Simulated Annealing (SA) and Whale Optimization Algorithm (WOA) | SA method improves classification accuracy by identifying most relevant attributes.<br>WOA is used to construct iterative feature selection in a SA algorithm-based large data optimization technique. |
| Neural Networks | Chronic disease diagnosis is the process of determining whether or not a patient has a disease with the help of neural networks [53]. |
| PSO | Remote sensing image registration, time-series prediction. |
| GreyWolf Optimization algorithm (GWO) | Used for selection of best features, community detection. |
| Artificial Bee Colony (ABC) | A big data clustering strategy based on the ABC algorithm that finds the optimal cluster and optimizes it for varied dataset sizes.<br>Reduces execution time and improves clustering accuracy when used map/reduce-based Hadoop system. Has been used to train pattern recognition neural networks. |
| Improved ACO algorithm (IACO) | Managing medical data such as patient and operation data that allows clinicians to get the information they need in a short amount of time using big data analytics. |
| Ant Colony Optimization (ACO) | Missing value treatment, anomaly detection, and predictive control for nonlinear systems. |
| Cat Swarm Optimization (CSO) | To improve feature selection accuracy, the CSO method employs the term frequency-inverse document frequency. |
| Bacterial Foraging Optimization (BFO) algorithm | Characterizes medical information into actionable categories. |

**Table 7.2 (*Continued*) Different Techniques Used in Healthcare**

| *Techniques* | *Healthcare Applications* |
|---|---|
| Lion Optimization Algorithm (LOA) | Extracts liver location from CT images using data clustering. |
| Whale Optimization Algorithm | Feature selection and prediction of COVID-19 cases are now proposed. |
| Pattern Recognition | Public health surveillance improvement. |
| Spatial Analysis | Using visual data, advanced analytics to extract significant population-level insights. |

would help minimize wastage, freeing money to be spent elsewhere, and healthcare fraud would be minimized. The potential is truly unimaginable. For instance, using the huge amount of data available in the system, several outcomes could very easily be predicted and estimated with great precision. Surgery would be more effective, and precision guided. The accuracy of disease detection systems would be greatly increased, and so on. The following are some of the primary benefits, according to recently published studies [54–56]:

*Clinical operations*: Cost-effective strategies to diagnose disease quickly and thereby treating patients are being investigated through comparative effectiveness research.

*Healthcare providers*: Information gathered from medical organizations assists stakeholders in implementing innovative healthcare initiatives for patients in order to prevent unnecessary hospitalizations.

*Patients*: Patients can benefit from healthcare information by making the best decision at the right time, thereby improving their health and avoiding healthcare expenses.

*Public health:* Monitoring and analyzing healthcare data is a huge task, which can help to improve public health surveillance. The large amount of data available in public health systems can be converted into actionable information that identifies the need and predicts crises. BDA also contributes in different areas such as genomics, X-ray images, CT scan images, device monitoring and so on.

*Research and development*: Researchers and scientists can use healthcare data to improve services by enabling more precise and appropriate treatments, such as using different statistical algorithms and techniques to improve clinical structure and patient enrolment, minimizing structural failures and bringing rapid innovative therapies to market. Modeling structure can be predicted which reduce attrition then deliver faster, and finalized medication and device R&D.

## 7.7 Application of Big Data Analytics in Healthcare

The active digitization of literature from data is necessary since the majority of healthcare data is unstructured and predominantly in printed form, making it difficult for clinicians and politicians alike to build service delivery and public policy based on health recommendation systems and economic-based data [57, 58].

### 7.7.1 Healthcare Monitoring

Users' (patients') health could be tracked over time using healthcare data analytics to improve their quality of life [59]. Workers are connected to their healthcare records using big data analytics. Most of the hospital are using Hadoop-based systems such as HDFS, Pig, Apache and so on, which converts the unstructured data formats generated by sensors, analyzes blood pressure, and monitors patient signs, heartbeats, into structured form.

### 7.7.2 Healthcare Risk Prediction

Deep analysis of healthcare data aids the development of risk prediction solutions by healthcare stakeholders and medical practitioners. Clinicians can also use system predictions to make patient-related decisions [60, 61]. Two issues, high-risk and high-cost patients, are also identified with help of data analytics [62].

### 7.7.3 Behavioral Monitoring

A home healthcare system in was suggested by some 2005 research to record patients' behavioral data for the purpose of identifying their illnesses [63]. Monitoring of patients with anomalous behavior [64] is another potential application of BDA in healthcare.

### 7.7.4 Treatment of Cancer and Genomics

Three billion base pairs are known to exist in human DNA. Large amounts of data must be efficiently arranged in order to combat cancer. Individual genetics influence the patterns of cancer mutations and their responses, which explains why some cancers are incurable. When it comes to spotting cancer patterns, oncologists have learned that providing tailored treatment for distinct tumors depending on the patient's genetic composition is crucial. To find optimal cancer solution, two different platforms can used, Hadoop and MapReduce.

### 7.7.5 Detect and Prevent Fraud

Health insurance firms employ a variety of approaches to uncover fraudulent activities and develop different types of methods to prevent medical fraud. Companies use Hadoop apps that use data from earlier health claims, earnings, and demographics, among other data sources, to identify fraudsters. According to the authors [65], different technologies are also used in healthcare to detect fraud such as data mining and machine learning technologies.

### 7.7.6 Hospital Network

Several hospitals are now using technology effectively. Hadoop is frequently used in this context to collect and manage large amounts of real-time data from many sources. This procedure enables them to identify high-risk individuals while also reducing day-to-day expenses [66].

### 7.7.7 Clinical Decision Support System

To analyze a patient's health condition, a clinical decision support system is designed which facilitates input from healthcare professionals [67, 68].

### 7.7.8 Clinical Trials and Drug Development

For drug discovery, the pharmaceutical industry heavily relies on healthcare BDA to aid doctors, developers in the field of pharmaceuticals, and other healthcare experts in getting the right drug to the right patient at the right time [69, 70].

### 7.7.9 Telediagnosis and Image Informatics

Imaging informatics is one of the important methods, generating different types of biological data such as representation, organizing and generating image data. It is involved in the interchange and analysis of medical images across complicated healthcare systems [71, 72]. Authors of [73] describe a new tele-mammography system that uses image processing and machine learning approaches to detect breast cancer early. Computer-aided diagnosis (CAD) [74] is a critical component of medical imaging.

### 7.7.10 Healthcare Knowledge System

According to [75], an expert management system based on big data in healthcare is being developed to aid clinical decision making and health detection. EHR, medical images, and DNA information are all used in the "healthcare expert system".

## 7.8 Challenges and Recommendations

For AI-based technology interventions, the accuracy of diagnosis of COVID-19 cases is now a difficulty. Because AI algorithms have performance concerns,

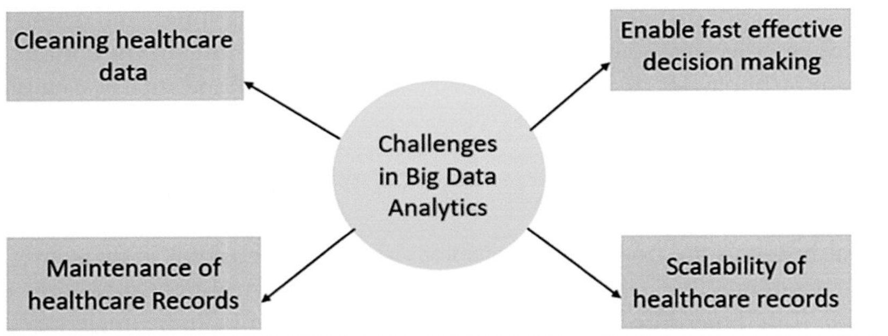


**Figure 7.6 Challenges in Big Data Analytics for Healthcare.**

implementing nature-inspired computing models could help to enhance performance. Furthermore, contact tracing on a larger scale is not only expensive but also tedious, mainly because contacts accumulate quickly, necessitating additional search efforts in tracing etc. Some challenges are presented in Figure 7.6. Various challenges are described in the following sections, with recommendations for tackling them.

### *7.8.1 Obtaining and Cleaning Huge Amounts of Health Data from Different Sources*

To make original data sets faultless, reduce the time it takes to process data and ensure integrity in healthcare data, several automated tools will have to work together and have to adapt themselves according to the latest trends. For data analysis, healthcare data is often obtained from external as well as internal records. The data sets that will be recorded will come in a range of sizes and formats. Data sets would be clean, thorough, correct, and in the proper format before being transferred to several medical systems or clinicians, because poor data quality can undermine big data analytics [76]. It must also entail the integration of organized, unstructured, and semi-structured data, as well as the removal of errors and disparities. To properly leverage big data, system designers must resolve errors quickly, maintain consistency, and try to minimize losses.

### *7.8.2 Maintaining the Storage and Quality of Large Amounts of Health Data*

Clinicians take more accurate decisions, owing to the insights that they have gained based on big data analysis. If the data being analyzed is inaccurate, it will lead to rash conclusions that are ultimately harmful to patients. Because of the importance of data quality, testing is a top concern. As a result, ensuring the accuracy of the information stored necessitates a significant investment of resources. In the healthcare industry, the range of data is rising at an exponential rate. For any healthcare worker, and/or anyone conducting a clinical study, storing and maintaining high-quality medical data has become a major concern. Some healthcare providers have lost control of their medical data centers and are unable to manage expenditure. Large amounts of data in diverse formats are frequently collected, stored, and analyzed using data lakes or data warehouses. Data mistakes, duplication, and inaccurate data linkage increase as a result of these coarse data from various sources, necessitating a dedicated data cleansing process [77].

### 7.8.3 Big Health Data Can Be Scaled Up or Down Depending on Need

Unlike other types of data, big health data is always growing and evolving. As a result, healthcare companies frequently overlook the reality that the volume and burden associated with big data are fast increasing. They will need to build an infrastructure that makes it easier to process new data on a frequent basis. Many hospitals have recently chosen cloud systems to efficiently store and handle large amounts of healthcare data by utilizing on-demand computing capabilities. Some large data solutions, on the other hand, will not work as well on a cloud server. As a result, the healthcare industry must face the difficulty of scaling medical data sets up and down in response to doctor or patient demand. Indeed, new processing tools and storage capacity will have an impact on the real analytical process. Consequently, system complexity and speed will immediately reduce the difficulty of scaling up large data sets [78]. The third critical factor is that owing to the speed and variety of data, algorithms that focus on tackling the difficulties of data growth or changes to data sets itself are required. The most critical matter is to transform a distributed medical server, with individual server storing and viewing local data flow.

### 7.8.4 Using Big Health Data to Make Faster and Better Decisions

When healthcare records contain complex and varied occurrences, the data set must be customized without an overly searching structure and converted into relevant measurements in real time for speedy analysis. Patients will receive lower-quality care if complicated medical datasets are processed too slowly [79]. After the clinical data has been analyzed, the big data analysts must seek help from clinicians to explain the results to patients, as a clear understanding of the medical report is essential for making generalized judgments. In addition, the computer must be capable of anticipating or recommending important and potential doctors and other experts to the user. They also have to analyze diverse geographic proximity questions and find a precise answer, which mandates the creation of a new indexing strategy to suit such medical inquiries. If the data volume continues to grow rapidly, medical practitioners' queries will be subject to strict response time limits.

## 7.9 Future Direction in Healthcare for Big Data

Three key limitations were highlighted in the existing research on BDA in healthcare that was evaluated here: assumptions of the study, collection of data, and constraints of technology. The research has highlighted scope for future research in several areas: growth of theoretical concepts, technological rigor, research design, and advances in technologies. These highlighted points reflect the four different sets of future research.

### 7.9.1 Issues in the Collection of Health Data

Big data in healthcare involves a number of issues, including data quality and quantity, according to previous studies. Data are collected from various sources such as hospital records, diagnostic reports, and patient details. Future research should concentrate on filling in the gaps in the literature as well as finding solutions to the problems that have been identified.

### 7.9.2 Data Governance

Future work can look at ways to better manage data. There is also a gap in cyber law research and policies for using healthcare data. Furthermore, researchers should pay more attention to privacy of patients. Future research agendas can therefore be divided into two categories: conceptual advances and study design.

### 7.9.3 The Importance of Recent Technologies

The technological research perspective is very important for improving future research in the field of healthcare. BDA's healthcare insights may benefit from new peripheral technologies. Future researchers should look at the potential benefits of cutting-edge technology in healthcare, such as augmented reality, quantum computing, and machine learning. Another interesting research topic is how upcoming technologies such as digital twins, 5G connectivity, and the physical internet can be leveraged to improve healthcare delivery.

### 7.9.4 Investigating the Success of Big Data Analytics

Big data analytics aids hospital administrators to increase their efficacy in healthcare. This is further enhanced by providing patients with personalized services and individualized treatment. The role of big data in improving hospital service quality should be studied empirically in future research. Scholars are also expected to look at new ways of offering help to individuals, particularly seniors and chronic disease sufferers.

## 7.10 Conclusion

Big data analytics has shown tremendous potential to transform healthcare. The use of current tools and technologies has further provided a framework that could indeed enhance patient care. Furthermore, from the information gathered from clinical and medical data repositories, previously undiscovered patterns have been found that should shape the future of the field. Naturally, we can expect a widespread implementation of these techniques in the healthcare industry. It is also expected that the literature will focus on the several challenges that the field of healthcare is facing. This article presented a study on using big data analytics, particularly in the healthcare area. Several models, techniques and challenges were discussed that could help pave the way for future work in this arena. We must point out that, although the field is still in its infancy, it is expected that the growth of healthcare will continue, and healthcare will be greatly improved for patients in the future.

## References

[1] Raghupathi, W., and Raghupathi, V. Big data analytics in healthcare: promise and potential, *Health Information Science and Systems*, vol. 2, no. 1, pp. 1–10, 2014.

[2] Manogaran, G., Lopez, D., Thota, C., Abbas, K.M., Pyne, S., and Sundarasekar, R., Big data analytics in healthcare Internet of Things, in Qudrat-Ullah, H. and Tsasis, P. (Eds.), *Innovative Healthcare Systems for the 21st Century* (pp. 263–284). Springer, Cham, 2017.

[3] Zanella, A., Bui, N., Castellani, A., Vangelista, L., and Zorzi, M., Internet of things for smart cities, *IEEE Internet of Things Journal*, vol. 1, no. 1, pp. 22–32, 2014.

[4] Bauer, H., Patel, M., and Veira, J., *The Internet of Things: Sizing Up the Opportunity*. McKinsey & Company, New York, 2016. Cited at 2016 Jul 1. Available from: http://www.mckinsey.com/industries/high-tech/our-insights/the-internet-of-things-sizing-up-the-opportunity.

[5] Scheen, A.J., Precision medicine: the future in diabetes care? *Diabetes Research and Clinical Practice*, vol. 117, pp. 12–21, 2016.

[6] van Leeuwen, N., Swen, J.J., Guchelaar, H.J., and Hart, L.M., The role of pharmacogenetics in drug disposition and response of oral glucose-lowering drugs, *Clinical Pharmacokinetics*, vol. 52, no. 10, pp. 833–854, 2013.

[7] Keeling, M.J., Hollingsworth, T.D., and Read, J.M., Efficacy of contact tracing for the containment of the 2019 novel coronavirus (COVID-19), *Journal of Epidemiology and Community Health*, vol. 74, pp. 861–866, 2020.

[8] Pham, Q.-V., Nguyen, D.C., Huynh-The, T., Hwang, W.-J., and Pathirana, P.N., Artificial intelligence (AI) and big data for coronavirus (COVID-19) pandemic: a survey on the state-of-the-arts, *IEEE Access*, vol. 8, p. 130820, 2020.

[9] Devakunchari, R., Analysis on big data over the years, *International Journal of Scientific and Research Publications*, vol. 4, pp. 383–389, 2014.

[10] Herland, M., Khoshgoftaar, T.M., and Wald, R., A review of data mining using big data in health informatics, *Journal of Big Data*, vol. 1, no. 1, pp. 2, 2014.

[11] Garcia, S., Luengo, J., and Herrera, F., *Data Preprocessing in Data Mining*. Springer, Basel, Switzerland, 2015.

[12] Mehmood, R., and Graham, G., Big data logistics: a healthcare transport capacity sharing model, *Procedia Computer Science*, vol. 64, pp. 1107–1114, 2015.

[13] Mehmood, R., and Graham, G., Big data logistics: a healthcare transport capacity sharing model, *Procedia Computer Science*, vol. 64, pp. 1107–1114, 2015.

[14] Tsai, C.-W., Lai, C.-F., Chao, H.-C., and Vasilakos, A.V., Big data analytics: a survey, *Journal Big Data*, vol. 2, p. 21, 2015.

[15] Longbottom, C., and Bamforth, R., Optimising the Data Warehouse, in *Dealing with Large Volumes of Mixed Data to Give Better Business Insights*. Quocirca, Maidenhead, UK, 2013. Available online: https://docplayer.net/11650848-Optimising-the-data-warehouse.html (accessed on 23 February 2020).

[16] Ren, Y., Monitoring patients via a secure and mobile healthcare system, in *IEEE Symposium on WIRELESS Communication*, 2011.

[17] Zikopoulos, P., Deroos, D., Parasuraman, K., Deutsch, T., Giles, J., and Corrigan, D., *Harness the Power of Big Data the IBM Big Data Platform*. McGraw Hill Professional, New York, 2012.

[18] Zikopoulos, P., and Eaton, C., *Understanding Big Data: Analytics for Enterprise Class Hadoop and Streaming Data*. McGraw-Hill Osborne Media, New York, 2011.

[19] Oussous, A., Benjelloun, F.-Z., Ait Lahcen, A., and Belfkih, S., Big data technologies: a survey, *Journal of King Saud University—Computer and Information Sciences*, vol. 30, no. 4, pp. 431–448, 2018.

[20] Rajaraman, V., Big data analytics, *Resonance*, vol. 21, no. 8, pp. 695–716, 2016.

[21] Oussous, A., Benjelloun, F.-Z., Ait Lahcen, A., and Belfkih, S., Big data technologies: a survey, *Journal of King Saud University—Computer and Information Sciences*, vol. 30, no. 4, pp. 431–448, 2018.

[22] Rajaraman, V., Big data analytics, *Resonance*, vol. 21, no. 8, pp. 695–716, 2016.

[23] https://www.datasciencecentral.com/profiles/blogs/thehadoop-ecosystem-hdfs-yarn-hivepig-hbase-and-growing.

[24] Khan, N., Yaqoob, I., Hashem, I.A.T. et al., Big data: survey, technologies, opportunities, and challenges, *The Scientific World Journal*, vol. 2014, p. 18, 2014.

[25] Bhadani, A.K., and Jothimani, D., Big data: challenges, opportunities, and realities, in *Effective Big Data Management and Opportunities for Implementation* (pp. 1–24). IGI Global, Pennsylvania, PA, 2016.

[26] van Leeuwen, N., Swen, J.J., Guchelaar, H.J., and Hart, L.M., The role of pharmacogenetics in drug disposition and response of oral glucose-lowering drugs, *Clinical Pharmacokinetics*, vol. 52, no. 10, pp. 833–854, 2013.

[27] Flores, M., Glusman, G., Brogaard, K., Price, N.D., and Hood L., P4 medicine: how systems medicine will transform the healthcare sector and society, *Personalized Medicine*, vol. 10, no. 6, 565–576, 2013.

[28] MyTomorrows, Amsterdam: MyTomorrows, 2016. Cited at 2016 Jul 1. Available from: https://mytomorrows.com.

[29] Fritchman, K., et al., Privacy-preserving scoring of tree ensembles: a novel framework for AI in healthcare, in *2018 IEEE International Conference on Big Data (Big Data)*. IEEE, 2018.

[30] LeCun, Y., Bengio, Y., and Hinton, G., Deep learning, *Nature*, vol. 521, pp. 436–444, 2015.

[31] Hu, D., Zhou, X.,Yu, X., and Hou, Z., Study on deep learning and its application in visual tracking, in *Proceedings of the 2015 10th International Conference on Broadband and Wireless Computing*. Communication and Applications, Krakow, Poland, pp. 240–246.

[32] Ma, J., Sheridan, R.P., Liaw, A., Dahl, G.E., and Svetnik, V., Deep neural nets as a method for quantitative structure–Activity relationships, *Journal of Chemical Information and Modeling*, vol. 55, pp. 263–274, 2015.

[33] Leung, M.K., Xiong, H.Y., Lee, L.J., and Frey, B.J., Deep learning of the tissue-regulated splicing code, *Bioinformatics*, vol. 30, pp. i121–i129, 2014.

[34] Kumar, A., Gupta, P.K., and Srivastava, A., A review of modern technologies for tackling COVID-19 pandemic, *Diabetes and Metabolic Syndrome: Clinical Research and Reviews*, vol. 14, pp. 569–573, 2020.

[35] Ma, F., Chitta, R., Zhou, J., You, Q., Sun, T., and Geo, J., Dipole: diagnosis prediction in healthcare via attention-based bidirectional recurrent neural networks, in *Proceedings of the 23rd ACM SIGKDD International Conference on Knowledge Discovery and Data Mining*, Halifax, NS, Canada (pp. 1903–1911). ACM, Halifax, NS, 13–17 August 2017.

[36] Lipton, Z.C., Kale, D.C., Elkan, C., and Wetzel, R., Learning to diagnose with LSTM recurrent neural networks, arXiv, arXiv:1511.03677, 2015.

[37] Pham, T., Tran, T., Phung, D., and Venkatesh, S., Deepcare: a deep dynamic memory model for predictive medicine, in *Proceedings of the Pacific-Asia Conference on Knowledge Discovery and Data Mining*, Auckland, New Zealand (pp. 30–41). Springer, Cham, 19–22 April 2016.

[38] Sayalee, P., *Deep Learning-Based Computational Drug Discovery to Inhibit the RNA Dependent RNA Polymerase: Application to SARS-CoV and COVID-19*. Adlai E. Stevenson High School, Lincolnshire, IL, 2020.

[39] Krizhevsky, A., Sutskever, I., and Hinton, G.E., Imagenet classification with deep convolutional neural networks, *Advances in Neural Information Processing Systems*, vol. 25, pp. 1097–1105, 2012.

[40] Liu, W., Anguelov, D., Erhan, D., Szegedy, C., Reed, S., Cheng-Yang, F., and Berg, A.C., Ssd: single shot multibox detector, in *European Conference on Computer Vision* (pp. 21–37). Springer, 2016.

[41] Redmon, J., Divvala, S., Girshick, R., and Farhadi, A., You only look once: united, real time object detection, in *Proceedings of the IEEE Conference on Computer Vision and Pattern Recognition* (pp. 779–788), 2016.

[42] Badrinarayanan, V., Kendall, A., and Cipolla, R., Segnet: a deep convolutional encoder-decoder architecture for image segmentation, *IEEE Transactions on Pattern Analysis and Machine Intelligence*, vol. 39, no. 12, pp. 2481–2495, 2017.

[43] Ronneberger, O., Fischer, P., and Brox, T., U-net: convolutional networks for biomedical image segmentation, in *International Conference on Medical Image Computing and Computer-Assisted Intervention* (pp. 234–241). Springer, 2015.

[44] Goodfellow, I., Pouget-Abadie, J., Mirza, M., Xu, B., Warde-Farley, D., Ozair, S., Courville, A., and Bengio, Y., Generative adversarial nets, in *Advances in Neural Information Processing Systems* (pp. 2672–2680). 2014.

[45] Choudhary, T., Mishra, V., Goswami, A., and Sarangapani, J., A transfer learning with structured filter pruning approach for improved breast cancer classification on point-of-care devices, *Computers in Biology and Medicine*, vol. 134. p. 104432, 2021.

[46] Qummar, S., Khan, F.G., Shah, S., Khan, A., Shamshirband, S., Ur Rehman, Z., Ahmed Khan, I., and Jadoon, W., A deep learning ensemble approach for diabetic retinopathy detection, *IEEE Access*, vol. 7, pp. 150530–150539, 2019.
[47] Sumithra, R., Suhil, M., and Guru, D.S., Segmentation and classification of skin lesions for disease diagnosis, *Procedia Computer Science*, vol. 45, pp. 76–85, 2015.
[48] Hochreiter, S., and Schmidhuber, J., Long short-term memory, *Neural Computation*, vol. 9, no. 8, pp. 1735–1780, 1997.
[49] Chung, J., Gulcehre, C., Cho, K.H., and Bengio, Y., Empirical evaluation of gated recurrent neural networks on sequence modeling, arXiv preprint arXiv:1412.3555, 2014.
[50] Elman, J.L. Finding structure in time. *Cognitive Science*, vol. 14, no. 2, pp. 179–211, 1990. DOI:10.1207/s15516709cog1402_1
[51] Abdel-Basset, M., Mohamed, R., Elhoseny, M., Chakrabortty, R.K., and Ryan, M., A hybrid COVID-19 detection model using an improved marine predators algorithm and a ranking-based diversity reduction strategy, *IEEE Access*, 8, 79521–79540, 2020.
[52] Chen, J., Cai, H., and Wang, W., A new metaheuristic algorithm: car tracking optimization algorithm, *Soft Computing*, vol. 22, pp. 3857–3878, 2017.
[53] Zikopoulos, P., and Eaton, C., *Understanding Big Data: Analytics for Enterprise Class Hadoop and Streaming Data*. McGraw-Hill Osborne Media, New York, 2011.
[54] Wang, Y., Kung, L., and Byrd, T.A., Big data analytics: understanding its capabilities and potential benefits for healthcare organizations, *Technological Forecasting and Social Change*, vol. 126, pp. 3–13, 2018.
[55] Mehta, N. and Pandit, A., Concurrence of big data analytics and healthcare: a systematic review, *International Journal of Medical Informatics*, vol. 114, pp. 57–65, 2018.
[56] Bahri, S., Zoghlami, N., Abed, M., and Tavares, J.M.R.S., Big data for healthcare: a survey, *IEEE Access*, vol. 7, pp. 7397–7408, 2019.
[57] Sukumar, S.R., Natarajan, R., and Ferrell, R.K., Quality of big data in health care, *International Journal of Health Care Quality Assurance*, vol. 28, no. 6, pp. 621–634, 2015.
[58] Cleland, B., Wallace, J., Bond, R. et al., Insights into antidepressant prescribing using open health data, *Big Data Research*, vol. 12, pp. 41–48, 2018.
[59] Oussous, A., Benjelloun, F.-Z., Ait Lahcen, A., and Belfkih, S., Big data technologies: a survey, *Journal of King Saud University—Computer and Information Sciences*, vol. 30, no. 4, pp. 431–448, 2018.
[60] Phillips-Wren, G., Iyer, L.S., Kulkarni, U., and Ariyachandra, T., Business analytics in the context of big data: a roadmap for research, *Communications of the Association for Information Systems*, vol. 37, no. 1, p. 23, 2015.
[61] Watson, H.J., Tutorial: big data analytics: concepts, technologies, and applications, *Communications of the Association for Information Systems*, vol. 34, no. 1, p. 65, 2014.
[62] Bates, D.W., Saria, S., Ohno-Machado, L., Shah, A., and Escobar, G., Big data in health care: using analytics to identify and manage high-risk and high-cost patients, *Health Affairs*, vol. 33, no. 7, pp. 1123–1131, 2014.
[63] Nambu, M., Nakajima, K., Noshiro, M., and Tamura, T., An algorithm for the automatic detection of health conditions, *IEEE Engineering in Medicine and Biology Magazine*, vol. 24, no. 4, pp. 38–42, 2005.
[64] Mehta, N., and Pandit, A., Concurrence of big data analytics and healthcare: a systematic review, *International Journal of Medical Informatics*, vol. 114, pp. 57–65, 2018.

[65] Platt, R., Carnahan, R., Brown, J.S. et al., The U.S. Food and Drug Administration's mini-sentinel program, *Pharmacoepidemiology and Drug Safety*, vol. 21, pp. 1–303, 2012.
[66] Kos, A., and Umek, A., Wearable sensor devices for prevention and rehabilitation in healthcare: swimming exercise with real-time therapist feedback, *IEEE Internet of Things Journal*, vol. 6, no. 2, pp. 1331–1341, 2018.
[67] Sahoo, A.K., Mallik, S., Pradhan, C., Mishra, B.S.P., Barik, R.K., and Das, H., Intelligence-based health recommendation system using big data analytics, in *Big Data Analytics for Intelligent Healthcare Management* (pp. 227–246). Academic Press, Cambridge, MA, 2019.
[68] Hoens, T.R., Blanton, M., Steele, A., and Chawla, N.V., Reliable medical recommendation systems with patient privacy, *ACM Transactions on Intelligent Systems and Technology*, vol. 4, no. 4, pp. 1–31, 2013.
[69] Hamburg, M.A., and Collins, F.S., The path to personalized medicine, *New England Journal of Medicine*, vol. 363, no. 4, pp. 301–304, 2010.
[70] Wang, G., Jung, K., Winnenburg, R., and Shah, N.H., A method for systematic discovery of adverse drug events from clinical notes, *Journal of the American Medical Informatics Association*, vol. 22, no. 6, pp. 1196–1204, 2015.
[71] Luo, J., Wu, M., Gopukumar, D., and Zhao, Y., Big data application in biomedical research and health care: a literature review, *Biomedical Informatics Insights*, vol. 8, 2016.
[72] Saheb, T., and Izadi, L., Paradigm of IoT big data analytics in healthcare industry: a review of scientific literature and mapping of research trends, *Telematics and Informatics*, vol. 41, pp. 70–85, 2019.
[73] Syed, L., Jabeen, S., and Manimala, S., Telemammography: A novel approach for early detection of breast cancer through wavelets based image processing and machine learning techniques, in *Advances in Soft Computing and Machine Learning in Image Processing* (pp. 149–183). Springer, Cham, Switzerland, 2018.
[74] Doi, K., Computer-aided diagnosis in medical imaging: historical review, current status and future potential, *Computerized Medical Imaging and Graphics*, vol. 31, no. 4–5, pp. 198–211, 2007.
[75] Manogaran, G., Thota, C., Lopez, D., Vijayakumar, V., Abbas, K.M., and Sundarsekar, R., Big data knowledge system in healthcare, in *Internet of Things and Big Data Technologies for Next Generation Healthcare* (pp. 133–157). Springer, Cham, Switzerland, 2017.
[76] Das, N., Das, L., Rautaray, S.S., and Pandey, M., Big Data Analytics for Medical Applications, *International Journal of Modern Education and Computer Science*, vol. 2, pp. 35–42, 2018.
[77] Pramanik, M.I., Lau, R.Y.K., Demirkan, H., and AbulKalam Azad, M., Smart health: big data enabled health paradigm within smart cities, *Journal of Expert Systems with Applications*, vol. 87, pp. 370–383, 2017.
[78] Assuncao, M.D., Calheiros, R.N., Bianchi, S., Netto, M.A.S., and Buyya, R., Big data computing and clouds: trends and future directions, *Journal of Parallel and Distributed Computing*, pp. 3–15, 2015.
[79] Mehta, N., and Pandit, A., Concurrence of big data analytics and healthcare: a systematic review, *International Journal of Medical Informatics*, vol. 114, pp. 57–65, 2018.

*Chapter 8*

# Reliable Biomedical Applications Using AI Models

Shambhavi Mishra, Tanveer Ahmed and Vipul Mishra

*Bennett University, Greater Noida, India*

## Contents

8.1 Introduction ....................................................................................... 148
8.2 Artificial Intelligence ............................................................................. 149
  8.2.1 The Benefits of Artificial Intelligence in the Biomedical Field ....................................................................................... 150
  8.2.2 Machine Learning ........................................................................ 150
    8.2.2.1 Supervised Learning .......................................................... 150
    8.2.2.2 Unsupervised Learning ...................................................... 151
    8.2.2.3 Semi-Supervised Learning .................................................. 151
    8.2.2.4 Reinforcement Learning ...................................................... 152
  8.2.3 Popular Machine Learning Techniques ............................................ 152
    8.2.3.1 K-Nearest Neighbor (KNN) ................................................. 152
    8.2.3.2 Naïve Bayes ......................................................................... 153
    8.2.3.3 Support Vector Machines .................................................... 153
    8.2.3.4 Decision Tree Ensembles .................................................... 153
    8.2.3.5 Logistic Regression ............................................................. 153

DOI: 10.1201/9781003322597-8

8.2.4 Deep Learning ....................154
8.2.4.1 Convolutional Neural Networks ....................154
8.2.4.2 Recurrent Neural Networks ....................154
8.3 Applications ....................155
8.3.1 Omics ....................156
8.3.1.1 AI for Genomics ....................157
8.3.1.2 AI For Protein Analysis ....................159
8.3.2 AI in Drug Discovery ....................160
8.3.3 AI for Bio and Medical Imaging ....................160
8.3.4 AI in Radiology ....................161
8.3.5 AI for surgery optimization ....................161
8.3.6 Brain and Body Interface ....................162
8.4 Discussion and Challenges ....................163
8.5 Future Directions in Healthcare Using AI ....................164
8.5.1 Integrative Analysis ....................165
8.5.2 Federated Learning ....................165
8.5.3 Model Transparency ....................165
8.5.4 Model Security ....................166
8.5.5 Data Bias ....................166
8.6 Conclusion ....................166
References ....................167

## 8.1 Introduction

Biomedicine is a diverse field that has applications in various domains. Technological advances in the medical and biological arenas have resulted in a massive amount of physiological and biological data, including protein sequences, genomics, electroencephalography, and medical images. The availability of increasingly large amounts of data has created a lot of opportunities for automated computer-aided diagnosis. However, as expected, it has also created a lot of challenging issues. A vast volume of unstructured data is available in an unorganized format. Storing, analyzing, and understanding this deluge of biological data requires effective and efficient computing methods [1], [2]. The examination and interpretation of the biomedical data also require skilled technicians and well-equipped laboratories. Further, manual examination of the data is time-consuming, tedious, and error prone. It has also been found that manual diagnosis and examination suffer from inter- and intra-observation variability among practitioners [3], [4]. Diagnostic, surgical, rehabilitative, clinical and predictive practices, decision making, and disease diagnosis are some of the key areas where automated technologies can help with early identification and treatment.

In this regard, recently automated biomedical methods have become popular and shown superior performance. Specifically, artificial intelligence (AI)-based methods have attracted much attention from researchers in every domain [5]. The AI community has seen a tremendous improvement in the performance of various machine and deep learning models on numerous tasks such as classification [6], detection [7], segmentation [8], and generation [9]. AI-based methods have also attracted significant attention from the healthcare domain and have shown significant improvement on several tasks [10], [11]. Two of the important sub-fields of AI that are gaining in popularity are machine learning and deep learning. Traditional methods of machine learning require hand-crafted features and have shown superior performance on several tasks.

The data available in the biomedical field suffers from imbalance, creating a major bottleneck while training the AI methods [12]. Specifically, more samples can be found for the negative (a person has cancer) class and comparatively fewer for the positive (a person does not have cancer). Therefore, in recent years, deep learning-based algorithms based on artificial neural networks have been offering a significant improvement over traditional machine learning methods [13]. Deep learning methods can extract and reuse complicated patterns from data automatically. Deep learning models trained on existing datasets, a paradigm known as transfer learning, can offer another alternative for improving performance compared to existing machine learning algorithms. In this article, we try to cover the broad range of AI that uses automated machine-driven algorithms in healthcare. We also seek to explore the importance of AI-based methods from the perspective of biomedical applications. In particular, the paper provides an idea of the two of the important AI fields in biomedicine: machine learning and deep learning.

The paper is structured as follows. Section 8.2 provides an overall idea of artificial intelligence and its popular methods, machine learning and deep learning. In Section 8.3, we summarize biomedical applications and the various state-of-the-art methods that have been proposed for different kinds of biomedical applications. Section 8.4 discusses the challenges encountered in this field. Section 8.5 summarizes the future direction of biomedical applications and Section 8.6 provides a conclusion.

## 8.2 Artificial Intelligence

It has been hypothesized that artificial intelligence is expected to revolutionize practically every aspect of medicine in the near future. AI can assist physicians in making more informed clinical decisions and improving patient outcomes. This section summarizes the benefits that AI can bring in various biomedical tasks and provides an overview of the AI methods that have been widely applied in biomedical and healthcare systems. We focus in particular on machine and deep learning techniques.

### 8.2.1 The Benefits of Artificial Intelligence in the Biomedical Field

- Checking for abnormalities and recommending medical action.
- Predicting the onset of new diseases.
- Accurate and efficient diagnosis.
- A good outcome for the patient.
- Improving the experience of doctors and surgeons.
- Improving the quality of medical care.
- Pathological outcome improvement.
- Maintaining clinical records.
- Providing the patient with outstanding service.
- Assisting doctors and patients by providing comfort.
- Improving training for medical students.
- Enhancing hospital security.
- Helpful in the treatment of complex and novel conditions.
- Balancing patients' blood glucose levels.
- Patient monitoring.

### 8.2.2 Machine Learning

Machine learning is an important field of AI which is becoming increasingly popular. A large amount of data is available in every domain and the biomedical field is no exception. In the context of the paradigm of machine learning, the computer itself can learn from the vast amount of data available to the user. Machine learning can be supervised (using labeled data) and unsupervised (unlabeled). In the former, each input sample has an associated ground truth target label, while in the latter, the model learns useful patterns from the data itself without the ground truth data. Popular machine learning methods include linear regression, logistic regression, support vector regression (SVR), decision trees, and deep learning methods (discussed in Sections 8.2.3 and Section 8.2.4). These methods can further be classified into two categories, depending on the outcome of the task: classification or regression problems. In classification problems, the aim is to predict a discrete label for new data, for example, with a chest X-ray image as input, the task is to classify whether the patient is COVID-19 positive or not. Regression problems, on the other hand, try to predict a continuous value. For example, given heartbeat, cholesterol, and blood pressure as inputs, a regression model can predict the chance of having a cardiac arrest. Figure 8.1 illustrates different types of machine learning.

#### 8.2.2.1 Supervised Learning

A supervised learning problem can be a classification or a regression problem. In a supervised problem, the labeled value is a discrete value. For raw data classification,

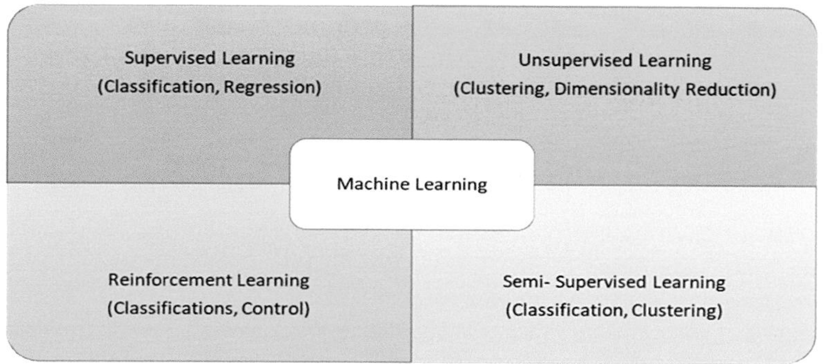


**Figure 8.1 Different Types of Machine Learning.**

the data must first be selected, then preprocessing must be conducted to remove any missing information. The data is then normalized using Z-score or min-max normalization, following which the best features are selected using an automated extraction procedure. After the best features have been chosen, raw data is classified using supervised approaches [14]. Supervised regression learning [15] uses models to predict outcomes with the help of continuous (numeric) data. Supervised learning entails training the model on labeled data before applying it to new data to make predictions. Basically, there are two different sets: a training set and a testing set. Training is usually done on the training set. The performance of the trained model is then evaluated on the testing set. Evaluation metrics [15] can be used to assess model performance. Different types of evaluation metrics are used for both problems. In classification F1 score, precision recall and accuracy of the model are evaluated and for regression problem models, performance is evaluated with the help of mean square error (MSE), root mean square error (RMSE), and mean absolute error (MAE), among others.

#### 8.2.2.2 Unsupervised Learning

The performance of the model cannot be assessed in unsupervised learning since the label value is missing or unknown. The labels receive no training at all. Clustering, including hierarchical clustering, association rule mining of the algorithm, are among the techniques utilized for unsupervised learning [15]. A cluster is produced based on the presence of training data with unknown labels. With the use of data samples, these algorithms are employed to create a developing framework.

#### 8.2.2.3 Semi-Supervised Learning

This is a technique for determining the best classifier from a set of unlabeled and labeled data. Labeled data can lose a little more information than unlabeled data. Semi-supervised learning uses both unlabeled and labeled data, and combines supervised and unsupervised learning. It performs classification very effectively using unlabeled data. The effectiveness of this strategy is entirely dependent on a number of assumptions.

#### 8.2.2.4 Reinforcement Learning

Reinforcement learning is accomplished by creating a system that improves its performance by incorporating feedback from the environment and taking appropriate actions to improve it. The software receives feedback in the form of incentives and punishments, learning from the environment by interacting with it without the assistance of humans. It is a step-by-step procedure.

### 8.2.3 Popular Machine Learning Techniques

#### 8.2.3.1 K-Nearest Neighbor (KNN)

The distance measure used to locate the K-nearest neighbor query points has a significant impact on the KNN classifier's performance [16]. In practice, the usual Euclidean distance is frequently utilized. [17] makes use of a large amount of data to make diagnoses depend on historical data. It focuses on employing a unique algorithm to calculate the chance of a specific condition occurring. The accuracy of such diagnoses is improved by applying the KNN algorithm. The KNN method can be used to improve automated diagnostics, such as those that detect several diseases with identical symptoms. KNN is used for the causes of common chronic diseases, for example diabetes, cancer and heart disease in the biomedical domain. Figure 8.2 describes different algorithms used in the healthcare sector.

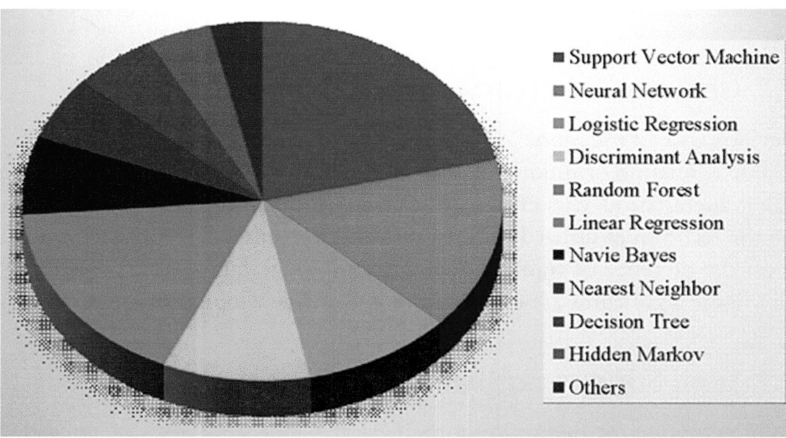


**Figure 8.2 Different Algorithms Used in Healthcare Sector.**

#### 8.2.3.2 Naïve Bayes

One of the most frequently used data machine learning is naïve Bayes [18]. Its efficiency comes from the assumption of attribute independence, which in many real-world data sets may be violated. The naïve Bayes technique is employed in a variety of applications. The primary goal is to create a cost-effective and easily accessible healthcare system that will benefit medical professionals [19].

#### 8.2.3.3 Support Vector Machines

Support vector machines (SVM) are one of the most commonly used machine learning tools in classification and regression [20]. Linear and nonlinear SVM classifiers are the two main models used to develop SVM classifiers. The first assumes that there is an optimum hyperplane that divides objects into two classes. The second method employs the kernel trick to identify the best way to separate non-linear linear hyperplanes in higher dimensions. SVM is also applied heavily in the biomedical field with such various purposes as protein classification [21], analysis of gene expression profiles [22], detection of splice sites [23], and breast cancer detection [10].

#### 8.2.3.4 Decision Tree Ensembles

One of the simple and straightforward machine learning algorithms is decision trees [24]. Tree-based classifiers are faster in training and classification than neural networks and require fewer tuning parameters. They are simple to parallelize and robust to noise. Common decision tree ensemble techniques are AdaBoost, Multi-Boost, and random forest. The target class of a decision tree is determined by a series of queries, i.e., comparisons to a threshold, on input features that begin at the root node and end in a leaf node. Clinical decision analysis (CDA) has been used to solve medical problems that are complex and unclear. The development and growth of clinical treatment standards, the approval of new pharmaceuticals, drug prescriptions, the applicability of medical insurance for treatments, and healthcare policy are all examples of CDA [25].

#### 8.2.3.5 Logistic Regression

In academia and industrial research, logistic regression is used extensively across multiple problems [26]. The main objective of this model is to quantify and identify the relationship between multiple independent variables. In the biomedical field, breast cancer, heart disease and tumor detection are among the areas where logistic regression is applied [27].

### 8.2.4 Deep Learning

Machine learning algorithms are known to suffer from the curse of dimensionality. Another important limitation is that these methods require hand-crafted features for learning. Today's deep learning methods are useful to overcome this. The field is primarily focused on methods and algorithms designed for artificial neural networks (ANN) [28]. The basic idea of ANN is inspired by the biological neural network, i.e., the brain. Deep learning has gained a great deal of popularity in recent years. These methods automatically learn the discriminating feature, eliminating the need for hand-crafted features [29].

Feed-forward neural networks are also known as completely connected networks. Early architectures were based on feed-forward models that generally consisted of an input layer, an output layer, and a few hidden layers. Nowadays, the number of layers in deep learning architectures has expanded; deep architectures (networks with more hidden layers) are now referred to as deep neural networks (DNNs). Further, there are various variants of the DNN models, such as convolutional neural networks (CNN) designed primarily for images and video data. In recent years, CNNs have gained more popularity due to their ability to learn complex patterns from the data and parameter sharing. CNNs with more than 150 layers have been successfully trained and achieved superior performance on the benchmark datasets [30]. Recurrent neural networks (RNN) designed to deal with time-varying sequence data, and generative models for generating new data are some of the other variants of deep learning models.

#### 8.2.4.1 Convolutional Neural Networks

The evolution of deep network architectures gave birth to CNNs. CNNs are a special kind of neural network and have shown improved performance over feed-forward neural networks. Since the superior performance on the ImageNet dataset achieved in 2012 by AlexNet [6] CNN, many different deep architectures have been proposed. The earlier CNNs such as AlexNet and VGG16 were sequential networks wherein the output of one layer was fed into the next layer. Other models use CNNs as a base model or feature extractions such as object detection models: SSD [7], YOLO [31], segmentation models; SegNet [8] and Unet [32], generative models; GAN [9]. CNN are also used heavily in the biomedical field for different purposes such as disease classification [11], detection [33], and segmentation [34].

#### 8.2.4.2 Recurrent Neural Networks

Another popular deep learning variant is the recurrent neural network (RNN), which deals with sequence data and is primarily used in applications such as financial time-series, speech recognition, music generation, natural language processing

(NLP), and language translation. Traditional RNNs have the limitation that they cannot preserve long-term dependency when used in NLP applications, and they suffer from the gradient vanishing problem. To address the limitations of traditional RNNs, nowadays, more advanced sequence models i.e., long short-term memory (LSTM) [35] and gated recurrent units (GRU) [36] have evolved and are used more frequently than traditional RNNs. Sequence models are the backbone networks behind the success of Google Translate, Siri, and Alexa. Sequence models have been used in the biomedical field for DNA and gene analysis [37], [38].

## 8.3 Applications

Biomedical informatics combine biology, medicine, and computer science to aid in the effective organization, analysis, management, and use of data in healthcare. Medical informatics has enormous opportunities and challenges as a result of the massive amount of biomedical data. Artificial intelligence is widely used in biomedical informatics, as well as dealing with massive amounts of data, such as protein structure, biological sequencing, drug discovery, and medical imaging. Different components of AI applications in the biomedical domain are shown in Figure 8.3. Recent development ideas in biomedical applications using AI are listed in Table 8.1.

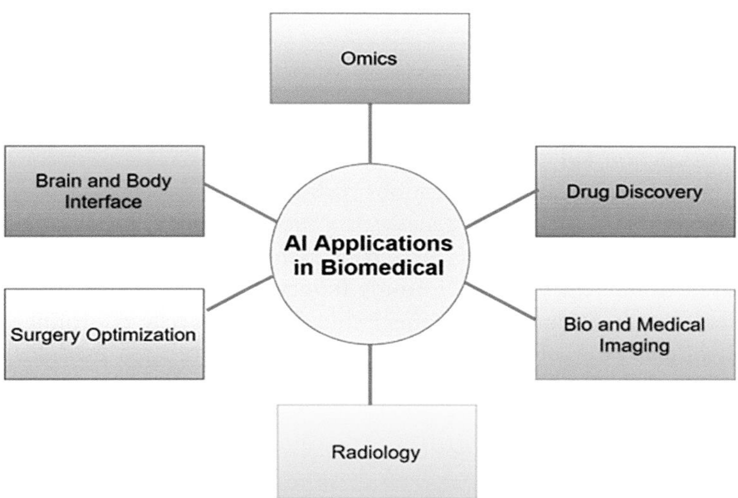


**Figure 8.3 Reliable AI applications in biomedicine, including omics, drug discovery, bio and medical imaging, radiology, surgery optimization, and brain and body interface.**

**Table 8.1 Recent Developments in Biomedical Applications Using AI**

| *Applications* | *Representative recent work* |
|---|---|
| Omics | Zeng et al. [39], Holzinger et al. [40], Biswas et al. [41], D'Adamo et al. [42], Li et al. [43]. |
| AI for genomics | Williams et al. [44], Xu et al. [45], Salto-Tellez et al. [46], D'Adamo et al. [47], Kumar et al. [48]. |
| Around the protein structure | Zimmeret et al. [49], Yu et al. [50], Raza et al. [51], Park et al. [52], Haimed et al. [53]. |
| AI in drug discovery | Fleming et al. [54], Batool et al. [55], David et al. [56], Arora et al. [57], Bender et al. [58]. |
| AI for bio and medical imaging | Chakraborty et al. [59], Nakata et al. [60], Suri et al. [61], Shi et al. [62], Born et al. [63]. |
| AI for surgery optimization | Hashimoto et al. [64], Haleem et al. [65], Bashir et al. [66], Buchlak et al. [67], Gumbs et al. [68]. |
| Brain and body interface | Silva et al. [69], Wang et al. [70], Papakostas et al. [71], Cao et al. [72], Olsen et al. [73]. |

### *8.3.1 Omics*

Studies based on genomics sequencing and gene expression directed towards protein structure prediction fall under the biomedical sector. Several studies show omics work on genomics, but other applications such as biomedicine and bioinformatics can also be found. Omics covers genetic data such as protein, metabol, gen, transcript, and epigen. It also concerns protein–protein interactions (PPIs). The authors of [39] studied different statistical learning framework methods that are integrated with different multidisciplinary areas including biology, machine learning, and AI. In the literature, PCA, clustering methods, regularization-based methods, regression methods, and knowledge enhancement learning have all been investigated and analyzed. The limitations and strengths of multiple standard ML methods are also discussed. According to [40]'s research, image data alone is insufficient for analyzing complicated disorders and obtaining an appropriate diagnosis. In parallel with large, high-quality data sets, domain knowledge and the requirement for multiple networks is also important. While high-dimensional data will always yield better results, all three components are crucial for providing robust ML model training and validation. The authors of one of the studies[41] looked at various AI-based approaches to analyzing different types of cancer.

AI-based analysis for assessing diseases and patient care is also mentioned. The authors of [42] conclude that AI-based methods can quickly generate and analyze information but have some limitations. The term "omics" is now being used in clinical practice. It is suggested [43] that harnessing big data for "precision" or "personalized" treatment has almost endless possibilities. The author focuses on future techniques such as natural language understanding (NLU), artificial intelligence (AI), and transparency. The NLU model permits researchers to collaborate with the "brain" in a simple dialog, as well as examining issues with bioinformatics partners, and the social media element promotes teamwork by making idea sharing, tool sharing, and data sharing easier. Figure 8.4 describes omics information, in terms of genomics and protein structures.

#### 8.3.1.1 AI for Genomics

Human genome data is interpreted using prior knowledge of key genetic variants and inferences about their impact on functional genomic components. AI systems can improve the application of this prior knowledge by guiding phenotype-to-genotype mapping, because many of the AI methods for predicting the presence of a functional element from primary DNA and RNA sequence data are also used to anticipate the impact of genetic variations on those functional elements. Genome research is divided into three different types.

*Protein Binding Prediction*. Interactions between proteins and DNA are essential for a range of cell functions, including transcription, translation, repair, and replication [74]. In numerous fields, such as drug discovery and development, pinpointing the exact position of these binding sites is critical.

*DNA RNA-binding proteins*. Protein binding studies the chemical interaction between DNA and RNAs. These types of binding involve a great deal of complexity in a variety of biological processes including DNA repair, mutations and gene regulation.

*Enhancer and promoter deification*. Enhancers are DNA sequences that are bordered by a specific type of protein called transcription factors. RNA polymerase machinery is defined by promoters at transcription initiation sites. It is identified during the characterization of genes at the molecular level.

The three basic steps in the biological process for gene expression are transcription, RNA processing, and translation.

*Transcription* makes RNA molecules (also known as RNA (premRNA)), which are basically replicas of the DNA reproduced in gene structure.

*In RNA processing*, RNA (pre-mRNA) goes into a new RNA module known as messenger RNA(mRNA).

*In translation*, the mRNA sequence is translated into a protein molecule.

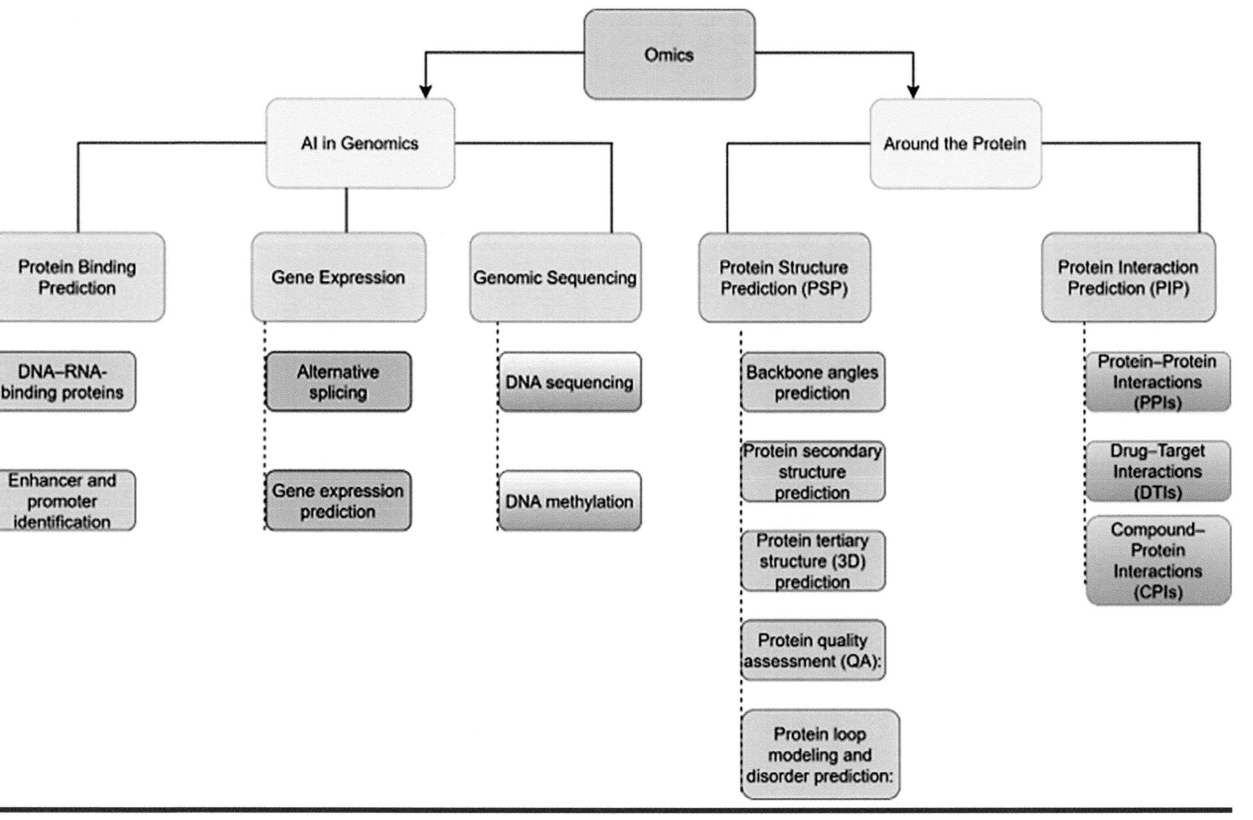


**Figure 8.4 Omics information in terms of genomics and protein structures.**

#### 8.3.1.1.1 Genomic Sequencing

This application is used in various fields of biology such as medical diagnosis, virology, biological research, medical diagnosis and biological systematics. Genomic sequencing is one of the basic processes that determine the exact order of nucleotides in the DNA molecule.

#### 8.3.1.1.2 DNA Sequencing

Fundamental difficulties in omics applications include investigation of the functional activity [75], calculating the functions [76], and finding the functional non-coding variation effects [77] of DNA sequences with the help of genomics data.

#### 8.3.1.1.3 DNA Methylation

This is one of the methods of introducing methyl groups to the DNA molecules. It can change DNA segment activities without changing their sequence structuring.

### *8.3.1.2 AI For Protein Analysis*

In the analysis of proteins, protein structure prediction (PSP) and protein interaction prediction (PIP) are two different research topics. PSSM (protein position specific scoring matrix), secondary structure, and protein disorder are among the challenges that can be encountered.

#### 8.3.1.2.1 Protein Structure Prediction (PSP)

Obtaining the best modeling knowledge of the protein folding process is currently one of the most difficult topics in omics [78]. During the gene expression process, each protein fold goes into a special type of 3-D structure which specifies its biological functionalities. The majority of these studies are focused on predicting protein secondary and tertiary structures.

#### 8.3.1.2.2 Protein Interaction Prediction (PIP)

One of the advantages in the field of drug target identification, network pharmacology, drug discovery, and protein activity elucidation is understanding the interactions between chemical compounds and protein structures. In order to uncover molecular pathways in biological processes, several machine learning methods are now being used to predict protein interactions. PIP is of three types: 1) compound protein interactions (CPIs), 2) drug target interactions (DTIs), and 3) protein–protein interactions (PPIs).

### 8.3.2 AI in Drug Discovery

Artificial intelligence is becoming increasingly effective in drug research. Hundreds of new opportunities and targets have evolved due to proteomic, genomic, and structural studies. Dealing with microscopic images can be difficult because the results of any given experiment can vary greatly from batch to batch. Temperature fluctuations and exposure period variations can all provide false results that are unrelated to the study or the action of a prospective therapeutic molecule. In addition, a large number of factors can be used in the research. In data-driven drug discovery, keeping track of and differentiating the effects is a major challenge. Fortunately, AI can assist in overcoming these obstacles, particularly during the virtual high throughput screening phase, resulting in a more efficient, less expensive, and speedier drug discovery process. In [54], the authors show how AI is rapidly changing the drug discovery field. Structure-based drug design (SBDD) is also becoming popular. The authors of [55] focus on methods and algorithms for SBDD, including de novo and virtual screening drug design. They also emphasize AI methods used for drug discovery and discuss the challenges of handling the large data created by combinatorial chemistry. The authors state that AI and deep learning are important components of statistical machine learning approaches for integrating and analyzing enormous data sets. They also point out that although SBDD has seen a visible improvement in drug discovery, more consistent solutions need to be developed.

Many electronic molecular and macromolecular representations utilized in drug development are based on graph representations. In [56], the authors provide an overview of the popular macromolecular and molecular representations utilized in drug discovery, and describe their application in AI-assisted drug discovery. The authors of the research [57] focus on various drug discoveries for COVID-19 using AI, the three main components of the work being protein synthesis, time management in the laboratory, and molecular changes to accelerate the process of drug discovery.

### 8.3.3 AI for Bio and Medical Imaging

Bio and medical imaging are employed for accurate diagnosis from both image interpretation and image acquisition in the field of AI. Clinicians mainly perform medical image interpretation, which can be subject to considerable differences between interpreters. Tiredness is also a factor. With technological advances, image acquisition has significantly improved in recent years. Medical imaging includes the study and analysis of different (clinical/medical/health) images. Large medical high-resolution image acquisition systems, such as digital positron emission tomography (PET), 2-D/3-D X-ray, and parallel magnetic resonance imaging (MRI), are now available.

AI methods are showing significant performance improvements in bio and biomedical imaging analysis and the interpretation of computer-aided images or digital pathology. The majority of AI research in bio and medical imaging utilizes a number of image modalities at various stages of treatment, for example, tumor delineation and therapy monitoring. A variety of AI-based automated biomedical image analysis techniques are discussed in the literature [49]. In a study [60], deep learning is found to result in significant advances in diagnostic medical imaging. The authors of the research in [61] also agreed that AI has infiltrated medicine, particularly radiology. The research by [62] also shows that AI-assisted image acquisition can help to automate scanning and reconstruction processes. Furthermore, computer-assisted platforms assist radiologists in making clinical judgments. AI can enhance work efficiency by accurately analyzing X-ray and CT images, allowing for subsequent quantification. During the COVID-19 pandemic there was increased demand for medical imaging (CT, X-ray, ultrasound) due to speed, low cost, and precision in patient treatment. Medical imaging has taken a quantum leap because of the digitization of modern medicine and the emergence of AI [63].

### 8.3.4 AI in Radiology

In radiology, skilled clinicians visually examine medical images to detect, monitor, and report disease findings. The reliability of these evaluations depends on experience, and they can be subjective at times. When AI is integrated into the clinical process as a tool to assist clinicians, more accurate and reproducible radiological assessments can be made. Examples in the field of radiology include thoracic imaging, mammography, brain imaging, and radiation oncology. According to researchers, [79], artificial intelligence systems that use continuous learning and retrain themselves are less error prone. Radiology departments are working together to co-develop and test AI algorithms, provide continuous data feeds, and integrate more diversified data sources in order to execute continuous learning AI. Another study looked at how AI monitoring tools could assist radiologists in prioritizing their patient lists by detecting suspicious or positive cases that need to be reviewed immediately. Current constraints in technical competence and even processing capacity will be alleviated with time, and remote access technologies will be able to help [80].

### 8.3.5 AI for surgery optimization

Synergy between domains is also required for AI to improve its applications. A Google Image search can provide relevant images in response to a textual query such as a word or phrase, thanks to a combination of computer vision and natural language processing. Furthermore, machine learning and neural networks, particularly deep learning, are now an integral part of the architecture of many AI systems. AI applications in the surgery include machine learning, deep learning, and natural language processing, to name a few. Each set of data can be assessed separately or in combination with all other types of algorithms to generate new ideas. While fully autonomous robotic surgery is still a long way off, synergy between sectors will undoubtedly improve AI's potential as a surgical therapy supplement. AI has the ability to examine both structured and unstructured data, such as test results, EMR notes, video, and other types of big data, in order to produce clinical decision support [64].

Researchers [65] describe different AI-based technologies such as machine learning, ANN, NLP, SVM, and heuristic analysis for the medical domain. By recording data from all phases of surgery, doctors and surgeons are effectively incorporating AI in surgery. The authors claim that AI has a bright future in terms of providing the best patient care possible and making a clinical choice based on evidence to improve patient care and surgeon workflow; thus it efficiently delivers difficult surgical outcomes. In the surgical domain, the use of AI methods is often criticized as ethically ambiguous, biased, inscrutable, or opaque. However, authors in [67] showed that human decisions are also equally criticized. Further, during stress or fatigue, humans are more susceptible to the influence of heuristics. The use of AI in aortic surgery is explored by [66], the authors of which also show how AI systems will impact surgeons' learning skills and adaptability, and patient outcomes.

### *8.3.6 Brain and Body Interface*

The four components of a brain and body interface (BBIM) are a sensor device, amplifier, filter, and control system. This interface encompasses the signals generated by the brain and muscles, which are recorded using appropriate sensors. The technology decodes and analyzes data from complex brain systems to provide a digital link between the brain and the computer. Techniques utilized in the literature include electroencephalography (EEG), magnetoencephalography (MEG), and functional near-infrared spectroscopy (FNIRS). BBIMs are also employed for automated identification of myocardial infarction using ECG signals and for seizure diagnosis utilizing electroencephalography data with AI techniques [81].

To enable "smart" nano-engineered brain–machine interfaces, machine learning and AI are used. The author of [69] focuses on neurological functions such as neural prosthesis, as well as non-invasive technology allowed by signals like electroencephalography (EEG). Author [70] also focuses on brain research and brain-inspired AI, presenting accomplishments and trends as well as highlighting certain obstacles in brain-inspired computing and computation using spiking neural networks (SNNs). In another research [71], the authors focus on human–computer interaction, addressing two different issues: 1) What are the needs of the user? and 2) What options are available to the user? In this case, the multi-model system gave a satisfactory performance with the help of electroencephalogram (EEG) and electromyogram (EMG) analysis using minimally invasive sensors. Brain–computer interface (BCI) is one of the interdisciplinary research areas where computer methods give the human brain the opportunity to communicate and interact with the environment. [71] also explored BCI-inspired AI applications such as robotic control, computer vision and natural language processing. In one of the researches [73], the authors used a closed-loop BCI simulator to test AI-BCI with nine human subjects performing a typing task, and found a variety of results, including categorically higher information communication rates, improved precision control to "dial in" on targets, and faster ballistic movements between targets.

## 8.4 Discussion and Challenges

Needless to say, intelligent AI-based methods will introduce a lot of advances to the biological field in the near future and play an important role in various tasks. Further, in upcoming years, significant progress will be made in early detection, diagnosis, and recommendation systems. The data collected through small devices offers a lot of opportunity for personalized care. The development of personalized intelligent devices will be another point of innovation. It is expected that precision medicine will also receive significant attention in the near future.

Despite the advances in the biomedical domain and in AI technology, there remain some challenges that need to be addressed. Biomedical data are obstructing the development of AI-based applications and limiting advances in healthcare and medical science. In clinical settings, AI currently has limitations. Even the most efficient unsupervised algorithms cannot make decisions about an unprecedented incident as well or as quickly as a skilled clinician. Even at times like the current COVID-19 pandemic, data-sharing restrictions have hindered researchers working on a wide spectrum of infectious diseases from gaining access to vital data. While recognizing the importance of maintaining confidentiality and privacy, it is critical to find a solution to this problem. Establishing rules, standards, techniques, and definitions to protect the confidentiality and privacy of data while allowing sharing will permit a fast and effective scientific response in the future. In reality, the COVID-19 pandemic emphasized the crucial need for teamwork, sharing resources, and exchanging data and knowledge to achieve significant scientific advances. The major challenges are the following [64]:

- *Data quality and interpretability:* Sometimes, metadata and clinical information are at variance in the real world because of the quality and lack of datasets. Publicly available datasets were (partially) collected using antiquated systems, giving low-quality image data, expert labeling is lacking, or the sample size produced is too small where researchers have used high-quality algorithms. Furthermore, several publicly available datasets are only available for non-commercial (research) use. This is a significant barrier for academics who want to build algorithms that are commercially viable, as for clinical implementation.
- *Lack of balanced datasets:* Most research organizations now have limited access to medical images, and the applicability and accuracy of created solutions are hampered by a reduced number of samples in the data and a lack of geographical diversity. In the world of AI, industries or in research organizations,

large amounts of datasets containing annotations and high-quality images are required to achieve best implementation in the clinical domain with the help of supervised training, validation, and testing. Although modest datasets may suffice for the training of AI algorithms in the academic environment, this is scarcely the case in the clinical setting.

- *Clinical data collection biases:* When we used data from a single or a few institutions in a small geographic area to train AI algorithms, sampling bias was one of the biggest problems. If an AI system is educated in this way and then deployed to a different geographical location, the algorithm's results may be erroneous due to differences between the sample and target populations. Differences in size, age and race, imaging machine use (vendors, kinds, acquisition techniques), and disease prevalence are all sources of bias. There may even be unconscious biases, such as differences in local practice, that researchers are unaware of. In clinical practice, because labels and segmentations are manually produced, there is a significant difference among specialists who analyze images for numerous medical applications.
- *Supervised learning relies on data labeling:* For example, identifying criteria now used in surgery-specific patient registries, which can take longer to collect, and data that is wrongly labeled can lead to unsatisfactory findings.

## 8.5 Future Directions in Healthcare Using AI

We believe that artificial intelligence (AI) will play a significant role in future healthcare products. It is the key capability behind the creation of precision medicine, which is universally acknowledged as a much needed advance in care. Although early attempts at diagnosis and therapy recommendations have been difficult, we believe AI will eventually master this domain as well.

Given the significant advances in AI for imaging analysis, most radiology and pathology images are expected to be reviewed by a computer at some time. Patient communication and clinical note capture, and this trend will continue with the help of speech and text. The most difficult hurdle for AI in many healthcare fields is not whether the technology is capable enough to be useful, but ensuring its acceptance in daily clinical practice. AI systems must be approved by regulators, integrated with electronic heath record (EHR) systems, standardized to the point that similar products perform in a similar way, taught to clinicians, paid for by public or private payer organizations, and updated in the field over time in order for widespread adoption to occur. These obstacles will be overcome in the end, but it will take considerably longer than the technologies themselves to mature.

Human physicians may eventually evolve toward activities and job designs that rely on uniquely human abilities such as empathy, persuasion, and big-picture understanding. It is also becoming evident that AI systems will not, on a large

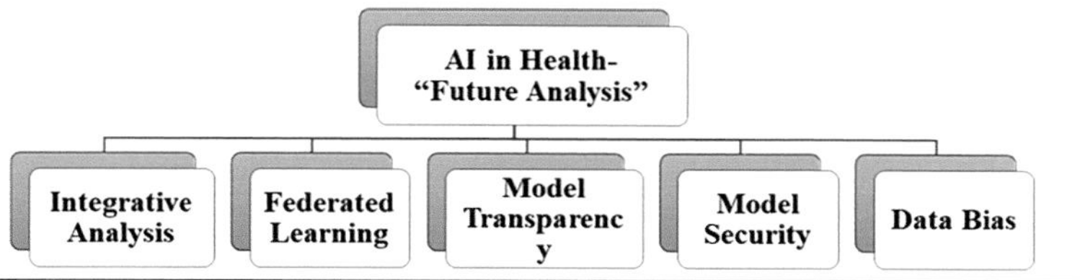


**Figure 8.5 Different Future Directions in Healthcare Using AI.**

scale, replace human clinicians, but rather will supplement their efforts to care for patients. Figure 8.5 describes the different future directions in healthcare using AI, which are summarized in the following subsections.

## 8.5.1 Integrative Analysis

Future scientists will devise novel methods for monitoring and interpreting a wide range of biological data, including genetic, genomic, cellular, clinical, behavioral, physiological, and environmental factors. Integrative mining can provide a holistic view and therefore give comprehensive insights into healthcare. In contrast to other computers, where enormous data sets can be acquired, patient data is typically limited here.

## 8.5.2 Federated Learning

The purpose of federated learning is to create models that provide excellent results. There is an increasing amount of patient-generated data nowadays, in addition to clinical data. Wearable devices or mobile phones, for example, can generate these data on a constant basis. Patients may hesitate to submit their private details over a public cloud in order to train a prediction model for their future state of health. Every person can then use the most recent version of the model and update it using their own data. The model changes will be compiled into a targeted update. The model will then be improved by averaging the focused updates from different users. The data will then be sent to local devices during the process. No intermittent data will be saved at any server.

## 8.5.3 Model Transparency

Rule-based systems are highly interpretable in traditional AI technology. Deep learning models, for example, are recent AI technologies that can achieve outstanding quantitative performance but are still usually viewed as black boxes. Ownership is a related issue when it comes to model transparency. According to the author [82], there is a concerning tendency toward proprietary algorithms that are opaque, with developers "reluctant to clearly publish" model specifics. When these models are used in clinical practice, this may increase the risk of injury [83]. Concerning predictive analytics in medicine [84], "regulatory and professional authorities should guarantee the advanced algorithms meet acknowledged standards of clinical benefit, just as they do for clinical medicines and predictive biomarkers."

### 8.5.4 Model Security

We talk a lot about how crucial it is to keep health data secure and private, especially data about individual patients. As the field of AI matures, there are several security threats to be dealt with. For example, attacks are available that can confuse an algorithm by injecting data that results in a poor decision-making process. Many authors believe that 1) people must be made aware of the possible risk; 2) policymakers should consider this risk while developing regulatory models; and 3) AI researchers should integrate effective defense mechanisms within their work.

### 8.5.5 Data Bias

In AI, all models need data to train themselves. Typically, the training sample size is insufficient to capture patient variations and the complexities of their health conditions. This issue is known as data bias. It remains one of the most important issues in AI-based healthcare. A straightforward solution is to collect a large amount of data. Diversity in the dataset can also be maintained. The issue can be dealt with throughout the model-building process [85] by employing techniques like the counterfactual Gaussian Process for risk prediction and customized treatment planning.

## 8.6 Conclusion

Artificial intelligence is one of the popular fields in the area of biomedical applications, including omics, brain–body machine interfaces, and medical imaging. This study explored several existing methods used in the domain, seeking to analyze the work to improve upon the suitability of methods in practice. Guidelines that could pave the way for future work in the field were also presented. Although research has achieved tremendous breakthroughs in this arena, there is scope for improvement. In other words, although AI-based methods have brought visible advances to the field, the true potential of AI is yet to be revealed. Technological advances will bring improvements in AI-assisted robotic surgery, drug discovery, disease risk prediction, virtual nursing assistants, medical diagnosis, and medical image analysis. Despite the great success of AI techniques in biomedical applications, many limitations such as bias, interpretability and imbalance are yet to receive much needed attention.

## References

[1] Krzysztof J. Cios, Hiroshi Mamitsuka, Tomomasa Nagashima, and Ryszard Tadeusiewicz. Computational intelligence in solving bioinformatics problems. 2005.

[2] Chensi Cao, Feng Liu, Hai Tan, Deshou Song, Wenjie Shu, Weizhong Li, Yiming Zhou, Xiaochen Bo, and Zhi Xie. Deep learning and its applications in biomedicine. *Genomics, Proteomics & Bioinformatics*, 16(1):17–32, 2018.

[3] Azzam F. G. Taktak and Anthony C. Fisher. *Outcome prediction in cancer*. Elsevier, 2006.

[4] William H. Wolberg, W. Nick Street, and Olvi L. Mangasarian. Machine learning techniques to diagnose breast cancer from image-processed nuclear features of fine needle aspirates. *Cancer Letters*, 77(2–3):163–171, 1994.

[5] Fei Jiang, Yong Jiang, Hui Zhi, Yi Dong, Hao Li, Sufeng Ma, Yilong Wang, Qiang Dong, Haipeng Shen, and Yongjun Wang. Artificial intelligence in healthcare: Past, present and future. *Stroke and Vascular Neurology*, 2(4), 2017. doi: 10.1136/svn-2017-000101

[6] Alex Krizhevsky, Ilya Sutskever, and Georey E. Hinton. Imagenet classification with deep convolutional neural networks. *Advances in Neural Information Processing Systems*, 25:1097–1105, 2012.

[7] Wei Liu, Dragomir Anguelov, Dumitru Erhan, Christian Szegedy, Scott Reed, Cheng-Yang Fu, and Alexander C. Berg. SSD: Single shot multibox detector. In *European Conference on Computer Vision*, pages 21–37, Springer, 2016.

[8] Vijay Badrinarayanan, Alex Kendall, and Roberto Cipolla. Segnet: A deep convolutional encoder-decoder architecture for image segmentation. *IEEE transactions on pattern analysis and machine intelligence*, 39(12):2481–2495, 2017.

[9] Ian Goodfellow, Jean Pouget-Abadie, Mehdi Mirza, Bing Xu, David Warde-Farley, Sherjil Ozair, Aaron Courville, and Yoshua Bengio. Generative adversarial nets. In *Advances in Neural Information Processing Systems*, pages 2672–2680, 2014.

[10] Rishav Singh, Tanveer Ahmed, Abhinav Kumar, Amit Kumar Singh, Anil Kumar Pandey, and Sanjay Kumar Singh. Imbalanced breast cancer classification using transfer learning. *IEEE/ACM Transactions on Computational Biology and Bioinformatics*, 18(1):83–93, 2020.

[11] Tejalal Choudhary, Vipul Mishra, Anurag Goswami, and Jagannathan Sarangapani. A transfer learning with structured filter pruning approach for improved breast cancer classification on point-of-care devices. *Computers in Biology and Medicine*, 134:104432, 2021.

[12] Long Gao, Lei Zhang, Chang Liu, and Shandong Wu. Handling imbalanced medical image data: A deep-learning-based one-class classification approach. *Artificial Intelligence in Medicine*, 108:101935, 2020.

[13] Dieu Tien Bui, Paraskevas Tsangaratos, Viet-Tien Nguyen, Ngo Van Liem, and Phan Trong Trinh. Comparing the prediction performance of a deep learning neural network model with conventional machine learning models in landslide susceptibility assessment. *Catena*, 188:104426, 2020.

[14] Alpaydin, Ethem. "Introduction to Machine Learning, edition." (2009).

[15] Kathryn P. Linthicum, Katherine Musacchio Schafer, and Jessica D. Ribeiro. Machine learning in suicide science: Applications and ethics. *Behavioral sciences & the law*, 37(3):214–222, 2019.

[16] Thomas Cover and Peter Hart. Nearest neighbor pattern classification. *IEEE Transactions on Information Theory*, 13(1):21–27, 1967.

[17] Hassan Shee Khamis, Kipruto W. Cheruiyot, and Stephen Kimani. Application of knearest neighbour classification in medical data mining. *International Journal of Information and Communication Technology Research*, 4(4):121–128, 2014.
[18] Irina Rish et al. An empirical study of the naive bayes classifier. In *IJCAI 2001 workshop on empirical methods in artificial intelligence*, volume 3, pages 41–46, 2001.
[19] Subasish Mohapatra, Prashanta Kumar Patra, Subhadarshini Mohanty, and Bhagyashree Pati. Smart health care system using data mining. In *2018 International Conference on Information Technology (ICIT)*, pages 44–49, IEEE, 2018.
[20] Bernhard E. Boser, Isabelle M. Guyon, and Vladimir N. Vapnik. A training algorithm for optimal margin classifiers. In *Proceedings of the Fifth Annual Workshop on Computational Learning Theory*, pages 14–152, 1992.
[21] Taishin Kin, Tsuyoshi Kato, Koji Tsuda, and Kiyoshi Asai. Protein classification via kernel matrix completion. *Genome Informatics*, 14:516–517, 2003.
[22] Chen Liao, Shutao Li, and Zhiyuan Luo. Gene selection using wilcoxon rank sum test and support vector machine for cancer classification. In *International Conference on Computational and Information Science*, pages 57–66, Springer, 2006.
[23] Gunnar Ratsch and Soren Sonnenburg. 13 accurate splice site detection for Caenorhabditis elegans. *Kernel methods in computational biology*, page 277, MIT Press, 2004.
[24] J. Ross Quinlan. Induction of decision trees. *Machine Learning*, 1(1):81–106, 1986.
[25] Alan Jovic, Karla Brkic, and Nikola Bogunovic. Decision tree ensembles in biomedical time-series classification. In *Joint DAGM (German Association for Pattern Recognition) and OAGM Symposium*, pages 408–417. Springer, 2012.
[26] David W. Hosmer Jr, Stanley Lemeshow, and Rodney X. Sturdivant. *Applied logistic regression*, volume 398. John Wiley & Sons, 2013.
[27] Maria Esther Urrutia-Aguilar, Ruth Fuentes-Garcia, Vargas Danae Mirel Martnez, Edward Beck, Silvia Ortiz Leon, Rosalinda Guevara-Guzman, et al. Logistic regression model for the academic performance of first-year medical students in the biomedical area. *Creative Education*, 7(15):2202, 2016.
[28] Ian Goodfellow, Yoshua Bengio, and Aaron Courville. *Deep learning*. MIT press, 2016.
[29] Dinggang Shen, Guorong Wu, and Heung-Il Suk. Deep learning in medical image analysis. *Annual review of biomedical engineering*, 19:221–248, 2017.
[30] Kaiming He, Xiangyu Zhang, Shaoqing Ren, and Jian Sun. Deep residual learning for image recognition. In *Proceedings of the IEEE Conference on Computer Vision and Pattern Recognition*, pages 770–778, 2016.
[31] Joseph Redmon, Santosh Divvala, Ross Girshick, and Ali Farhadi. You only look once: United, real time object detection. In *Proceedings of the IEEE Conference on Computer Vision and Pattern Recognition*, pages 779–788, 2016.
[32] Olaf Ronneberger, Philipp Fischer, and Thomas Brox. U-net: Convolutional networks for biomedical image segmentation. In *International Conference on Medical Image Computing and Computer-Assisted Intervention*, pages 234–241, Springer, 2015.
[33] Sehrish Qummar, Fiaz Gul Khan, Sajid Shah, Ahmad Khan, Shahaboddin Shamshirband, Zia Ur Rehman, Iftikhar Ahmed Khan, and Waqas Jadoon. A deep learning ensemble approach for diabetic retinopathy detection. *IEEE Access*, 7:150530–150539, 2019.
[34] R. Sumithra, Mahamad Suhil, and D. S. Guru. Segmentation and classification of skin lesions for disease diagnosis. *Procedia Computer Science*, 45:76–85, 2015.

[35] Sepp Hochreiter and Jurgen Schmidhuber. Long short-term memory. *Neural computation*, 9(8):1735–1780, 1997.
[36] Junyoung Chung, Caglar Gulcehre, KyungHyun Cho, and Yoshua Bengio. Empirical evaluation of gated recurrent neural networks on sequence modeling. arXiv preprint arXiv:1412.3555, 2014.
[37] Rahul Sarkar, Chandra Churh Chatterjee, Sayantan Das, and Dhiman Mondal. Splice junction prediction in dna sequence using multilayered RNN model. In *Advances in Decision Sciences, Image Processing, Security and Computer Vision*, pages 39–47, Springer, 2020.
[38] R. Rajeev, J. Abdul Samath, and N. K. Karthikeyan. An intelligent recurrent neural network with long short-term memory (LSTM) based batch normalization for medical image denoising. *Journal of Medical Systems*, 43(8):1–10, 2019.
[39] Irene Sui Lan Zeng and Thomas Lumley. Review of statistical learning methods in integrated omics studies (an integrated information science). *Bioinformatics and Biology Insights*, 12:1177932218759292, 2018.
[40] Andreas Holzinger, Benjamin Haibe-Kains, and Igor Jurisica. Why imaging data alone is not enough: AI-based integration of imaging, omics, and clinical data. *European Journal of Nuclear Medicine and Molecular Imaging*, 46(13):2722–2730, 2019.
[41] Nupur Biswas and Saikat Chakrabarti. Artificial intelligence (AI)-based systems biology approaches in multi-omics data analysis of cancer. *Frontiers in Oncology*, 10:588221, 2020.
[42] Gemma L. D'Adamo, James T. Widdop, and Edward M. Giles. The future is now? Clinical and translational aspects of "omics" technologies. *Immunology and Cell Biology*, 99(2):168–176, 2021.
[43] Jun Li, Hu Chen, Yumeng Wang, Mei-Ju May Chen, and Han Liang. Next-generation analytics for omics data. *Cancer Cell*, 39(1):3–6, 2021.
[44] Anna Marie Williams, Yong Liu, Kevin R. Regner, Fabrice Jotterand, Pengyuan Liu, and Mingyu Liang. Artificial intelligence, physiological genomics, and precision medicine. *Physiological Genomics*, 50(4):237–243, 2018.
[45] Jia Xu, Pengwei Yang, Shang Xue, Bhuvan Sharma, Marta Sanchez-Martin, Fang Wang, Kirk A. Beaty, Elinor Dehan, and Baiju Parikh. Translating cancer genomics into precision medicine with artificial intelligence: applications, challenges and future perspectives. *Human Genetics*, 138(2):109–124, 2019.
[46] Manuel Salto-Tellez, Perry Maxwell, and Peter Hamilton. Artificial intelligence – The third revolution in pathology. *Histopathology*, 74(3):372–376, 2019.
[47] A. B. M. Asadullah, Alim Al Ayub Ahmed, and Praveen Kumar Donepudi. Artificial intelligence in clinical genomics and healthcare. *European Journal of Molecular & Clinical Medicine*, 7(11):1194–1202, 2020.
[48] Kumar, R., Al-Turjman, F., Anand, L., Kumar, A., Magesh, S., Vengatesan, K., Sitharthan, R. and Rajesh, M. Genomic sequence analysis of lung infections using artificial intelligence technique. *Interdisciplinary Sciences: Computational Life Sciences*, 13(2):192–200, 2021.
[49] David Zimmer, Kevin Schneider, Frederik Sommer, Michael Schroda, and Timo Muhlhaus. Artificial intelligence understands peptide observability and assists with absolute protein quantification. *Frontiers in Plant Science*, 9:1559, 2018.
[50] Chi-Hua Yu, Zhao Qin, Francisco J. Martin-Martinez, and Markus J. Buehler. A self-consistent sonification method to translate amino acid sequences into musical compositions and application in protein design using artificial intelligence. *ACS Nano*, 13(7):7471–7482, 2019.

[51] Khalid Raza. Artificial intelligence against covid-19: A meta-analysis of current research. In Aboul Ella Hassanien, Nilanjan Dey, Sally Elghamrawy (Eds.), *Big Data Analytics and Artificial Intelligence Against COVID-19: Innovation Vision and Approach*, pages 165–176, Springer, 2020.
[52] Yurim Park, Daniel Casey, Indra Joshi, Jiming Zhu, and Feng Cheng. Emergence of new disease: How can artificial intelligence help? *Trends in Molecular Medicine*, 26(7):627–629, 2020.
[53] Ahmad M. Abu Haimed, Tanzila Saba, Ayman Albasha, Amjad Rehman, and Mahyar Kolivand. Viral reverse engineering using artificial intelligence and big data covid-19 infection with long short-term memory (LSTM). *Environmental Technology & Innovation*, 22:101531, 2021.
[54] Nic Fleming. How artificial intelligence is changing drug discovery. *Nature*, 557(7706):S55–S55, 2018.
[55] Maria Batool, Bilal Ahmad, and Sangdun Choi. A structure-based drug discovery paradigm. *International journal of molecular sciences*, 20(11):2783, 2019.
[56] Laurianne David, Amol Thakkar, Rocro Mercado, and Ola Engkvist. Molecular representations in AI-driven drug discovery: A review and practical guide. *Journal of Cheminformatics*, 12(1):1–22, 2020.
[57] Kawal Arora and Ankur Singh Bist. Artificial intelligence-based drug discovery techniques for covid-19 detection. *Aptisi Transactions on Technopreneurship (ATT)*, 2(2):120–126, 2020.
[58] Andreas Bender and Isidro Cortes-Ciriano. Artificial intelligence in drug discovery: what is realistic, what are illusions? Part 2: A discussion of chemical and biological data used for AI in drug discovery. *Drug Discovery Today*, 2021.
[59] Shouvik Chakraborty, Sankhadeep Chatterjee, Amira S. Ashour, Kalyani Mali, and Nilanjan Dey. Intelligent computing in medical imaging: A study. In Nilanjan Dey (Ed.), *Advancements in Applied Metaheuristic Computing*, pages 143–163. IGI global, 2018.
[60] Norio Nakata. Recent technical development of artificial intelligence for diagnostic medical imaging. *Japanese Journal of Radiology*, 37(2):103–108, 2019.
[61] Jasjit S. Suri, Anudeep Puvvula, Mainak Biswas, Misha Majhail, Luca Saba, Gavino Faa, Inder M. Singh, Ronald Oberleitner, Monika Turk, Paramjit S. Chadha, et al. Covid-19 pathways for brain and heart injury in comorbidity patients: A role of medical imaging and artificial intelligence-based covid severity classification: A review. *Computers in Biology and Medicine*, 124:103960, 2020.
[62] Feng Shi, Jun Wang, Jun Shi, Ziyan Wu, Qian Wang, Zhenyu Tang, Kelei He, Yinghuan Shi, and Dinggang Shen. Review of artificial intelligence techniques in imaging data acquisition, segmentation, and diagnosis for covid-19. *IEEE Reviews in Biomedical Engineering*, 14:4–15, 2020.
[63] Jannis Born, David Beymer, Deepta Rajan, Adam Coy, Vandana V. Mukherjee, Matteo Manica, Prasanth Prasanna, Deddeh Ballah, Michal Guindy, Dorith Shaham, et al. On the role of artificial intelligence in medical imaging of covid-19. *Patterns*, 2:100269, 2021.
[64] Daniel A. Hashimoto, Guy Rosman, Daniela Rus, and Ozanan R. Meireles. Artificial intelligence in surgery promises and perils. *Annals of Surgery*, 268(1):70, 2018.
[65] Abid Haleem, Mohd Javaid, and Ibrahim Haleem Khan. Current status and applications of artificial intelligence (AI) in medical field: An overview. *Current Medicine Research and Practice*, 9(6):231–237, 2019.

[66] Mohamad Bashir and Amer Harky. Artificial intelligence in aortic surgery: the rise of the machine. In *Seminars in thoracic and cardiovascular surgery*, 31:635–637. Elsevier, 2019.

[67] Quinlan D. Buchlak, Nazanin Esmaili, Jean-Christophe Leveque, Christine Bennett, Massimo Piccardi, and Farrokh Farrokhi. Ethical thinking machines in surgery and the requirement for clinical leadership. *The American Journal of Surgery*, 220(5):1372–1374, 2020.

[68] Andrew A. Gumbs, Silvana Perretta, Bernard d'Allemagne, and Elie Chouillard. What is artificial intelligence surgery? *Artificial Intelligence Surgery*, 1(1):1–10, 2021.

[69] Gabriel A. Silva. A new frontier: The convergence of nanotechnology, brain machine interfaces, and artificial intelligence. *Frontiers in Neuroscience*, 12:843, 2018.

[70] Lidong Wang and Cheryl Ann Alexander. Brain science and brain-inspired artificial intelligence: Advances and trends. *Journal of Computer Sciences and Applications*, 7(1):56–61, 2019.

[71] Michalis Papakostas. From body to brain: Using artificial intelligence to identify user skills & intentions in interactive scenarios. PhD thesis, The University of Texas at Arlington, 2019.

[72] Zehong Cao. A review of artificial intelligence for EEG-based brain-computer interfaces and applications. *Brain Science Advances*, 6(3):162–170, 2020.

[73] Sebastian Olsen, Jianwei Zhang, Ken-Fu Liang, Michelle Lam, Usama Riaz, and Jonathan C. Kao. An artificial intelligence that increases simulated brain–computer interface performance. *Journal of Neural Engineering*, 18(4):046053, 2021.

[74] Yi Xiong, Xiaolei Zhu, Hao Dai, and Dong-Qing Wei. Survey of computational approaches for prediction of DNA binding residues on protein surfaces. In *Computational systems biology*, pages 223–234, Humana Press, 2018.

[75] David R. Kelley, Jasper Snoek, and John L. Rinn. Basset: Learning the regulatory code of the accessible genome with deep convolutional neural networks. *Genome Research*, 26(7):990–999, 2016.

[76] Daniel Quang and Xiaohui Xie. Danq: A hybrid convolutional and recurrent deep neural network for quantifying the function of DNA sequences. *Nucleic Acids Research*, 44(11): e107–e107, 2016.

[77] Jian Zhou and Olga G. Troyanskaya. Predicting effects of noncoding variants with deep learning-based sequence model. *Nature Methods*, 12(10):931–934, 2015.

[78] Amarda Shehu, Daniel Barbara, and Kevin Molloy. A survey of computational methods for protein function prediction. In *Big data analytics in genomics*, pages 225–298, Springer, 2016.

[79] Oleg S. Pianykh, Georg Langs, Marc Dewey, Dieter R. Enzmann, Christian J. Herold, Stefan O. Schoenberg, and James A. Brink. Continuous learning AI in radiology: Implementation principles and early applications. *Radiology*, 297(1):6–14, 2020.

[80] James H. Thrall, Xiang Li, Quanzheng Li, Cinthia Cruz, Synho Do, Keith Dreyer, and James Brink. Artificial intelligence and machine learning in radiology: Opportunities, challenges, pitfalls, and criteria for success. *Journal of the American College of Radiology*, 15(3):504–508, 2018.

[81] Bojan Kerous and Fotis Liarokapis. Brain-computer interfaces – A survey on interactive virtual environments. In *2016 8th International Conference on Games and Virtual Worlds for Serious Applications (vs-games)*, pages 1–4. IEEE, 2016.

[82] Nilay D. Shah, Ewout W. Steyerberg, and David M. Kent. Big data and predictive analytics: Recalibrating expectations. *JAMA*, 320(1):27–28, 2018.

[83] Eric J. Topol. High-performance medicine: The convergence of human and artificial intelligence. *Nature medicine*, 25(1):44–56, 2019.
[84] Ravi B. Parikh, Ziad Obermeyer, and Amol S. Navathe. Regulation of predictive analytics in medicine. *Science*, 363(6429):810–812, 2019.
[85] Peter Schulam, and Suchi Saria. Reliable decision support using counterfactual models. *Advances in Neural Information Processing Systems*, 30:1697–1708, 2017.

## Chapter 9

# Plant Disease Detection Using Imaging Sensors, Deep Learning and Machine Learning for Smart Farming

Chanchal Upadhyay
*B.R. Ambedkar University, Agra, India*

Hemant K Upadhyay
*BM Institute of Engineering and Technology, Sonepat, India*

Sapna Juneja, Abhinav Juneja
*KIET Group of Institutions, Delhi NCR, India*

## Contents

9.1 Introduction ....................174
9.2 Imaging Sensors for Plant Disease Detection ....................175
9.3 Machine Learning in Plant Disease Detection ....................175
9.3.1 Deep Learning in Plant Disease Detection ....................176
9.3.2 RGB Imaging ....................177
9.3.3 Multispectral Sensors ....................177

DOI: 10.1201/9781003322597-9

9.3.4 Infrared Thermography (IRT) ....................177
9.3.5 Hyperspectral Sensors ....................177
9.4 Sensor Mechanisms ....................178
9.5 Statistical Analysis for Monitoring Plant Diseases ....................178
9.6 A General Framework for Monitoring Plant Diseases ....................179
9.7 Application of Sensors to Detection of Plant Diseases....................180
9.8 Conclusion ....................181
References ....................182

## 9.1 Introduction

Both population and food consumption are increasing rapidly around the world, while the consequences of global warming have broadened the food security agenda towards increased sustainability (Villa-Henriksen et al., 2020). Agriculture is the primary occupation for Indian villagers. Many mechanical and chemical advances have been made to improve yields and help farmers deal with issues such as crop diseases. In addition to crop losses through natural disasters like earthquakes, diseases and pests, fungi and bacteria are affecting crop yields worldwide (Oerke, 2006). Diseases may be transmitted to almost parts of the plant. Traditional evaluation methodologies for the detection of plant diseases include visual monitoring and microbiological methods (Martinelli et al., 2014).

Farm owners are not sufficiently resourceful to respond to the complexities of diseases. In addition, the use of large amounts of fungicides greatly increases farmers' costs. In some cases, it has been observed that the discovery and focusing on diseases and their vector pests showed huge strength in numerous applications (Huang et al., 2007; Yang et al., 2010) and estimation of losses in investigations of agricultural insurance (Zhang et al., 2005).

New information tools like IoT, cloud computing, remote sensors, etc. have led to big-data production, and the era of artificial intelligence has accelerated the progress of society (Borgia, 2014, Thakura et al., 2020, Fan et al., 2021, Thorat et al., 2017). Bio computing requires large amounts of information to be handled, leading to the development of better computational models to address specific tasks in some application issues. Deep learning is a subset of several machine-learning algorithms used exclusively for the analysis of signals and images (Hernández and López, 2020).

At a time when the human eye cannot accurately detect plant disease, technologies such as image processing, machine learning and sensors will be useful. An image sensor detects and searches for data used to create an image of a particular thing. It converts the transformative changes of light waves into useful signals. New technologies for the detection of plant diseases use machine learning-based classification techniques rather than conventional methodologies (Nagaraju and Chawla, 2020, Kulkarni et al., 2012, Jasim and Tuwaijari, 2020, Sun et al., 2020). These help farmers improve crop quality, as well as reducing disease by pre-detection and early treatment (Sinha and Shekhawat, 2020). Today an increasing number of non-invasive imaging sensors support the detection and discovery of plant disease in various fields of application as well as the study of complicated host–pathogen structures.

Reducing diseases makes crops more nutritious, as well as reducing health problems for consumers and farmers. Sensor networks are used to continuously monitor crop development parameters, protect crops from diseases and improve irrigation, so that farmers can manage resources, enhance crop quality, and react faster to increasing adversity. Internet-based tools may be instrumental in improved productivity and the dynamics of crop development. Efficient imaging sensors are being used extensively in recent techniques where the pixels of an image are used to detect current plant diseases. In this technology, a broad light range is utilized to assess the pixels of every image. High-definition images assist microscopic analysis of various leaves at different levels.

This chapter discusses the use of imaging sensors in relation to plant disease, and comprehensively reviews research regarding plant disease detection using new and efficient tools like machine learning, AI, IoT and deep learning. The challenges ahead and future directions are outlined.

## 9.2 Imaging Sensors for Plant Disease Detection

Image sensors are used to create an image of an object that detects relevant information and converts the variable attenuation of light waves into signals, which transmit information by short bursts of current (Mishra et al., 2020, Zhang et al., 2019). Image sensors are used in both analog and digital imaging devices such as camera phone, optical mouse, digital camera, medical imaging modules, radar and sonar. The first digital cameras used charge-coupled devices, which facilitated the movement of electric charge through the device so that it could be modified and used in the same way as above. Image sensors work in a similar way, converting input photons into a signal that can be read and interpreted.

Sensors can be categorized into CCD and CMOS, color and monochromatic, global and rolling. They can be further categorized according to resolution, pixel size and format. Integrated cameras typically use CMOS sensors, because of low cost and ease of use, and consume less power than CCDs. CCD sensors have been in demand for video cameras.

In a typical CMOS sensor (Figure 9.1), the chip is organized as a set along protective glass. The set consists of contact pads that attach the sensor to the PCB. The chip consists of pixels of micro lenses and micro components. Wire bond transfers signals from the dye to the contact pad behind the sensor. Several considerations affect the efficacy of an image sensor, including signal-to-noise ratio and low-light sensitivity. For comparable types of sensors, the dynamic range is improved, increasing the image size to make it appear larger and clearer.

## 9.3 Machine Learning in Plant Disease Detection

Next-generation technology is used to increase the acknowledgment rate and accuracy of the results so that they can be used in real time. Machine-learning investigations

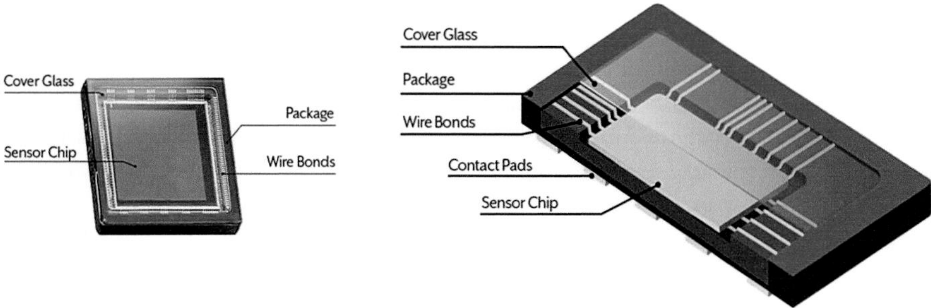


**Figure 9.1 CMOS Image Sensor.**

into plant diseases have been conducted using various methods including random forest, K-instrument systems, convolutional neural networks (CNNs), SVMs, fuzzy logic, etc. (Sujatha et al., 2021).

## 9.3.1 Deep Learning in Plant Disease Detection

Deep learning architecture stacks multiple convolution that develops solid representations out of basic input values. This enhances complication of the model, also increasing the frequency of label instances required for efficient learning. Unconventional computer vision tools can be developed for automated crop investigation by deep learning tools. These methodologies permit the creation of end-to-end structures that visualize leaf images and eliminate the possibility of particular disease of the plant (Kamilaris et al., 2018).

In-depth learning has been proposed to determine the amount of uncertainty in the categorization of medical imaging. The value of the amount of uncertainty in medical imaging categorization, combining it with probability-based interpretations, abortions, and providing a wrong decision, point to prediction of subversion results, innate confidence, inadequate understanding of output models, and overfitting in building neural networks. Most estimation algorithms related with deep learning under ADI have been on the basis of stochastic gradient descent (SGD) (Robbins and Monro, 1951).

Unlike animals in the plant, past infection lacks a favorable immune set limiting the capability for adaption to memory-based diseases (Singla and Krattinger, 2016). First, symptoms may be recognized locally, while the vector invades the host tissue, reflecting deviations in photosynthetic activity with early anatomical and structural changes. Locally developed symptoms may be changes in intensity of photosynthetic pigments, modifications in water content and enhanced plant defense response metabolites. Some years ago, scientists succeeded in connecting a wireless sensor network with ZigBee protocol and used the internet for transfer of online accessed data. This enabled farmers to limit irrigation of the area by logging into a particular web account and diseases on pods were detected.

### 9.3.2 RGB Imaging

Digital photographic images have been a useful simple technique for assessing plant health, recognizing and eliminating diseases. The technical characteristics of these handheld systems, such as spatial resolution and sensor photosensitization, have improved considerably. An RGB color image set is used for investigation of biological stress in plants (Bock et al., 2008).

The prime concern of the RGB image model has been image display in electronic systems. Many of the issues faced in the automatic reorganization of elements in color images arise with the theory of fluorophores display because of the unwanted overlap between the fluorophore spectra of emission and camera sensitivity. The results shows the red color appears in the other color channel images, and others are also shown in the three color channels.

### 9.3.3 Multispectral Sensors

Spectral sensors are usually classified on the basis of the quantity and dimension of the measured waveform and non-imaging sensorb system. Multispectral sensors, which are the best-known spectral sensors, particularly analyze the spectral data of elements in many relatively wide waves. Multispectral imaging cameras, for example, can access information in R, G and B waves. Multispectral sensors are used in drone-based agricultural mapping and analytics (Singh et al., 2020).

The ability to capture data at extraordinary spatial resolution and determine reflections in the infrared makes these sensors efficient for both farmers and scientists. Collection of multispectral information is an important tool in conducting efficient crop health assessment. To produce powerful figures on leaf areas, plant wedges, and canopy cover, several bands of light design precision analytics tools and mapping for farming. Without multispectral data, it is impossible to capture early indicators of disease, pests and weeds, and it can be difficult to obtain accurate measurements of the vegetative biomass of densely planted crops.

### 9.3.4 Infrared Thermography (IRT)

Infrared thermography (IRT) analyzes the temperature of plants and relates it to the state of the plant water. The miniclimate in the crop (Lenthe et al., 2007) and modified transpiration because of early infection by plant pathogens (Oerke et al., 2006) are detected. Infrared radiation may be investigated by thermographic cameras. In plant study, IRT is utilized on a variety of spatial scales and in a variety of applications, but it is dependent on climate factors.

### 9.3.5 Hyperspectral Sensors

Hyperspectral data are connected to physiological processes in plants. Special characteristics of hyperspectral reflection patterns have been assessed and confirmed by complex methodologies (Zhao et al., 2016). This botanical explanation of hyperspectral reflectance may be obtained during plant pathogenesis interactions that affect the plant physiology. The spectral effect of fungal pathogens is related to their nutritional type (Thomas et al., 2017). The development of unconventional hyperspectral sensors increases complications with the measured data and potentially low spectral resolution.

## 9.4 Sensor Mechanisms

When implementing imaging sensors for assessment of plant pests, it is important to first identify efficient and specific sensor characteristics. To date, many types of sensor characteristics have been identified for detecting plant symptoms because of disease or habitat destruction, including vision NIR spectral characteristics, and image characteristics including imaging sensors. Not all plant diseases are suitable for remote sensory identification because of a lack of specific characteristics. But some diseases which have a specific effect on plant physiology can be considered. The process of identifying and managing plant diseases by remote sensing arises with a particular response which is capable of detection by a particular sensing system (Zhang et al., 2019; Khattaba et al., 2019).

Various types of imaging sensor systems to identify and manage plant diseases are now on the market. Efforts to implement various sensor sets to successfully detect and monitor plant diseases, and to capture physiological changes and structural changes, are reported by Hahn (2009), Mahlein (2015), Sankaran et al. (2010), and Subashini et al. (2018). Based on sensory theories and evolving technology, sensory systems for monitoring plant diseases and pests can generally be classified into three types: (1) visible and near-infrared (VISSWIR) spectral systems; (2) fluorescence and thermal systems; and (3) synthetic aperture radar (SAR) and light detection and instrumentation (LIDAR) systems.

On the farm, soil moisture sensors, temperature and humidity sensors are deployed to detect diseases on a plant. The data obtained from the sensor is sent to the computer via wired or wireless devices and is confirmed and checked with relevant figures such as moisture values in the server-side data. If there is any difference in price, information is conveyed to the farmer electronically. The outputs of the sensor are created electronically and the farmer receives the complete crop and environment data online. Crop disease is detected by the image. The camera system remains around the crop to get an image of the leaves. The images obtained are sent to the server and then back to the farmer using image processing techniques, web pages on the app and leaf positions on mobile phones (Figure 9.2).

## 9.5 Statistical Analysis for Monitoring Plant Diseases

Once appropriate images have been extracted from the plant disease-monitoring sensor data, different algorithms or a combination are used to enable the following

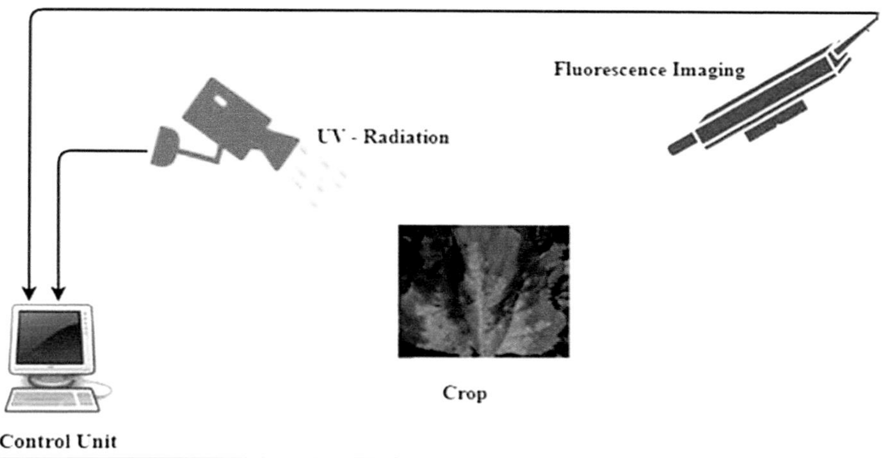


**Figure 9.2 Sensor mechanisms at remote location.**

*(Singh et al., 2020.)*

tasks: (1) detection of a particular insect, (2) isolation of diseases, and (3) limiting the severity of infection. Here we review the available algorithms, and examine their research status.

The discrimination model achieved an overall accuracy of 0.7. Further, logistic regression has been efficient in successfully detecting rhizomania in sugar beet and apple scabs (Delalieux et al., 2007).

Diseases and the damage from their vectors have demonstrated opposite and distinct characteristics at a specific stage. Related studies have been on the basis of airborne (Yang et al., 2010) or high-resolution satellite images (Yuan et al., 2015). Yang et al. (2010) found that a clear spectral response to symptoms of diseases such as cotton root rot was efficient and accurate in monitoring for hyperspectral as well as multispectral RS images.

## 9.6 A General Framework for Monitoring Plant Diseases

Given the considerable differences between growth procedures and symptoms of disease in host plants, there is no common imaging sensor facility or management model. However, strategy and methodology for plant diseases present some specific characteristics. On the basis of our review of imaging sensor characteristics, a usual set of algorithms can be created that may provide support in the context of unknown diseases (see flowchart in Figure 9.3).

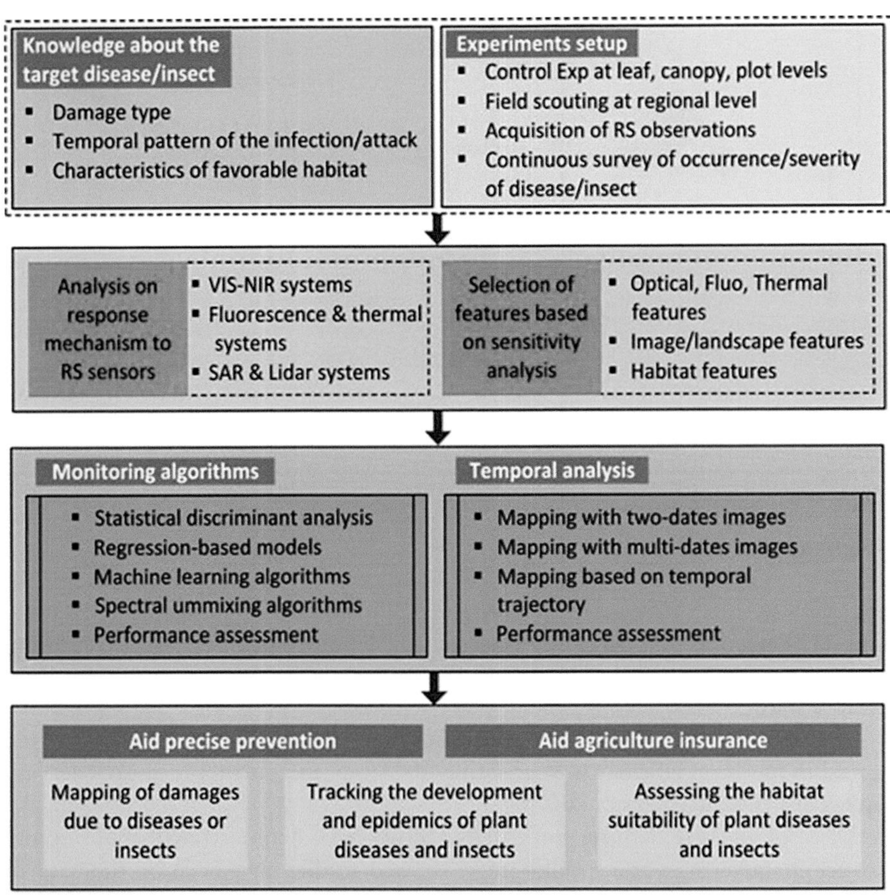


**Figure 9.3 A Framework for Plant Diseases by Imaging Sensor Observations.** *(Zhang et al., 2019.)*

## 9.7 Application of Sensors to Detection of Plant Diseases

With the development of machine-learning tools, feasible solutions for the largest problems, the most complicated regression and categorization issues have been enabled. Several statistics and methods are available to be shared across various devices dedicated to sharing tools (Pedregosa et al., 2011) such as Tensor-Flow (Abadi et al., 2015). Basic know-how is required for application of machine-learning tools. Improving the reach of strong machine-learning techniques has clear advantages for the research community. Imaging sensor technology is being applied for minute control of plant diseases in various areas and under usual conditions.

Newer fungicidal compounds to tackle diseases can be investigated. Low-range imaging sensor sets and spectro-radiometry can be utilized to examine the effects of pathogenesis at the cellular level. Hyperspectral imaging microscopy provides newer spatial data on chemical changes in plant tissue during host–pathogen interactions. The technical capabilities of the sensors are improving. But the application of sensors to support decisions and the use of fungicides in the field depends on the data available about the spread of the disease.

**CASE STUDY**

The research in this case study aimed to automate the process of detecting plant disease. CNN was used for image classification. Research shows that deep learning architecture and image processing outperform other machine-learning tools. The researchers applied and trained five CNN models – Inception Resnet V2, VGG 16, VGG 19, ResNet 50 and Exception – to village plant datasets of tomato leaf images. Researchers analyzed images of 18,160 tomato leaves spread across 10 square labels, and after comparing their performance measures, ResNet50 proved to be the most accurate forecasting tool. It was employed to create a mobile application to successfully classify and identify diseases of tomato plants (Verma et al., 2019).

## 9.8 Conclusion

This work summarizes and critically reviews the numerous sensor tools that are utilized to detect plant disease. Early identification of pathogenic infections is important for the management of polycyclic diseases. The work of detecting plant diseases used to be done using traditional nucleic acids and serological assessments, but nowadays other innovative methods such as remote sensing and precision agriculture applications are used for quick and efficient diagnosis of diseases. Many aspects of crop management have already started to benefit from the application of remote sensing and other technologies. The present work concludes that an instrumental and effective sensor used to meet the appropriate plant health criteria will also promote progress in farming. Future research work could establish a more effective set for timely automated tracking and could be expanded to recognize a greater number of diseases. In the last couple of years, several sensor technologies for monitoring plant diseases and pests have come into the picture, and considerable ability is developing to complement traditional manual inspection. Deep learning and machine learning tools exemplify this, with high levels of accuracy to assist botanists in database monitoring and disease diagnosis. The precision obtained in classification of leaf diseases is in the range between 95% and 100%, and this can be further improved as the database expands. A number of researchers have published reviews of big-data applications in smart farming and sustainable development in Smart Society 5.0, while field data has been available from artificial satellites.

## References

Abadi, M., Agarwal, A., Barham, P., Brevdo, E., Chen, Z., Citro, C., Corrado, G.S., Davis, A., Dean, J., Devin, M., Ghemawat, S., Irving, G., Isard, M., Kudlur, M., Levenberg, J., Monga, R., Moore, S., Murray, D.G., Steiner, B., Tucker, P., Vasudevan, V., Warden, P., Wicke, M., Yu, Y and Zheng, X (2015) Tensor flow: Large-scale machine learning on heterogeneous systems. *Software Proceeding 12th USENIX Symposium on Operating Systems Design and Implementation*, pp. 265–283.

Bock, C. H., Parker, P. E., Cook, A. Z. and Gottwald, T. R. (2008) Visual rating and the use of image analysis for assessing different symptoms of citrus canker on grapefruit leaves, *Plant Diseases*, vol. 92, pp. 530–541.

Borgia, E. (2014) The Internet of Things vision: Key characteristics, applications and open issues, *Computer Communications*, doi: 10.1016/j.comcom.2014.09.008.

Delalieux, S., Van Aardt, J., Keulemans, W., Schrevens, E. and Coppin, P. (2007) Detection of biotic stress (*Venturia inaequalis*) in apple trees using hyperspectral data: Non-parametric statistical approaches and physiological implications, *European Journal of Agronomy*, vol. 27, pp. 130–143.

Delwiche, S. R. and Kim, M. S. (2000) Hyperspectral imaging for detection of scab in wheat, *Proceedings of SPIE*, vol. 4203, pp: 13–20.

Fan, J., Zhang, Y., Wen, W., Gu, S., Lu, X. and Guo, X. (2021) The future of Internet of Things in agriculture: Plant high-throughput phenotypic platform, *Journal of Cleaner Production*, vol. 280, pp: 1–15.

Foughalia, K., Fathallahb, K. and Frihidab, A. (2018) Using cloud IoT for disease prevention in precision agriculture, *Procedia Computer Science*, vol. 130, pp. 575–582.

Furbank, R. T. and Tester, M. (2011) Phenomics–technologies to relieve the phenotyping bottleneck, *Trends in Plant Science*, vol. 16, pp. 635–644.

Glawe, D. A. (2008) The powdery mildews: A review of the world's most familiar (yet poorly known) plant pathogens, *Annual Review of Phytopathology*, vol. 46, 27–51.

Huang, W., Lamb, D.W., Niu, Z., Zhang, Y., Liu, L. and Wang, J. (2007) Identification of yellow rust in wheat using in-situ spectral reflectance measurements and airborne hyperspectral imaging, *Precision Agriculture*, vol. 8, pp. 187–197.

Hahn, F. (2009) Actual pathogen detection: Sensors and algorithms—A review, *Algorithms*, vol. 2, pp. 301–338.

Hernández, S. and López, J. L. (2020) Uncertainty quantification for plant disease detection using Bayesian deep learning, *Applied Soft Computing Journal*, vol. 96, pp. 1–9.

Huang, W., Lamb, D. W., Niu, Z., Zhang, Y., Liu, L. and Wang, J. (2007) Identification of yellow rust in wheat using in-situ spectral reflectance measurements and airborne hyperspectral imaging, *Precision Agriculture*, vol. 8, pp. 187–197.

Jasim, M. A. and Tuwaijari, J. M. A. L. (2020) Plant leaf diseases detection and classification using image processing and deep learning tools, *International Conference on Computer Science and Software Engineering (CSASE)*, Duhok, Iraq, vol. 2020, pp. 259–265, doi: 10.1109/CSASE48920.2020.9142097

Kamilaris, A., Francesc, X. and Prenafeta-Boldu (2018) Deep learning in agriculture: A survey, *Computers and Electronics in Agriculture*, vol. 147, pp. 70–90.

Kansara, K., Zaveri, V., Shah, S., Delwadkar, S. and Jani, K. (2015) Sensor based automated irrigation system with IOT: A technical review, *International Journal of Computer Science and Information Technologies*, Vol. 6, no. 6, pp. 5331–5333.

Khattaba, A., Habiba, S. E. D., Ismailb, H., Zayanc, S., Fahmya, Y. and Khairya, M. M. (2019) An IoT-based cognitive monitoring system for early plant disease forecast, *Computers and Electronics in Agriculture*, vol. 166, pp. 1–13.

Kulkarni, R. K., Anand, H. and Patil, A. (2012) Applying image processing technique to detect plant diseases, *International Journal of Modern Engineering Research*, vol. 2, no. 5, pp. 3661–3664.

Lenthe, J. H., Oerke, E. C. and Dehne, H. W. (2007) Digital infrared thermography for monitoring canopy health of wheat, *Precision Agriculture*, vol. 8, pp. 15–26.

Mahlein, A. K. (2015) Plant disease detection by imaging sensors – Parallels and specific demands for precision agriculture and plant phenotyping, *Plant Diseases*, vol. 100, pp. 241–251.

Martinelli, F., Scalenghe, R., Davino, S., Panno, S., Scuderi, G., Ruisi, P., Villa, P., Stroppiana, D., Boschetti, M., Guolart, L. R., Davis, C. E. and Dandekar, A. M. (2014) Advanced methods for plant disease detection, *Agronomy for Sustainable Development*, vol. 35, pp. 1–25.

Mishra, P., Polder, G. and Vilfan, N. (2020) Close range spectral imaging for disease detection in plants using autonomous platforms: A review on recent studies, *Current Robotics Reports*, vol. 1, pp. 43–48.

Moshou, D., Bravo, C., Wahlen, S., West, J., McCartney, A., De Baerdemaeker, J. and Ramon, H. (2006) Simultaneous identification of plant stresses and diseases in arable crops using proximal optical sensing and self-organising maps, *Precision Agriculture* vol. 7, no. 3, pp: 149–164.

Nagaraju, M. and Chawla, P. (2020) Systematic review of deep learning tools in plant disease detection, *International Journal of Systems Assurance Engineering and Management*, vol. 11, pp. 547–560.

Naidu, R. A., Perry, E. M., Pierce, F. J. and Mekuria, T. (2009) The potential of spectral *Computers and Electronics in Agriculture*, vol. 165.

Oerke, E. C. (2006) Crop losses to pests, *Journal of Agriculture Science (Cambridge)*, vol. 144, pp. 31–43.

Oerke, E. C., Steiner, U., Dehne, H. W. and Lindenthal, M. (2006) Thermal imaging of cucumber leaves affected by downy mildew and environmental conditions, *Experimental Botany*, vol. 57, pp. 2121–2132.

Pachayappana, M., Ganeshkumarb, C. and Sugundan, N. (2020) Technological implication and its impact in agricultural sector: An IoT based collaboration framework, *Procedia Computer Science*, vol. 171, pp. 1166–1173.

Pedregosa, F., Varoquaux, G., Gramfort, A., Michel, V., Thirion, B., Grisel, O., Blondel, M., Prettenhofer, P., Weiss, R., Dubourg, V., Vanderplas, J., Passos, A., Cournapeau, D., Brucher, M., Perrot, M. and Duchesnay, E. (2011) Scikit-learn: Machine learning in python, *Journal of Machine Learning Research*, vol. 12, pp. 2825–2830.

Qin, J., Burks, T. F., Kim, M. S., Chao, K. and Ritenour, M. A. (2008) Citrus canker detection using hyperspectral reflectance imaging and PCA-based image classification method, *Sensing and Instrumentation for Food Quality and Safety*, vol. 2, pp. 168–177.

Reddy, M. R., Srinivasa, K. G. and Reddy, B. E. (2018) Smart vehicular system based on the internet of things, *Journal of Organizational and End User Computing*, vol. 30, no. 3, pp. 45–62.

Robbins, H. and Monro, A. (1951) A stochastic approximation method, *Annals of Mathematical Statistics*, vol. 22, no. 3, pp. 400–407.

Sankaran, S., Mishra, A., Ehsani, R. and Davis, C. (2010) A review of advanced tools for detecting plant diseases, *Computers and Electronics in Agriculture*, vol. 72, pp. 1–13.

Sankarana, S., Mishraa, A., Ehsania, R. and Davis, C. (2010) A review of advanced tools for detecting plant diseases, *Computers and Electronics in Agriculture*, vol. 72, pp. 1–13.

Shakoor, N., Lee, S. and Mockler, T. C. (2017) High throughput phenotyping to accelerate crop breeding and monitoring of diseases in the field, *Current Opinion in Plant Biology*, vol. 38, pp. 184–192.

Sighicelli, M., Colao, F., Lai, A. and Patsaeva, S. (2009) Monitoring post-harvest orange fruit disease by fluorescence and reflectance hyperspectral imaging, *ISHS Acta Horticulturae*, vol. 817, pp. 277–284.

Singh, V., Sharma, N. and Singh, S. (2020) A review of imaging tools for plant disease detection, *Artificial Intelligence in Agriculture*, vol. 4, pp. 229–240.

Singla J. and Krattinger S. G. (2016) Biotic stress resistance genes in wheat, in: Geoffrey W. Smithers (Ed.), *Reference module in food science*. Amsterdam: Elsevier.

Sinha, R. S. and Shekhawat. (2020) Review of image processing approaches for detecting plant diseases, *IET Image Processing*, vol. 14, no. 8, pp. 1427–1439. doi: 10.1049/iet-ipr.2018.6210.

Subashini, M. M., Das, S., Heble, S., Raj, U. and Karthik, R. (2018) Internet of Things based wireless plant sensor for smart farming, *Indonesian Journal of Electrical Engineering and Computer Science*, vol. 10, no. 2, pp. 456–468.

Sujatha, R., Chatterjee, J. M., Jhanjhi, N. J. and Brohi, S. N. (2021) Performance of deep learning vs machine learning in plant leaf disease detection, *Microprocessors and Microsystems*, vol. 80, pp. 1–11.

Sun, J., Yang, Y., He, X. and Wu, X. (2020) Northern maize leaf blight detection under complex field environment based on deep learning, *IEEE Access*, vol. 8, pp. 33679–33688. doi: 10.1109/ACCESS.2020.2973658.

Thakura, D., Kumar, Y. and Vijendra, S. (2020) Smart irrigation and intrusions detection in agricultural fields using IoT, *Procedia Computer Science*, vol. 167, pp. 154–162.

Thomas, S., Kuska, M. T., Bohnenkamp, D., Brugger, A., Alisaac, E., Wahabzada, M., Behmann, J. and Mahlein, A. K. (2017) Benefits of hyperspectral imaging for plant disease detection and plant protection: A technical perspective, *Journal of Plant Diseases and Protection*. doi: 10.1007/s41348-017-0124-6.

Thorat, A., Kumari, S. and Valakunde, N. D. (2017) An IoT based smart solution for leaf disease detection, *International Conference on Big Data, IoT and Data Science (BID)*, Vishwakarma Institute of Technology, Pune.

Villa-Henriksen, A., Edwards, G. T. C., Pesonen, L. A., Green, O. and Sørensen, C. A. G. (2020) Internet of Things in arable farming: Implementation, applications, challenges and potential, *Biosystems Engineering*, vol. 191, pp. 60–84.

Wang, W., Thai, C., Li, C., Gitaitis, R., Tollner, E.W. and Yoon, S. C. (2009) Detecting of sour skin diseases in Vidalia sweet onions using near-infrared hyperspectral imaging. In *ASABE Annual International Meeting*, Reno, NV, Paper No. 096364.

Yang, C. (2010) Assessment of the severity of bacterial leaf blight in rice using canopy hyperspectral reflectance, *Precision Agriculture*, vol. 11, pp. 61–81.

Yang, C., Everitt, J. H. and Fernandez, C. J. (2010) Comparison of airborne multispectral and hyperspectral imagery for mapping cotton root rot, *Biosystems Engineering*, vol. 107, pp. 131–139.

Yang, X. and Guo, T. (2017) Machine learning in plant disease research, *European Journal of BioMedical Research*, vol. 3, no. 1, pp. 6–9.

Yuan, L., Pu, R., Zhang, J., Wang, J. and Yang, H. (2015) Using high spatial resolution satellite imagery for mapping powdery mildew at a regional scale, *Precision Agriculture*, 17, pp. 1–17.

Zhang, J., Huangb, Y., Puc, R., Gonzalez-Morenod, P., Yuane, L., Wua, K. and Huang, W. (2019) Monitoring plant diseases and pests through remote sensing technology: A review, *Computers and Electronics in Agriculture*, vol. 165, pp. 1–14.

Zhang, M., Qin, Z. and Liu, X. (2005) Remote sensed spectral imagery to detect late blight in field tomatoes, *Precision Agriculture* Vol. 6, no. 6, pp. 489–508.

Zhao, Y. R., Xiaoli, L., Yu K. Q., Cheng, F. and He, Y. (2016) Hyperspectral imaging for determining pigment contents in cucumber leaves in response of angular leaf spot disease, *Scientific Reports*, vol. 6, pp. 27790.

Chapter 10

# IoT Application for Healthcare

Monika Sharma
*Department of ECE, BMIET, Sonipat, India*

Hemant K Upadhyay
*BMIET, Sonipat, India*

Sapna Juneja
*Department of Computer Science, Krishna Institute of Engineering and Technology, Ghaziabad, India*

Abhinav Juneja
*Department of Computer Science, Krishna Institute of Engineering and Technology, Ghaziabad, India*

## Contents

10.1 Introduction ....................................................................................188
10.2 IoT-Based Solutions for Healthcare ........................................................190
10.2.1 Chest disease ..................................................................................190
10.2.2 Retinal Imaging................................................................................190
10.2.3 Heart Disease Monitoring System ......................................................190
10.2.4 Intelligent Ambulance and Traffic Clearance Based on Internet of Things..........................................................................................190
10.2.5 IoT and Mental Health Support .........................................................191

DOI: 10.1201/9781003322597-10

10.3 Smart Hospital Based on Internet of Things....191
10.4 Related Work....192
10.5 IoT Key Components....192
10.6 Data Monitoring by IOT....193
10.7 System Design....194
10.8 IoT in the COVID-19 Pandemic....195
10.8.1 IoT Applications during COVID-19....198
10.8.2 Contact-Tracing Mechanisms....198
10.8.2.1 Trace Together....198
10.8.2.2 Decentralized Privacy-Preserving Proximity Tracing (DP3T)....198
10.8.2.3 Efficient Privacy-Preserving Contact Tracing (EPIC)....199
10.8.2.4 Contact Categorization....199
10.8.2.5 Privacy-Sensitive Protocols and Mechanisms for Mobile Contact Tracing (PACT)....199
10.8.3 Internet of Things for COVID-19 Diagnosis....199
10.8.4 Internet of Things for Telemedicine Services during Coronavirus Disease....200
10.8.5 IoT-Enabled Wearable Technologies for Predicting Coronavirus Disease....200
References....200

## 10.1 Introduction

Technological advances mean the world has become smaller. Now people interact not only with other people but also with objects. IoT has made it possible to connect everything with everything else [4]. Billions of devices are connected using IoT. This concept makes life much easier.

Since the Stone Age, health has been one of the biggest issues faced by humans. With advances in technology, health issues are controlled and managed more easily than ever. Even though some major healthcare issues remain unresolved, we have come a long way from where we began. According to World Health Organization data, the world has recently been encountering greater health issues than in the previous decade. The WHO's Global Health Estimates provide the latest available data on causes of death and disability globally, by WHO region and country, by age, sex and by income group [1].

Even though health problems are rising worldwide, there are not enough health care professionals to combat them [1]. In developing countries, health care is a huge concern for the government and related institutions. Having enough facilities to offer in-house treatment is a major problem that has gained the attention of IoT researchers. The most promising solution we have is that with IoT, patients can manage their own health conditions and get help in emergency cases. On the other side, doctors can manage and consult with patients more easily. Over the years several advanced IoT applications have been developed to support patients and medical officers [9]. IoT helps healthcare to improve existing features by supporting patient management, medical records management, medical emergency management, treatment management and other facilities, increasing the quality of healthcare applications. As reported by Alam (2018), the number of connected devices is expected to reach 75.44 billion by the year 2021. The expansion of the internet and its collaboration with data science and artificial intelligence is making our machines ever smarter and able to communicate with us all the time.

Hospitals use IoT to monitor patients continuously and to provide real-time health care facilities. The internet of things has the potential to track people, services and objects accurately, so analyzing these data gives accurate results. In medicine, accurate information leads to the best treatment results. With IoT, doctors can measure vital signs and other biometric patient information through sensors attached to patients. Diseases and problems can therefore be diagnosed quickly. With the help of IoT, hospitals and ambulance services can be notified quickly when people need their services, roads and traffic lights can be controlled to support ambulances to reach hospital quickly. Remote healthcare systems have been receiving increasing attention in the last decade, which explains why intelligent systems with physiology signal monitoring for e-health care are an emerging area of development [3] (Figure 10.1).

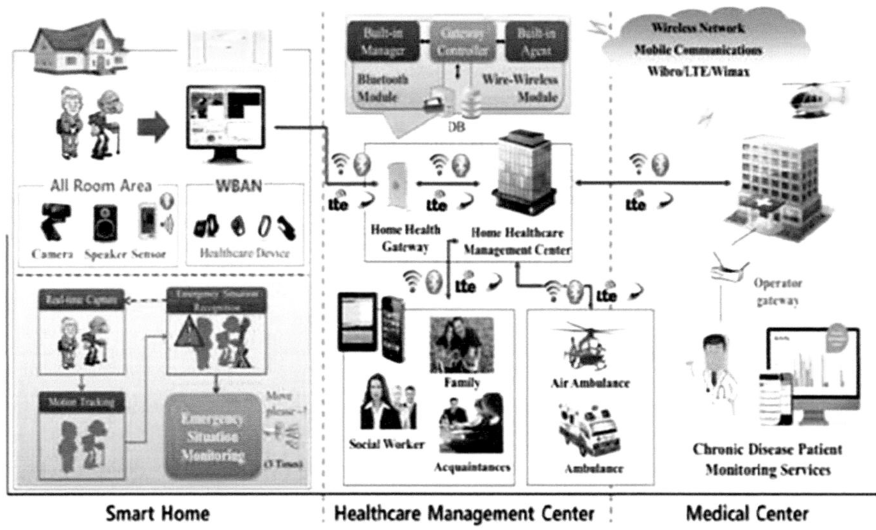


**Figure 10.1 IoT in Different Sectors.**

## 10.2 IoT-Based Solutions for Healthcare

### 10.2.1 Chest disease

The chest carries vital breath to be disseminated to other parts of the body, which provides for nearly all the basic survival needs of the body. A huge number of individuals globally have been detected annually as suffering from chest ailments of various types. Tuberculosis (TB), chronic obstructive aspiratory disease (COPD), pneumonia, asthma, and lung disease infections are the most significant chest illnesses, though they have also been regarded as extremely normal diseases. An LBPH (local binary pattern histogram) model uses the concept of sliding windows and applies the LBP operation to the image, which includes calculating the pixel values of the image, finding the threshold and then converting the image into binary.

### 10.2.2 Retinal Imaging

High-quality, wide-field retinal imaging is an effective screening method for retinal disease, which endangers vision but is preventable. Retinal smartphone-based cameras promise to increase access to retinal imagery, but variable image quality and restricted field of view can restrict their usefulness [54].

### 10.2.3 Heart Disease Monitoring System

Nowadays several cardiovascular diseases have become life-threatening even before the patient receives medication, because in case of heart failure patients are not able to call or get support from health care services by themselves. With IoT, observation of primary patient functioning can be done with ease anywhere in the world. A remote monitoring system is essential. Physical observations of sick people may be transferred to a remotely controlled medical app in real time by pervasive observation setting. With the help of the system, parameters related to hypertension, electrocardiography, heart rate, oxygen level, pulse, and glucose levels are computed by sensing devices.

### 10.2.4 Intelligent Ambulance and Traffic Clearance Based on Internet of Things

Huge traffic jams in metropolitan cities are a potential reason for taking a sick person to a local health center in time. Emergency services, including ambulances, have to face heavy traffic and that may cost a human life. These delays can be prevented with the help of intelligent ambulance setting. IoT-linked intelligent emergency vehicles utilize RFID techniques and sensing devices are applied to transmit signals to traffic lights. The traffic light-receiving device collects the signal and triggers the green light to clear the road for the ambulance. Emergency vehicles may also control traffic lights at cross-roads [21]. A transmitter placed on an emergency vehicle transmits a signal to the receivers installed at the traffic lights whenever it is in emergency mode. Using the proposed system ambulances can reach hospitals more quickly, potentially saving many lives.

EEG represents brain activities in the form of electrical signals. Due to the non-stationary nature of the EEG signals, nonlinear parameters like approximate entropy, wavelet entropy and Higuchi fractal dimensions are used to assess the variations in EEG rest as well as during Tratak *Sadhana*, i.e., at a rest state with eyes closed and during Tratak meditation.

### 10.2.5 IoT and Mental Health Support

Research has been conducted on how IoT-powered wearables can assist patients with depression symptoms. Since patients with mental health issues may be reluctant to regularly visit doctors, a wearable device is proposed that identifies unusual mood patterns in patients with depression, anxiety or stress. The wearable device uses the sensors to capture biological parameters experienced by patients in a critical condition. In an emergency, an alarm system is triggered and psychiatrists as well as relatives are notified.

Another mobile application proposed is automated to play music to reduce stress. The wrist-worn device has sensors to sense heart rate, temperature, SPO2 level, blood pressure, and galvanic skin response, gyroscope. Real-time daily routine data is analyzed and stored in the servers to be accessed by patients and clinicians.

## 10.3 Smart Hospital Based on Internet of Things

Even though hospital systems have the capability to maintain a certain level of information, they have some limitations, such as manual input systems for medical data, inter-departmental dependencies, single functions, etc. The proposed system has the ability to resolve these problems using IoT. It can implement information exchange, intelligent recognition, positioning, tracking, and monitoring. This system involves several key technologies. RFID technology is a wireless automatic identification technology for objects and other identification purposes [22]. In the IoT, a sensing network is the prime element. With sensor networks and RFID, the system can check the status of objects, such as their thermal parameters, geographical position, pressure, motion, etc. Wireless communication is used to transmit data using WIFI, UWB, Zigbee, or infrared.

The proposed technology can make hospitals smart, improve the patient experience and enable clinicians to manage information and patients conveniently. The system consists of three layers. The perception layer consists of smart objects embedded with sensors that collect and process real-time information of the physical and digital worlds. These sensors help in the measurement of physical resources and monitor changes in the physical environment. Using this layer, the system can identify assets, collect clinical information about patients and their surroundings, track doctors and other clinicians. The transportation layer is used for real-time regular transmissions from the database to the server [2]. The application layer has two elements: hospital information and an app for managing decisions [25]. The mobile network is the main tool for accessing smart healthcare centers as it is a convenient platform for all patients and medical staff.

## 10.4 Related Work

The internet of things has had a remarkable impact in a number of fields, and researchers across the globe have been exploring its uses. Rashmika Gamage (2020) presented a thorough study of health sector applications of IoT, with its increased sophistication in sensing, communication advances, actuations and vast amount of data. Dewangan and Mishra (2018) describe conventional methodologies for safety which may not be easily executed in the internet of things because of standardization and communicating stacks. According to Sathya et al. (2018), modern sensing devices may be embedded in the patient's body for regular observation of their health. The collected data may be assessed and utilized for developing timely predictive analysis of diverse diseases. Abu Adnan Abir et al. (2020) describe building flexibility against the coronavirus pandemic utilizing artificial intelligence, machine learning, and IoT. Su MyatTh aung et al. (2020) present an exploratory data analysis based on the Remote Health CareMonitoring System using IoT. Business intelligence (BI) incorporates business research, data mining, data visualization, data tools, infrastructure, and best practices to help businesses make more data-driven choices. BI's challenging characteristics include data breaches, difficulty in analyzing different data sources, and poor data quality.

## 10.5 IoT Key Components

The key components which enable any IoT device (as the example in Figure 10.2 shows) to function are given below (Abdur et al., 2017):

1. Sensors
2. Wired or wireless connection
3. Server for storage of data
4. Routers or switches for interconnection

The connected processor will control and monitor data from that IoT device (Ray, 2018). User interface can also be provided for IoT devices for ease of use. Further, all devices can be supported by either hard-wired or wireless connection

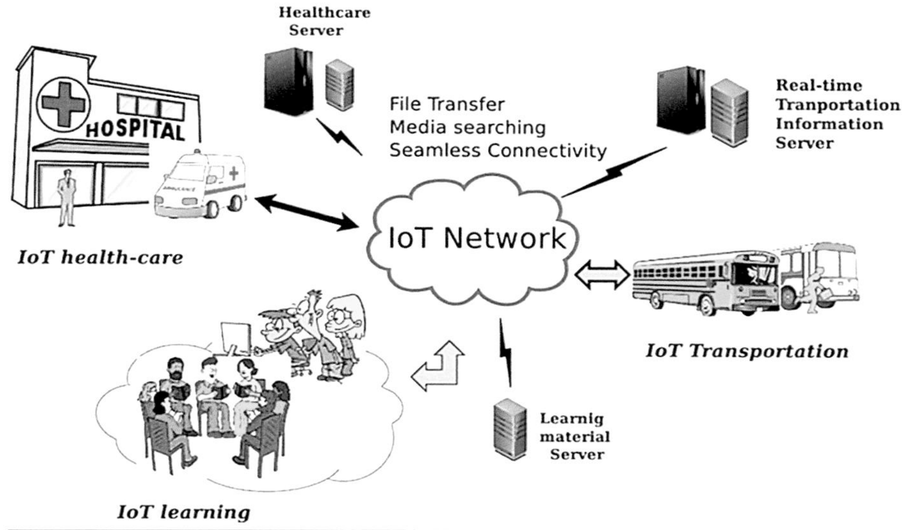


**Figure 10.2 IoT-Powered Wearable to Assist Individuals Facing Depression Symptoms.**

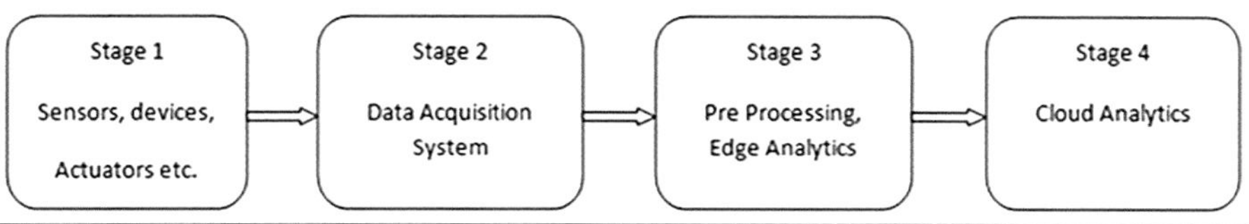


**Figure 10.3 Layered Structure of IoT Device.**

(Sánchez et al., 2017).The role of the server in the IoT device is to run the application program and store the overall data of the device (Figure 10.3).

## 10.6 Data Monitoring by IOT

Collected real-time health data obtained from sensors are displayed on the ThingSpeak and can be remotely monitored by computer and mobile devices. Figure 10.4 illustrates collection of health data relating to five different activities of 30 individuals, followed by exploratory data analysis (EDA). A normal healthy oxygen level range is between 95% to 100%. A normal healthy heart rate is between 60 and 100 bpm. Normal healthy human body temperature is 96°F to 99°F. The different BPM, SPO2 and temperature values for the five different activities are shown in the multivariate analysis in Figure 10.5.

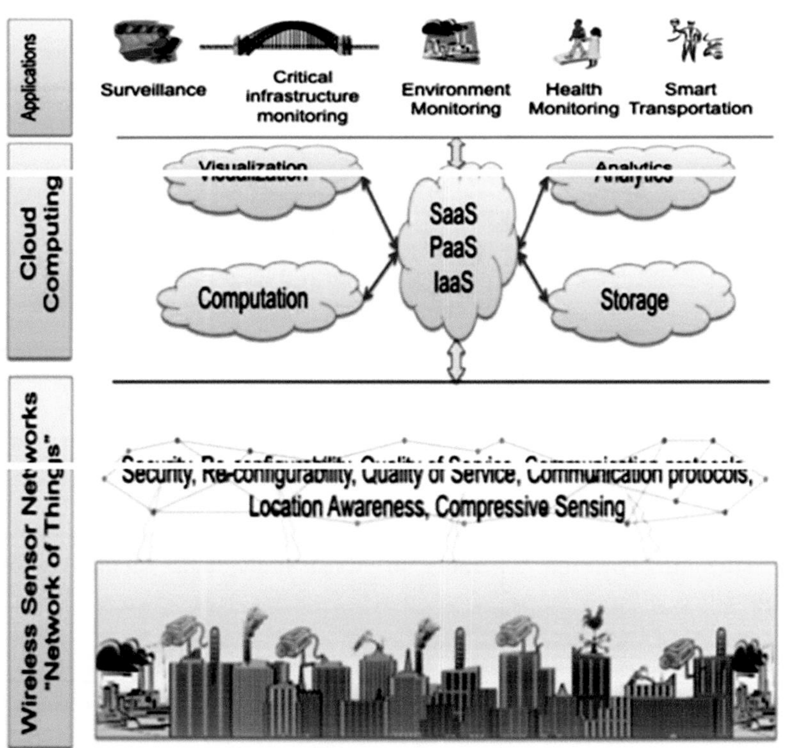


**Figure 10.4 Data monitoring by IoT.**

There have been many studies of the management of child health and development. An efficient real-time infant mortality analysis for improved health development using multi-feature covariance measures (MFCM) is illustrated in Figure 10.5.

Observation of patients' conditions using data analytics based on artificial intelligence and machine learning techniques helps understand how drug development and delivery may be achieved with these emerging technologies. Virus propagation can be modeled using AI and machine learning. Early prediction and timely detection may be instrumental to halting the spread of coronavirus, especially among healthcare workers who are at high risk of contracting it, and supporting the development of effective national policies. They may also assist with the enforcement of social distancing norms and increasing COVID-19 vaccinations.

## 10.7 System Design

Wearable technology, telemedicine, the use of drones and Covid tracing systems are examples of the importance of the IoT in healthcare. Customized monitoring of sick

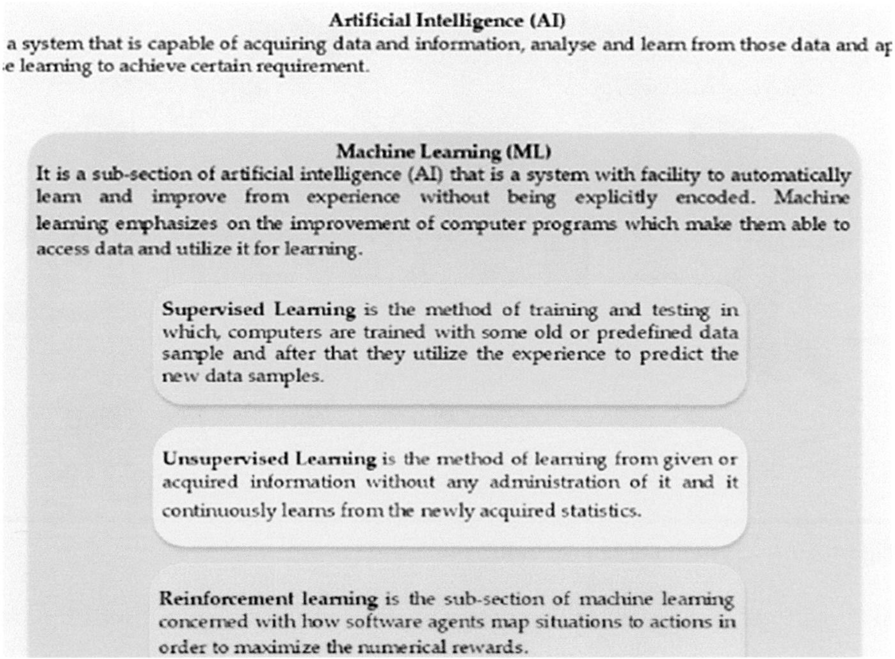

**Artificial Intelligence (AI)**

a system that is capable of acquiring data and information, analyse and learn from those data and ap
e learning to achieve certain requirement.

**Machine Learning (ML)**

It is a sub-section of artificial intelligence (AI) that is a system with facility to automatically learn and improve from experience without being explicitly encoded. Machine learning emphasizes on the improvement of computer programs which make them able to access data and utilize it for learning.

**Supervised Learning** is the method of training and testing in which, computers are trained with some old or predefined data sample and after that they utilize the experience to predict the new data samples.

**Unsupervised Learning** is the method of learning from given or acquired information without any administration of it and it continuously learns from the newly acquired statistics.

**Reinforcement learning** is the sub-section of machine learning concerned with how software agents map situations to actions in order to maximize the numerical rewards.

Figure 10.5 **The Relationship between Artificial Intelligence and its Elements.**

people is a complicated task. The proposed design method has two main steps: formulation of the problem and development of the product (Figure 10.6). The needs of stakeholders and would-be users are considered by the design team at every stage of the design process.

A sick person may be observed by a combination of small powered and compact wireless sensing nodes using the body sensor network (BSN) technique. However, it is important to consider security if advances in BSN techniques in healthcare are not to increase the vulnerability of patients. A secure IoT-based healthcare system, BSN-Care, has been proposed in recent research (Figures 10.7 and 10.9).

## 10.8 IoT in the COVID-19 Pandemic

The highly contagious nature of COVID-19 has exposed inadequacies in the conventional healthcare system. Artificial intelligence and machine learning have become the basis of newer mechanisms for efficient healthcare structures during the pandemic, with nations adopting many measures to develop resilience against coronavirus disease.

Artificial intelligence and machine learning have proved instrumental for the development of new effective diagnosis and predictive analysis of the spread of

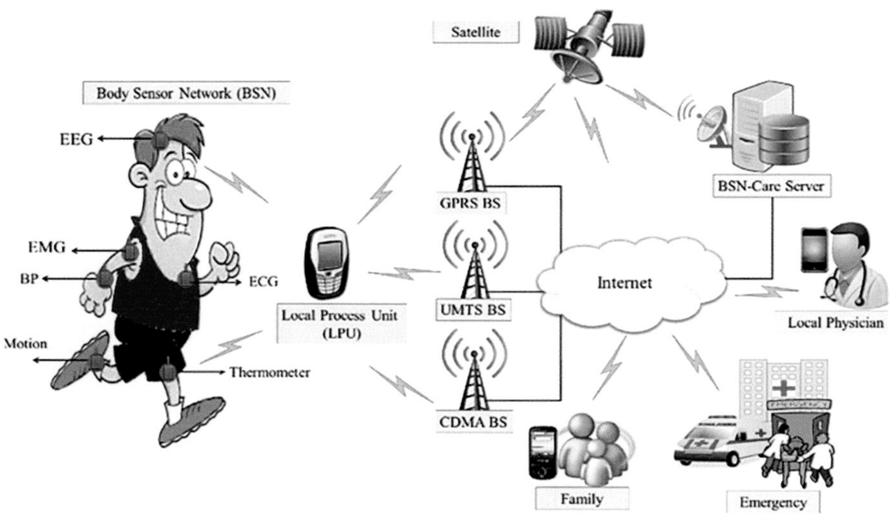


Figure 10.6 System Design Method.

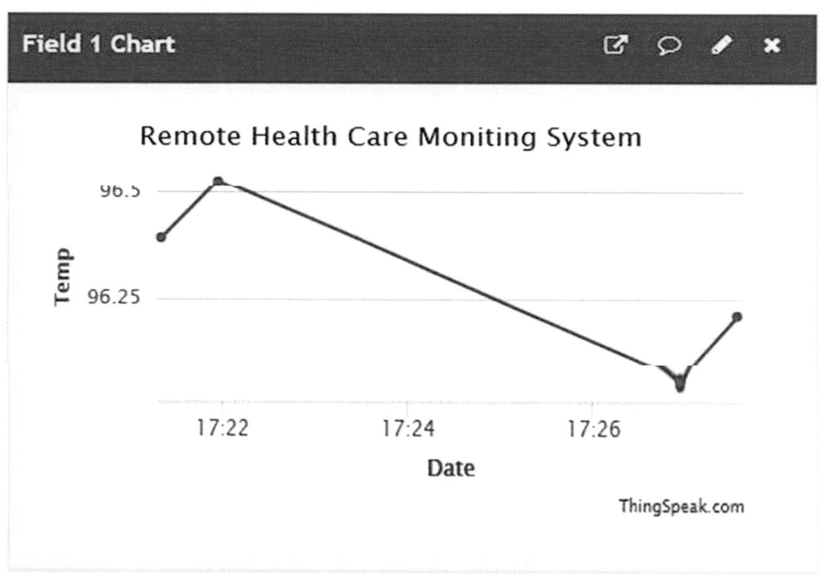


Figure 10.7 Body Temperature Fluctuation.

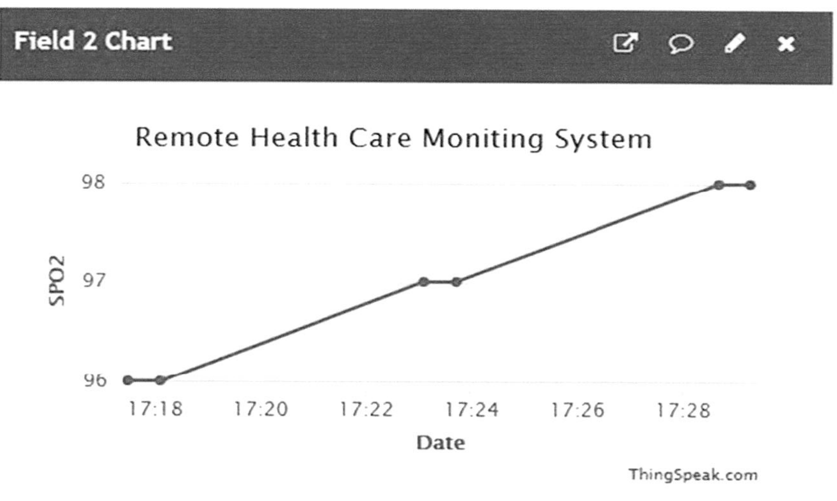


Figure 10.8 **Measured Oxygen Saturation Level Sensor Data Result of a Person.**

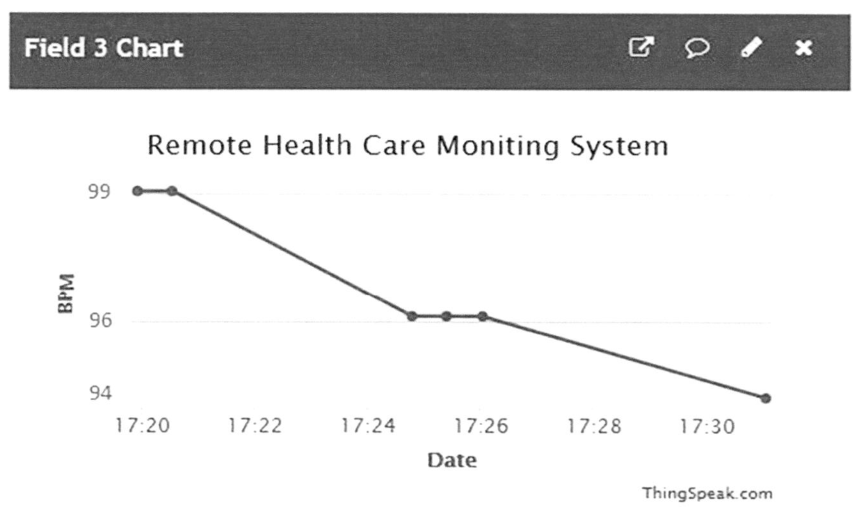


Figure 10.9 **Measured Heart Rate Sensor Data Result of a Person.**

COVID-19. These applications have been dependent on real-time observation of infected patients and efficient sharing of the data, in which the internet of things has a vital role. The IoT can also assist with such areas as automated delivery, responding to patient queries, and identifying factors responsible for the spread of the virus.

### *10.8.1 IoT Applications during COVID-19*

In the modern era of emerging ICT, IoT-related technologies are establishing an interest in healthcare applications. Technologies based on the internet of things have proved feasible alternative for coronavirus disease pandemic management. Internet of Things techniques may be used for tracing the spread of coronavirus infection spreading, diagnosing coronavirus-infected people, and managing telemedicine facilities.

### *10.8.2 Contact-Tracing Mechanisms*

IoT-linked contact tracing has become an efficient solution for managing coronavirus disease around the world. Contact tracing requires people infected with coronavirus to submit details of their travel history to public health officers so that testing or self-quarantine can be arranged for their contacts. The effectiveness of contact tracing may be improved by automated IoT-based processes.

Several IoT-based contact-tracing solutions have been proposed for the coronavirus pandemic.

#### *10.8.2.1 Trace Together*

This mobile phone application was developed by the Singapore government in March 2020. It uses Bluetooth to exchange randomly developed time-vary token systems in mobile phones that are in close proximity and the centralized server system The central server creates encrypted random tokens for every mobile phone which are broadcast at pre-determined time intervals.

#### *10.8.2.2 Decentralized Privacy-Preserving Proximity Tracing (DP3T)*

This tracing system was proposed by the Pan-European Privacy-Preserving Proximity Tracing project team. It allows each user to create random keys on a daily basis and do random broadcasting of ephemeral tracers. All users keep all identifiers near the device in the database of the device. The centralized administration can request any user's secret key as soon as that user becomes Covid positive. The secret key is shared with all the users, who may compute the identifiers of any particular time. Other users can thus verify if they have been a close contact of a Covid-positive user during the past couple of weeks.

#### 10.8.2.3 Efficient Privacy-Preserving Contact Tracing (EPIC)

In this system, sets of users are allowed to exchange Bluetooth communications with their locality devices and with the server. As soon as the server receives data about infected people, interested people can collect data about their own connection with the infected user by sharing time-related homomorphism-encrypted information with the server. The server responds with information about overlapping with an infected person. When other users share their timing with the server, the physical distance between the two parties is calculated and the relevant information made available.

#### 10.8.2.4 Contact Categorization

This methodology uses contact classifications instead of locations for infection-spreading identification. The devices of people store a quantum of contacts on the basis of incoming Bluetooth messages. This application recognizes the contact list with the set of infected persons, on the basis of data provided by the health ministry. If any matching is found, this application classifies the contact on the basis of the length of time that the uninfected person has been in close contact with the infected person. Category-wise analysis assists the health authorities to prioritize testing when the infection is spreading fast. Depending on the signal strength, the nearness of uninfected people may also be achieved like the other mechanisms.

#### 10.8.2.5 Privacy-Sensitive Protocols and Mechanisms for Mobile Contact Tracing (PACT)

This mechanism allows people to create randomly generated codes and share that code with people in their close proximity. Every person can store the incoming code and time note. Infected people share the codes and timing note with the server, which incorporates the data in the database of infected people. All users are entitled to download the database of infected people, check their own codes and time notes, and search for whether they have been in close proximity to an infected person.

### 10.8.3 Internet of Things for COVID-19 Diagnosis

Internet of Things techniques may improvise the speed, precision and effectiveness of coronavirus disease diagnosis and medication procedure. An integrated coronavirus disease smart diagnosis and medication help program may work through a cloud-based app that uses digital medical data and ML technologies for automated diagnosis. This may help the health authorities with data collection of infected people, coordinating and providing self-diagnosis. This application depends on 5G technology and large bandwidth.

### 10.8.4 Internet of Things for Telemedicine Services during Coronavirus Disease

To avoid the spread of COVID-19, appropriate healthcare should be made available remotely to infected people. Several health administration agencies have explored the development of chatbots for automated screening and scheduling follow-ups. Robotic telemedicine carts like IoT2020 and Viciln Touch can be used to remotely observe infected people in isolation in the absence of physical availability of health-sector practicing professionals. Numerous health care centers in the USA observe coronavirus-infected people in ICU using multi-directional audio-based and video-based communications.

### 10.8.5 IoT-Enabled Wearable Technologies for Predicting Coronavirus Disease

With IoT-based wearable technology, mobile applications can monitor physiologic parameters like heart rate, body temperature, and sleep cycles. Such devices or sensing systems may be utilized and incorporated with machine learning techniques for predictive analysis of the many phases of coronavirus disease infection. Automatic observation of body temperature and blood oxygen levels may alert health care workers and enable prioritization of patients.

## References

1. https://www.who.int/gho/mortality_Curden_disease/life_tables/situation_trends_text/en/
2. Abo-Zahhad, M., Ahmed, S.M., and Elnahas, O. (2014). A wireless emergency telemedicine system for patients monitoring and diagnosis. *International Journal of Telemedicine and Applications*, 2014, 380787.
3. Gotadki, S., Mohan, R., Attarwala, M., and Gajare, M.P. Intelligent Ambulance.
4. Lia, C., Hua, X., and Lili Zhang, B. (2017). The IoT-based heart disease monitoring system for pervasive healthcare service. In *International Conference on Knowledge Based and Intelligent Information and Engineering Systems, KES2017*, Marseilles, France.
5. Yu, L. (n.d.). Smart hospital based on internet of things. In *School of Computer and Information*, Hefei University of Technology, Hefei, China.
6. Minaam, D.S.A., and Abd-Elfattah, M. (2018). Smart drugs: Improving healthcare using smart pill box for medicine reminder and monitoring system. *Future Computing and Informatics Journal*, 3(2), 443–456.
7. Deepika Mathuvanthi, P., Suresh, V., and Pradeep, C. (2019). IoT powered wearable to assist individuals facing depression symptoms. *International Research Journal of Engineering and Technology (IRJET)*, 6, 1676–1681.
8. Haleem, A., Javaid, M., and Khan, I.H. (2019). Internet of things (IoT) applications in orthopaedics. *Journal of Clinical Orthopaedics and Trauma*, 11, S105–S106. https://doi.org/10.1016/j.jcot.2019.07.003.

9. Abo-Zahhad, M., Ahmed, S.M., and Elnahas, O. (2014). A wireless emergency telemedicine system for patients monitoring and diagnosis. *International Journal of Telemedicine and Applications*, 2014.
10. Alamr, A.A., Kausar, F., Kim, J., and Seo, C. (2016). A secure ECCbasedRFID mutual authentication protocol for internet of things. *The Journal of Supercomputing*, 1–14.
11. Atzori, L., Lera, A., and Morabito, G. (2010). The internet of things: a survey. *Computer Networks*, 54(15), 2787–2805.
12. Bagci, I.E., Raza, S., Roedig, U., and Voigt, T. (2016). Fusion: coalesced confidential storage and communication framework for the IoT. *Security and Communication Networks*, 9(15), 2656–2673.
13. Bandyopadhyay, D., and Sen, J. (2011). Internet of things: applications and challenges in technology and standardization. *Wireless Personal Communications*, 58(1), 49–69.
14. Benssalah, M., Djeddou, M., and Drouiche, K. (2016). Dual cooperative RFID-telecare medicine information system authentication protocol for health care environments. *Security and Communication Networks*, *9*(18),4924–4948.
15. Bruce, N., Sain, M., and Lee, H.J. (2014). A support middleware solution for e-healthcare system security. In *16th International Conference on Advanced Communication Technology*. https://doi.org/10.1109/ICACT.2014.6778919.
16. Chi, L., Hu, L., Li, H., Sun, Y., Yuan, W., and Chu, J. (2013). Improved energy-efficient access control scheme for wireless sensor networks based on elliptic curve cryptography. *Sensor Letters*, 11(5), 953–957.
17. Choi, J., In, Y., Park, C., Seok, S., Seo, H., and Kim, H. (2016). SecureIoT framework and 2D architecture for End-To-End security. *Journal of Super Computing*, 74(8), 3521–3535
18. Cvitic, I., Vujic, M., and Husnjak, S. (2016). Classification of security risks in the IoT environment. In *Proceedings of the 26th DAAAM International Symposium on Intelligent Manufacturing and Automation*, pp. 0731–0740.
19. Garkoti, G., Peddoju, S.K., and Balasubramanian, R. (2014). Detection of insider attacks in cloud based e-healthcare environment. In *International Conference on Information Technology (ICIT2014)*, pp. 195–200.
20. Gope, P., and Hwang, T. (2016). BSN-care: a secure IoT-based modern healthcare system using body sensor network. *IEEE Sensors Journal*, 16(5), 1368–1376.
21. Gordana, G., Mladen, V., Nebojsa, M., Dragan, V., Igor, R., Slavica, T., and Milutin, R. (2017). The IoT architectural framework, design issues and application domains. *Wireless Personal Communications*, *92*(1),127–148.
22. He, D., Kumar, N., Chen, J., Lee, C., Chilamkurti, N., and Yeo, S.S. (2015). Robust anonymous authentication protocol for health-care applications using wireless medical sensor networks. *Multimedia Systems*, 21(1), 49–60.
23. Redondi, A., Tagliasacchi, M., Cesana, M., Borsani, L., Tarrío, P., and Salice, F. (26–30 September 2010). LAURA—LocAlizationand ubiquitous monitoRing of pAtients for health care support. In *Proceedings of the 2010 IEEE 21st International Symposium on Personal, Indoor and Mobile Radio Communications Workshops (PIMRC Workshops)*, Istanbul, Turkey, 218–222.
24. Jachimczyk, B., Dziak, D., and Kulesza, W.J. (12–15 May 2014). RFID-hybrid scene analysis-neural network system for 3D indoor positioning optimal system arrangement approach. In *Proceedings of the 2014 IEEE International Instrumentation and Measurement Technology Conference (I2MTC) Proceedings*, Montevideo, Uruguay, 191–196.

25. Shen, X., Chen, Y., Zhang, J., Wang, L., Dai, G., and He, T. (19–22 October 2015). BarFi: Barometer-aidedWi-Fi floor localization using crowdsourcing. In *Proceedings of the 2015 IEEE 12th International Conference on Mobile Ad Hoc and Sensor Systems (MASS)*, Dallas, TX, pp. 416–424.
26. Kang, W., and Han, Y. (2015). SmartPDR: smartphone-based pedestrian dead reckoning for indoor localization. *IEEE Sensors Journal*, 15, 2906–2916.
27. Gjoreski, H., Lustrek, M., and Gams, M. (19–22 October 2011). Accelerometer placement for posture recognition and fall detection. In *Proceedings of the 2011 7th International Conference on Intelligent Environments (IE)*, Dallas, TX, 47–54.
28. Liu, X.Q., and Cai, W.M. (29–31 July 2011). The alarm system of elder tumble at the geracomium based on ZigBee. In *Proceedings of the 2011 International Conference on Electronics and Optoelectronics (ICEOE)*, Dalian, China, pp. 38–40.
29. Wang, L., Gu, T., Chen, H., Tao, X., and Lu, J. (23–25 August 2010). Real-time activity recognition in wireless body sensor networks: From simple gestures to complex activities. In *Proceedings of the 2010 IEEE 16th International Conference on Embedded and Real-Time Computing Systems and Applications (RTCSA)*, Macau, China, pp. 43–52.
30. Martin, H., Iglesias, J., Cano, J., Bernardos, A.M., and Casar, J.R. (19–23 March 2012). Towards a fuzzy-based multi-classifier selection module for activity recognition applications. In *Proceedings of the 2012 IEEE International Conference on Pervasive Computing and Communications Workshops (PERCOM Workshops)*, Lugano, Switzerland, pp. 871–876.
31. Aranki, D., Kurillo, G., Yan, P., Liebovitz, D.M., and Bajcsy, R. (2016). Real-time telemonitoring of patients with chronic heart-failure using a smartphone: Lessons learned. *IEEE Transactions on Affective Computing*, 7, 206–219.
32. Wu, C., Yang, Z., Xu, Y., Zhao, Y., and Liu, Y. (2015). Human mobility enhances global positioning accuracy for mobile phone localization. *IEEE Transactions on Parallel and Distributed Systems*, 26, 131–141.
33. Sun, L., Zhang, D., Li, B., Guo, B., and Li, S. (2010). Activity recognition on an accelerometer embedded mobile phone with varying positions and orientations. In *Ubiquitous Intelligence and Computing*. Springer, Berlin, Germany, pp. 548–562.
34. Millner, H., Ebelt, R., Hoffmann, G., and Vossiek, M. (24–25 September 2009). Wireless 3D localization of animals for trait and behaviour analysis in indoor and outdoor areas. In *Proceedings of the IEEE MTT-S International Microwave Workshop on Wireless Sensing, Local Positioning, and RFID*, Cavtat, Croatia, pp. 1–4.
35. Gonzalez, J., Blanco, J.L., Galindo, C., Ortiz-de-Galisteo, A., Fernandez-Madrigal, J.A., Moreno, F.A., and Martinez, J.L. (3–5 October 2007). Combination of UWB and GPS for indoor-outdoor vehicle localization. In *Proceedings of the 2007 IEEE International Symposium on Intelligent Signal Processing*, Alcala de Henares, Spain, pp. 1–6.
36. Kuo, W.H., Chen, Y.S., Jen, G.T., and Lu, T.W. (11–14 July 2010). An intelligent positioning approach: RSSI-based indoor and outdoor localization scheme in Zigbee networks. In *Proceedings of the 2010 International Conference on Machine Learning and Cybernetics*, Qingdao, China, pp. 2754–2759.
37. The ZigBee Alliance (2017). Control your world. *Applied Sciences*, 7, 596. Available online: http://www.zigbee.org/ (accessed on 6 June 2017).
38. Tabish, R., Ghaleb, A.M., Hussein, R., Touati, F., Mnaouer, A.B., Khriji, L., and Rasid, M.F.A. (17–20 February 2014). A 3G/WiFi-enabled 6LoWPAN-based U-healthcare system for ubiquitous real-time monitoring and data logging. In *Proceedings of the 2nd Middle East Conference on Biomedical Engineering*, Doha, Qatar, pp. 277–280.

39. Fielden, G.D.R. (1975). *Engineering Design*. HANSARD, London, UK.
40. Banzi, M. (2008). *Getting Started with Arduino*, 3rd ed. O'Reilly Media, Sebastopol, CA.
41. Dziak, D., Jachimczyk, B., and Kulesza, W.J. (2016). Wirelessly interfacing objects and subjects of healthcare system—IoTapproach. *ElektronikairElektrotechnika*, 22, 66–73.
42. Refaeilzadeh, P., Tang, L., and Liu, H. (2009). Cross-validation. In *Encyclopedia of Database Systems*, Liu, L., Özsu, M.T., Eds. Springer: New York, pp. 532–538.
43. Juneja, S., Juneja, A., Dhiman, G., Behl, S., and Kautish, S. (2021). An approach for thoracic syndrome classification with convolutional neural networks. *Computational and Mathematical Methods in Medicine*, 2021.
44. Upadhyay, H., Juneja, S., Juneja, A., Dhiman, G., and Kautish, S. (2021). Evaluation of ergonomics-related disorders in online education using fuzzy AHP. *Computational Intelligence and Neuroscience*, 2021. https://doi.org/10.1155/2021/2214971
45. Juneja, S., Gahlan, M., Dhiman, G., and Kautish, S. (2021). Futuristic cyber-twin architecture for 6G technology to support internet of everything. *Scientific Programming*, 2021. https://doi.org/10.1155/2021/9101782
46. Shao, C., Yang, Y., Juneja, S., and GSeetharam, T. (2022). IoT data visualization for business intelligence in corporate finance. *Information Processing & Management*, 59(1), 102736.
47. Juneja, S., Jain, S., Suneja, A., Kaur, G., Alharbi, Y., Alferaidi, A., Alharbi, A., Viriyasitavat, W., and Dhiman, G. (2021). Gender and age classification enabled blockschain security mechanism for assisting mobile application. *IETE Journal of Research*, 1–13. https://doi.org/10.1080/03772063.2021.1982418.
48. Uppal, M., Gupta, D., Juneja, S., Dhiman, G., and Kautish, S. (2021). Cloud-based fault prediction using IoT in office automation for improvisation of health of employees. *Journal of Healthcare Engineering*, 2021. https://doi.org/10.1155/2021/8106467.
49. Upadhyay, H.K., Juneja, S., Maggu, S., Dhingra, G., and Juneja, A. (2021). Multi-criteria analysis of social isolation barriers amid COVID-19 using fuzzy AHP *World Journal of Engineering*.
50. Dhankhar, A., Juneja, S., Juneja, A., and Bali, V. (2021). Kernel parameter tuning to tweak the performance of classifiers for identification of heart diseases. *International Journal of E-Health and Medical Communications (IJEHMC)*, 12(4), 1–16.
51. Juneja, A., Juneja, S., Soneja, A., and Jain, S. (2021). Real time object detection using CNN based single shot detector model. *Journal of Information Technology Management*, 13(1), 62–80.
52. Juneja, A., Juneja, S., Bali, V., and Mahajan, S. (2021). Multi-criterion decision making for wireless communication technologies adoption in IoT. *International Journal of System Dynamics Applications (IJSDA)*, 10(1), 1–15.
53. Juneja, S., Juneja, A., and Anand, R. (2020). Healthcare 4.0-digitizing healthcare using big data for performance improvisation. *Journal of Computational and Theoretical Nanoscience*, 17(9–10), 4408–4410.
54. Juneja, A., Juneja, S., Kaur, S., and Kumar, V. (2021). Predicting diabetes mellitus with machine learning techniques using multi-criteria decision making. *International Journal of Information Retrieval Research (IJIRR)*, 11(2), 38–52.
55. Tiwari, I., Juneja, S., Juneja, A., and Anand, R. (2020). A statistical-oriented comparative analysis of various machine learning classifier algorithms. *Journal of Natural Remedies*, 21(3), 139–144.

56. Juneja, S., Juneja, A., and Anand, R. (2019). Emerging role of big data as a tool for improving sustainability for the betterment of quality of life in metro cities, *International Journal of Control and Automation*, 12(5), 553–557.
57. Juneja, A., Bajaj, S., and Anand, R. (2020). Improvising green computing using multi criteria decision making. *Journal of Advanced Research in Dynamical and Control Systems*, 12(3), 1161–1165. https://doi.org/10.5373/JARDCS/V12SP3/20201362.

*Chapter 11*

# Machine Learning Techniques for Prediction of Diabetes

Tarun Jain
*Manipal University, Jaipur, India*

Payal Garg
*Ajay Kumar Garg Engineering College, Ghaziabad, India*

Jalak Yogesh Patel and Div Chaudhary
*Manipal University, Jaipur, India*

Horesh Kumar
*Ajay Kumar Garg Engineering College, Ghaziabad, India*

Vivek K. Verma and Rishi Gupta
*Manipal University, Jaipur, India*

## Contents

11.1 Introduction ....................................................................................206
11.2 Review of Work ..............................................................................207
11.3 Methodology ....................................................................................208

DOI: 10.1201/9781003322597-11

11.3.1 Dataset ....208
11.3.2 Predictive Indicators ....209
11.3.2.1 Confusion Matrix ....209
11.3.2.2 ROC curve ....210
11.3.2.3 True positive rate (TPR) ....210
11.3.2.4 False positive rate (FPR) ....210
11.3.2.5 Accuracy ....210
11.3.2.6 Precision ....210
11.3.2.7 Sensitivity (recall) ....211
11.3.2.8 F1 Score ....211
11.3.2.9 Specificity (true negative rate) ....211
11.3.2.10 False positive rate (FPR) ....211
11.3.2.11 False negative rate (FNR) ....212
11.3.2.12 False discovery rate (FDR) ....212
11.3.2.13 Negative predictive value (NPV) ....212
11.3.2.14 Matthews correlation coefficient (MCC) ....212
11.3.3 Method of analysis ....212
11.3.3.1 Number of Pregnancies ....215
11.3.3.2 Glucose level ....216
11.3.3.3 Blood pressure ....217
11.3.3.4 Skin thickness ....217
11.3.3.5 Insulin ....221
11.3.3.6 Body mass index (BMI) ....223
11.3.3.7 Diabetes pedigree function ....225
11.3.3.8 Age ....227
11.4 Machine Learning Algorithms ....228
11.4.1 Random forest algorithm ....228
11.4.2 XGBoost algorithm ....228
11.4.3 Support vector machine (SVM) ....229
11.4.4 Artificial neural network (ANN) ....229
11.5 Result and Analysis ....229
11.6 Conclusion ....234
References ....235


## 11.1 Introduction

Diabetes is a disease in which the individual's blood glucose or blood sugar is excessive. Blood glucose is the prime source of energy produced by food intake, as defined by the National Institute of Diabetes and Digestive and Kidney Diseases. The hormone insulin facilitates the transmission of glucose, which becomes the energy source, from food to cells. As time passes, the increased level of glucose in the blood can initiate health-related problems. Diabetes cannot be cured but it can be managed through a healthy lifestyle [1].

Irrespective of socio-economic status or national borders, diabetes is becoming a serious threat to the health of the world. It causes serious and life-threatening risks to develop, increasing the need for medical care. The management of diabetes and its complications is very poor, which can lead to premature death. At the world level diabetes is among the top ten causes of death. It is predicted that in 2030 nearly 578 million and in 2045, 700 million people will have to live with diabetes worldwide [2]. In South-east Asia, 88 million people were found to have diabetes in 2019 and it is predicted that this number will rise to 115 million and 153 million in 2030 and 2045 respectively. It shows a 74% increase in the number of people suffering from diabetes, which is alarming for India also [2].

Diabetes is becoming a major challenge in India. Nearly 8.7% of people between 20 and 70 years of age are diabetic [3]. Diabetes both significantly increases mortality and reduces life expectancy. The main problem for patients who may develop diabetes is lack of awareness about the high-risk factors associated with it. Late diagnosis increases the chances of developing other diseases. Early detection of the disease together with associated symptoms through machine learning may prove very supportive in its treatment.

Machine learning methods are acquiring popularity in the field of medical research, including in diabetes research [4]. A person can be classified as diabetic or non-diabetic based on their medical record or from a database. There are various statistical classification techniques for determining the occurrence of diabetes. The random forest classifier can be used to classify large data sets.

## 11.2 Review of Work

Various machine learning models have been used for diabetes classification. The work presented in [5] deals with the detection of diabetes using a hybrid model consisting of K-nearest neighbor (KNN) and light gradient boosting machine (LGBM). The model had an accuracy of 91%.

The work in [6] describes supervised machine learning algorithms. SVM and naïve Bayes were applied on a dataset of 520 patients aged between 16 and 90. The support vector machine gave the best results with an accuracy of 96.54%.

The work presented in [7] deals with diabetes classification through such constructs as long short-term memory (LSTM) and convolutional neural network (CNN) on HRV and ECG signals. SVM was used with CNN and LSTM to create a hybrid model. The model outputs an accuracy of 95.7%.

Furthermore, the work presented in [8] deals with Bayesian networks (BN) and artificial neural networks (ANN). The BN used is the naïve Bayesian network. The ANN used is a multilayer-feed forward neural network along with a Levenberg–Marquardt learning algorithm. It gives a maximum accuracy of 99%.

The work presented in [9] deals with removing noisy data and outliers using K-means and then using a support vector machine classifier for diabetes classification. The same dataset (Pima Indian Diabetes from the UCI repository) was used. The SVM gives high accuracy of 98.82%.

Iyer, Aiswarya, Jeyalatha et al. conducted research on diabetes diagnosis through classification mining techniques [10]. This research investigates the different aspects of decision tree for data mining techniques and naïve Bayes classifier to determine diabetes among women. The key aim of their research was to predict diabetic patients through data mining tools based on available medical data. The database deployed for patient classification of the type of data mining was collected from the Pima Indians Diabetes database from the National Institute of Diabetes and Digestive and Kidney Diseases. In their research paper, dual algorithms such as naïve Bayes and J48 (decision tree algorithm) have been taken to create diagnostic models. The data were classified into test sets and training sets using the percentage split and cross-validation techniques. Ten-fold cross-validation was executed to prepare testing as well as training data. Finally, data were divided into "tested negative" or "tested positive" based on the conclusion of the constructed decision tree. An accuracy level of 74.8698 % accuracy is ascertained by their research work.

The main objective of research paper [11] was to compare various kinds of machine learning classification algorithms for diabetic patients. The algorithms used are naïve Bayes, logistic regression, IBK, support vector machine, OneR, multilayer perceptron, decision tree (J48), Adaboostm1 bagging, and random forest. The ten-fold cross-validation was executed to avoid the problem of overfitting. The highest accuracy,78.01%, was given by logistic regression and the lowest, 70.99%, was given by IBK.

## 11.3 Methodology

A brief description of the dataset is given below. After analyzing and screening the data we split the data into two, one part for training and the other for testing the model. For training and testing purposes an 80: 20 ratio is used. We used both machine learning and deep learning models to maximize the accuracy of diabetes prediction. The machine learning and deep learning models used in the present research are random forest, XGBoost, SVM, and ANN [12,13].

### *11.3.1 Dataset*

The dataset was acquired from the UCI machine learning repository. Initially it was collected from the National Institute of Diabetes and Digestive and Kidney Diseases. All the patients in the dataset are females of Pima Indian heritage aged 21 years and above. The dataset contains 768 rows and nine columns. It contains eight independent variables and one dependent variable (see Table 11.1).

**Table 11.1 Variables Information**

| *Pregnancies* | *Frequency of Pregnancy* |
|---|---|
| Age | Age (in years) |
| BMI | Body mass index (weight in kg/(height in m)^2) |
| Glucose | Plasma glucose concentration through an oral glucose tolerance test of 2 hours' duration |
| Blood pressure | Diastolic (in mm Hg) |
| Skin Thickness | Thickness of triceps skin fold (in mm) |
| Insulin | Two-hour serum insulin (in mu U/ml) |
| Outcome | Class variable (0 or 1). Total 768. 268 are 1 and 500 are 0 |
| Diabetes Pedigree Function | Analysis of diabetes mellitus history in genetic relationships of the patient. |

## *11.3.2 Predictive Indicators*

The predictive indicators of different models are described below.

### *11.3.2.1 Confusion Matrix*

It is defined as a N × N matrix which is utilized to evaluate the performance and summarize the prediction results of a classification problem. N is the number of the targeted classes in our classification problem. It essentially shows how confused the classification model is while making predictions by maintaining a count of the number of predictions which are correct and/or incorrect. It provides insight not only into the errors being made by the classifier but also the types of errors that are made. After the model is trained with 80% of the data, it is to be run on the remaining 20% testing data and counted in four groups:

True Positive (TP)
The predicted value and the actual value are equal and are correctly identified as positive.

False Positive (FP)
Though the actual value is negative, the model falsely or incorrectly predicted it to be positive.

True Negative (TN)
The predicted value and the actual value are equal and are correctly identified as negative.

False Negative (FN)
Though the actual value is positive, the model falsely or incorrectly predicted it to be negative.

#### 11.3.2.2 ROC curve

To graphically analyze and measure the accuracy and performance of our classification model, a graph is plotted which shows how the false positive rate (FPR) and true positive rate (TPR) are correlated. This plot of TPR vs FPR is called the receiver operating characteristic (ROC) of our classification model.

#### 11.3.2.3 True positive rate (TPR)

TPR, the probability of an actual positive testing positive, is calculated as the ratio of the number of true positives to the sum of true positives and false negatives.

$$TPR = \frac{TP}{(TP + FN)}$$

#### 11.3.2.4 False positive rate (FPR)

The FPR is calculated as the ratio of the number of false positives to the sum of false positives and true negatives.

$$FPR = \frac{FP}{(FP + TN)} \tag{11.1}$$

#### 11.3.2.5 Accuracy

The correctness of the model indicates its accuracy – the probability of getting the correct results.

$$Accuracy = \frac{(TN + TP)}{(TN + FN + TP + FP)} \tag{11.2}$$

#### 11.3.2.6 Precision

Precision gives the number of the effectively anticipated cases that really ended up being positive. Wherever false positive is of a higher concern than false negative, it becomes a useful metric.

$$Precision = \frac{TR}{(TP + PN)} \tag{11.3}$$

#### *11.3.2.7 Sensitivity (recall)*

Sensitivity (recall) gives the number of the genuine positive cases we had the option to anticipate effectively with our model. Where false negative trumps false positive, recall is a useful metric.

$$Recall = \frac{TP}{(TP + FN)} \tag{11.4}$$

#### *11.3.2.8 F1 Score*

Generally, there is an inverse relationship between precision and recall. The F1-score incorporates values of precision and recall in itself. It is a harmonic mean of recall and precision, and therefore, it proposes an integrated idea about these two metrics. It reaches peak value when recall is equal to precision.

$$F1\ Score = \frac{2}{\left(\frac{1}{Precision} + \frac{1}{Recall}\right)} \tag{11.5}$$

#### *11.3.2.9 Specificity (true negative rate)*

The fraction where the correct negative predictions in numbers are the numerator and the total number of negatives are the denominator. It is also considered the true negative rate (TNR).

$$\mathrm{SP} = \mathrm{TNR}$$

$$SP = \frac{TN}{N} \tag{11.6}$$

$$SP = \frac{TN}{(TN + FP)} \tag{11.7}$$

#### *11.3.2.10 False positive rate (FPR)*

It is the fraction where incorrect positive predictions in numbers are the numerator and the total number of negatives are the denominator.

$$FPR = 1 - SP \tag{11.8}$$

$$FPR = \frac{FP}{(TN + FP)} \tag{11.9}$$

#### *11.3.2.11 False negative rate (FNR)*

False negative rate (FNR) is false negatives divided by actual positives.

$$FNR = \frac{FN}{(TP + FN)} \tag{11.10}$$

#### *11.3.2.12 False discovery rate (FDR)*

The false positives divided by total positives is the false discovery rate (FDR).

$$FDR = \frac{FP}{(FP + TP)} \tag{11.11}$$

#### *11.3.2.13 Negative predictive value (NPV)*

The number of correct negative predictions are the numerator and the sum of true negatives and false negatives are the denominator. The ratio obtained is the negative predicted value.

$$NPV = \frac{TN}{(TN + FN)} \tag{11.12}$$

#### *11.3.2.14 Matthews correlation coefficient (MCC)*

The Matthews correlation coefficient (MCC) is a correlation coefficient calculated by making use of all four values in the confusion matrix.

$$MCC = \frac{TP.TN - FP.FN}{\surd\{(TP + FP)(TN + FN)(TN + FP)(TP + FN)\}} \tag{11.13}$$

### *11.3.3 Method of analysis*

The machine learning algorithms used are random forest, SVM, ANN, and RNN. The relationship between the independent and its frequency were pictorially represented using histograms, a pie chart depicted the percentage of diabetic and non-diabetic patients, and a heatmap showed all the correlations between the variables (Figures 11.1–11.8).

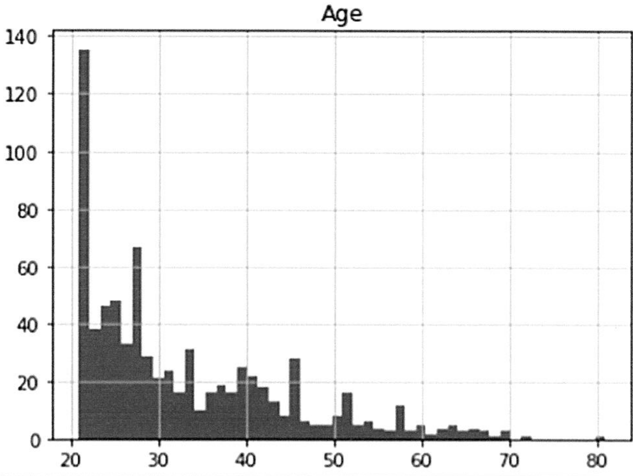


**Figure 11.1 Age histogram.**

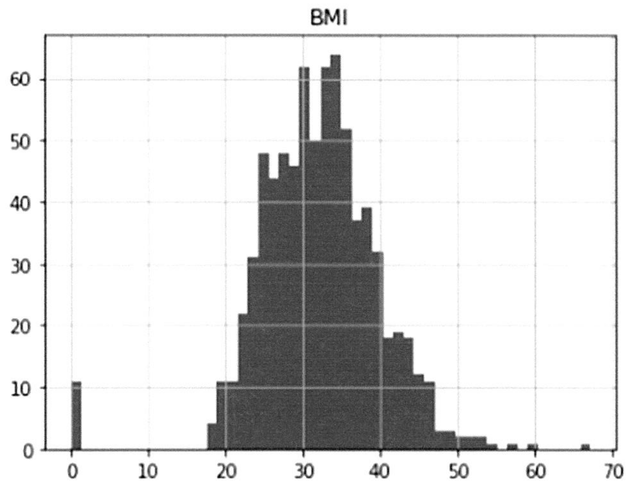


**Figure 11.2 BMI histogram.**

A total of 268 patients (34.8958%) were found to have diabetes and the remaining 500 (65.1041%) were found not to have diabetes (Figure 11.9).

Table 11.2 shows a correlation matrix with the significance level of the study variables (Figure 11.10).

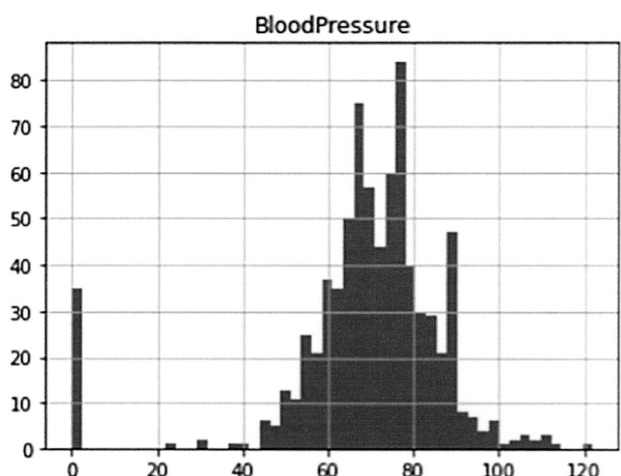


**Figure 11.3 Blood pressure histogram.**

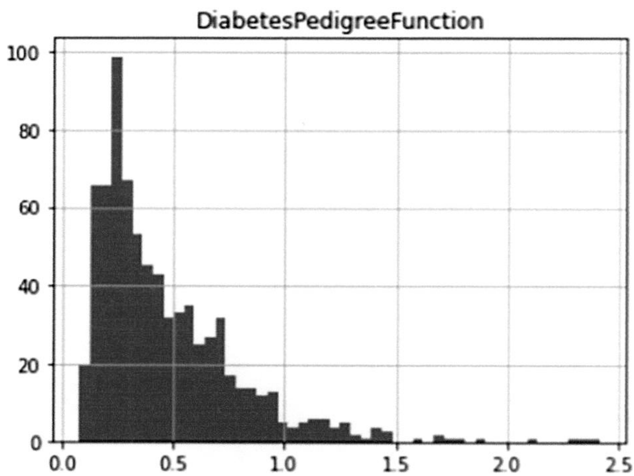


**Figure 11.4 Diabetes pedigree function histogram.**

Based on the algorithm outputs, the diabetics and non-diabetics are compared for number of pregnancies, glucose, blood pressure, skin thickness, insulin, BMI, diabetes pedigree function and age through an independent group t-test presented in Tables 11.3–11.10.

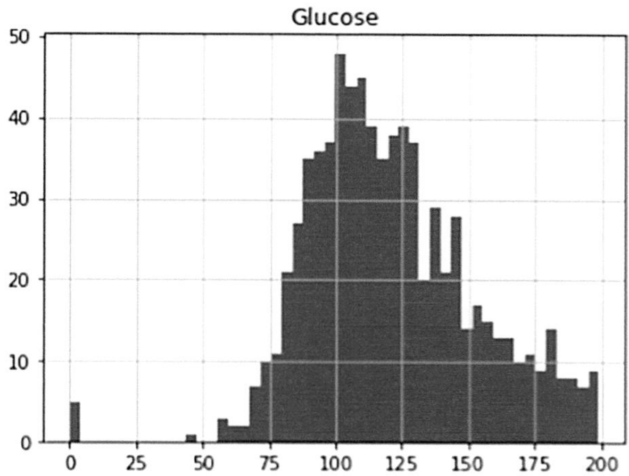


**Figure 11.5 Glucose histogram.**

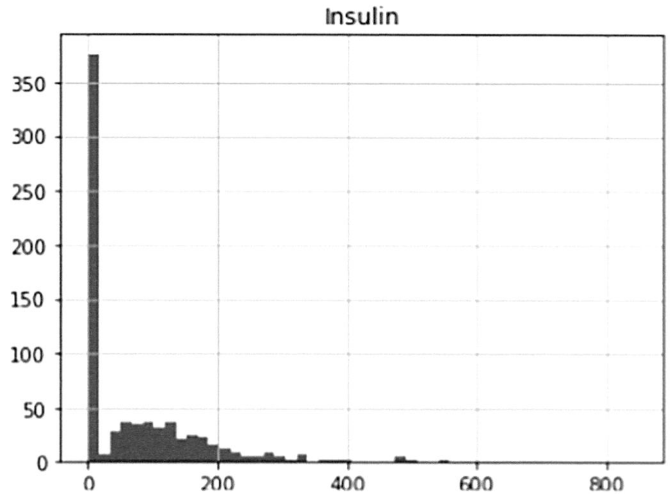


**Figure 11.6 Insulin histogram.**

### *11.3.3.1 Number of Pregnancies*

Table 11.3 and Figure 11.11 show that the mean number of pregnancies of the individuals without diabetes is 3.298 and with diabetes is 4.866. The mean difference is found to be 1.568 and the t-value is 6.298, which is significant at 0.01 level

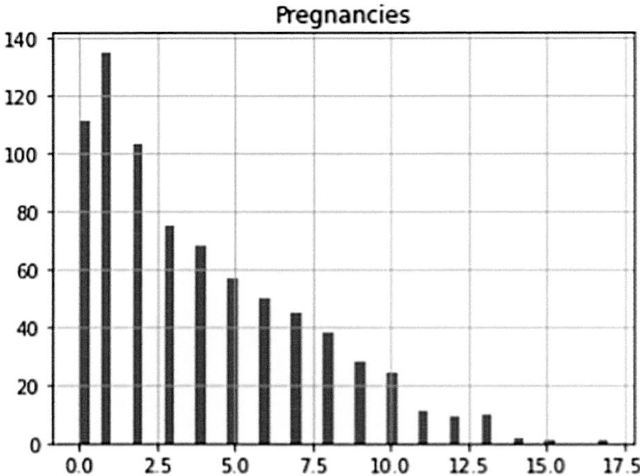


**Figure 11.7 Pregnancies histogram.**

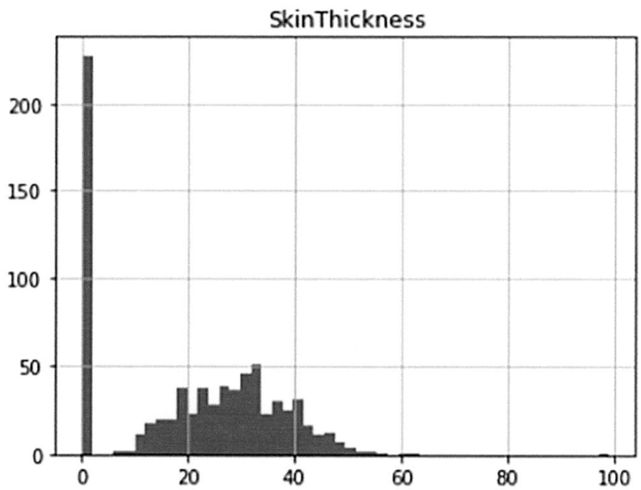


**Figure 11.8 Skin thickness histogram.**

($p < 0.01$). It infers that there is a significant difference in the number of pregnancies of individuals with and without diabetes. Furthermore, the mean score shows that the individuals with diabetes have significantly more pregnancies than those without diabetes.

#### *11.3.3.2 Glucose level*

Table 11.4 compares the glucose levels of individuals with and without diabetes.

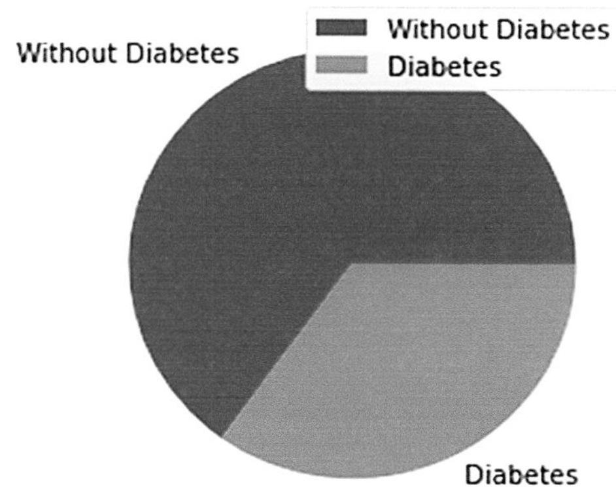


**Figure 11.9 Pie chart for diabetes prevalence.**

Table 11.4 and Figure 11.12 show that the mean glucose level of the individuals without diabetes is 109.980 and that of those with diabetes is 141.257. The mean difference is found to be 31.277 and t-value is found to be 14.600 which is significant at 0.01 level ($p < 0.01$). It infers that there is a significant difference in glucose level of individuals with and without diabetes. Furthermore, the mean score shows that the persons with diabetes have significantly higher glucose levels than those without diabetes.

### *11.3.3.3 Blood pressure*

Table 11.5 compares the blood pressure of individuals with and without diabetes.

Table 11.5 and Figure 11.13 show that the mean blood pressure of the individuals without diabetes is 68.184 and that of those with diabetes is 70.825. The mean difference is found to be 2.641 and the t-value is 1.805, which is insignificant at 0.05 level ($p > 0.05$). It infers that there is no significant difference in the blood pressure of individuals with and without diabetes. Furthermore, the mean score shows that the patients with diabetes and those without diabetes have similar blood pressure levels.

### *11.3.3.4 Skin thickness*

Table 11.6 compares the skin thickness of individuals with and without diabetes.

Table 11.6 and Figure 11.14 show that the mean skin thickness of the individuals without diabetes is 19.664 and that of those with diabetes is 22.164. The mean difference is found to be 2.500 and the t-value is found to be 2.075, which is significant at 0.05 level ($p < 0.05$). It infers that there is a significant difference in skin thickness of individuals with and without diabetes. Furthermore, the mean score shows that the persons with diabetes have significantly more skin thickness than those without diabetes.

**Table 11.2 Correlation Matrix of Study Variables**

| | | *Pregnancies* | *Glucose* | *Blood Pressure* | *Skin Thickness* | *Insulin* | *BMI* | *Diabetes Pedigree Function* | *Age* | *Outcome* |
|---|---|---|---|---|---|---|---|---|---|---|
| Pregnancies | r | 1 | 0.129** | 0.141** | −0.082* | −0.074* | 0.018 | −0.034 | 0.544** | 0.222** |
| | p | | 0.000 | 0.000 | 0.024 | 0.042 | 0.625 | 0.354 | 0.000 | 0.000 |
| | N | 768 | 768 | 768 | 768 | 768 | 768 | 768 | 768 | 768 |
| Glucose | r | 0.129** | 1 | 0.153** | 0.057 | 0.331** | 0.221** | 0.137** | 0.264** | 0.467** |
| | p | 0.000 | | 0.000 | 0.112 | 0.000 | 0.000 | 0.000 | 0.000 | 0.000 |
| | N | 768 | 768 | 768 | 768 | 768 | 768 | 768 | 768 | 768 |
| Blood Pressure | r | 0.141** | 0.153** | 1 | 0.207** | 0.089* | 0.282** | 0.041 | 0.240** | 0.065 |
| | p | 0.000 | 0.000 | | 0.000 | 0.014 | 0.000 | 0.253 | 0.000 | 0.072 |
| | N | 768 | 768 | 768 | 768 | 768 | 768 | 768 | 768 | 768 |
| Skin Thickness | r | −0.082* | 0.057 | 0.207** | 1 | 0.437** | 0.393** | 0.184** | −0.114** | 0.075* |
| | p | 0.024 | 0.112 | 0.000 | | 0.000 | 0.000 | 0.000 | 0.002 | 0.038 |
| | N | 768 | 768 | 768 | 768 | 768 | 768 | 768 | 768 | 768 |
| Insulin | r | −0.074* | 0.331** | 0.089* | 0.437** | 1 | 0.198** | 0.185** | −0.042 | 0.131** |
| | p | 0.042 | 0.000 | 0.014 | 0.000 | | 0.000 | 0.000 | 0.243 | 0.000 |
| | N | 768 | 768 | 768 | 768 | 768 | 768 | 768 | 768 | 768 |

*(Continued)*

| | | Pregnancies | Glucose | Blood Pressure | Skin Thickness | Insulin | BMI | Diabetes Pedigree Function | Age | Outcome |
|---|---|---|---|---|---|---|---|---|---|---|
| BMI | r | 0.018 | 0.221** | 0.282** | 0.393** | 0.198** | 1 | 0.141** | 0.036 | 0.293** |
| | p | 0.625 | 0.000 | 0.000 | .000 | 0.000 | | 0.000 | 0.316 | 0.000 |
| | N | 768 | 768 | 768 | 768 | 768 | 768 | 768 | 768 | 768 |
| Diabetes Pedigree Function | r | −0.034 | 0.137** | 0.041 | 0.184** | 0.185** | 0.141** | 1 | 0.034 | 0.174** |
| | p | 0.354 | 0.000 | 0.253 | 0.000 | 0.000 | 0.000 | | 0.353 | 0.000 |
| | N | 768 | 768 | 768 | 768 | 768 | 768 | 768 | 768 | 768 |
| Age | r | 0.544** | 0.264** | 0.240** | −0.114** | −0.042 | 0.036 | 0.034 | 1 | 0.238** |
| | p | 0.000 | 0.000 | 0.000 | 0.002 | 0.243 | 0.316 | 0.353 | | 0.000 |
| | N | 768 | 768 | 768 | 768 | 768 | 768 | 768 | 768 | 768 |
| Outcome | r | 0.222** | 0.467** | 0.065 | 0.075* | 0.131** | 0.293** | 0.174** | 0.238** | 1 |
| | p | 0.000 | 0.000 | 0.072 | 0.038 | 0.000 | 0.000 | 0.000 | 0.000 | |
| | N | 768 | 768 | 768 | 768 | 768 | 768 | 768 | 768 | 768 |

** Correlation is significant at the 0.01 level.
* Correlation is significant at the 0.05 level.

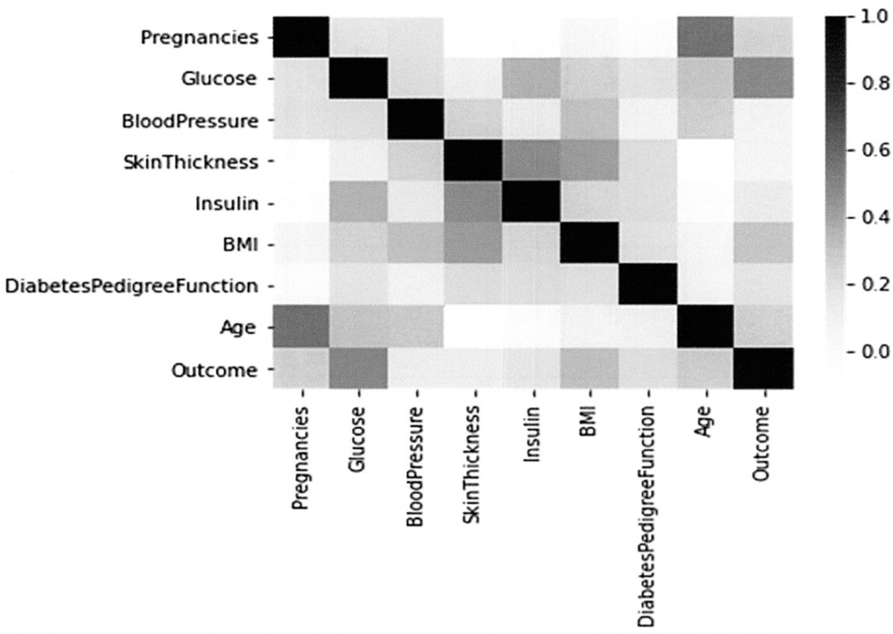


Figure 11.10 Correlation heat map of study variables.

**Table 11.3 Comparison of Number of Pregnancies of individuals with and without diabetes**

| | *Pregnancies* | |
|---|---|---|
| | *No Diabetes* | *Diabetes* |
| N | 500 | 268 |
| Mean | 3.298 | 4.866 |
| Std. Deviation | 3.017 | 3.741 |
| Std. Error Mean | 0.135 | 0.229 |
| Mean Difference | –1.568 | |
| t′ | 6.298 | |
| p value | 0.000 | |

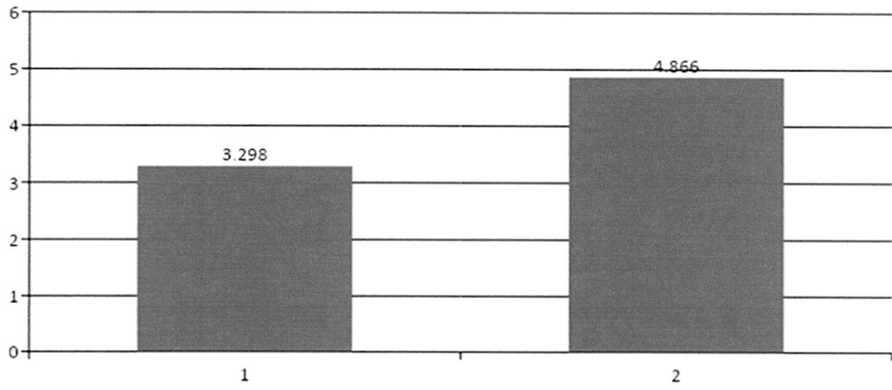


**Figure 11.11 Comparison of number of pregnancies of individuals with and without diabetes.**

**Table 11.4 Comparison of Glucose Level of Individuals with and without Diabetes**

| | *Glucose Level* | |
|---|---|---|
| | *No Diabetes* | *Diabetes* |
| N | 500 | 268 |
| Mean | 109.980 | 141.257 |
| Std. deviation | 26.141 | 31.940 |
| Std. error mean | 1.169 | 1.951 |
| Mean difference | –31.277 | |
| t′ | 14.600 | |
| p value | 0.000 | |

### *11.3.3.5 Insulin*

Table 11.7 compares insulin levels of individuals with and without diabetes.

Table 11.7 and Figure 11.15 show that the mean insulin level of individuals without diabetes is 68.792 and that of those with diabetes is 100.336. The mean difference is found to be 31.544 and the t-value is found to be 3.644 which is

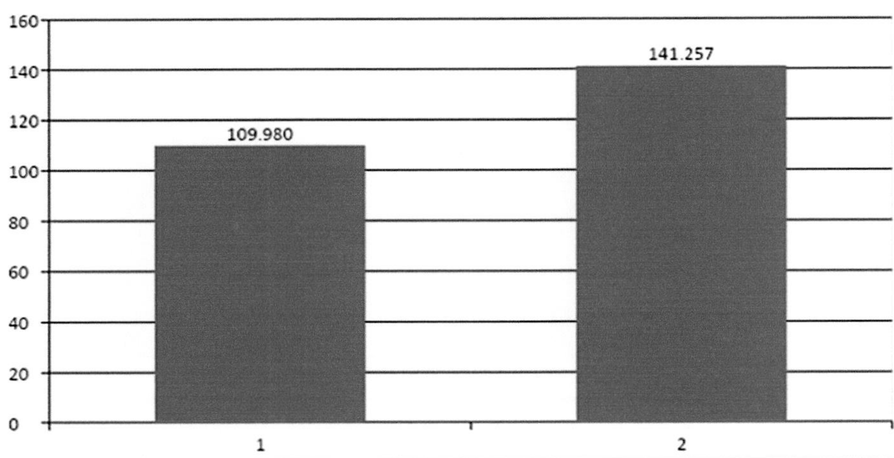


**Figure 11.12 Comparison of glucose level of individuals with and without diabetes.**

**Table 11.5 Comparison of Blood Pressure of Individuals with and without Diabetes**

| | *Blood Pressure* | |
|---|---|---|
| | *No Diabetes* | *Diabetes* |
| N | 500 | 268 |
| Mean | 68.184 | 70.825 |
| Std. deviation | 18.063 | 21.492 |
| Std. error mean | 0.808 | 1.313 |
| Mean difference | –2.641 | |
| t′ | 1.805 | |
| p value | 0.072 | |

significant at 0.01 level ($p < 0.01$). It infers that there is a significant difference in insulin levels of individuals with and without diabetes. Furthermore, the mean score shows that the persons with diabetes have significantly higher insulin levels than those without diabetes.

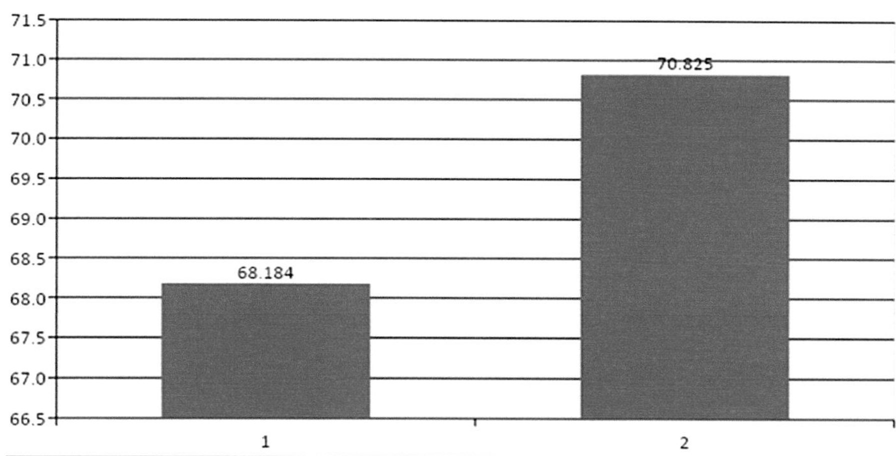


**Figure 11.13 Comparison of blood pressure of individuals with and without diabetes.**

**Table 11.6 Comparison of Skin Thickness of Individuals with and without Diabetes**

| | *Skin Thickness* | |
|---|---|---|
| | *No Diabetes* | *Diabetes* |
| N | 500 | 268 |
| Mean | 19.664 | 22.164 |
| Std. deviation | 14.890 | 17.680 |
| Std. error mean | 0.666 | 1.080 |
| Mean difference | –2.500 | |
| t′ | 2.075 | |
| p value | 0.038 | |

### *11.3.3.6 Body mass index (BMI)*

Table 11.8 compares the body mass index (BMI) of individuals with and without diabetes.

Table 11.8 and Figure 11.16 show that the mean BMI of the individuals without diabetes is 30.304 and with diabetes it is 34.143. The mean difference is found

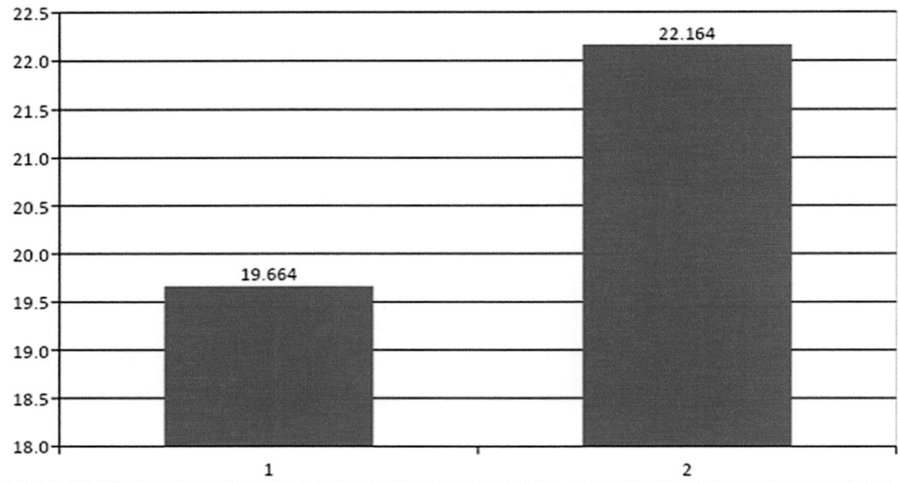


**Figure 11.14 Comparison of skin thickness of individuals with and without diabetes.**

**Table 11.7 Comparison of Insulin Levels of Individuals with and without Diabetes**

| | *Insulin* | |
|---|---|---|
| | *No Diabetes* | *Diabetes* |
| N | 500 | 268 |
| Mean | 68.792 | 100.336 |
| Std. deviation | 98.865 | 138.689 |
| Std. error mean | 4.421 | 8.472 |
| Mean difference | –31.544 | |
| t′ | 3.644 | |
| p value | 0.000 | |

to be 4.838 and the t-value is found to be 8.472 which is significant at 0.01 level ($p < 0.01$). It infers that there is significant difference in BMI between individuals with and without diabetes. Furthermore, the mean score shows that the persons with diabetes have a significantly higher BMI than those without diabetes.

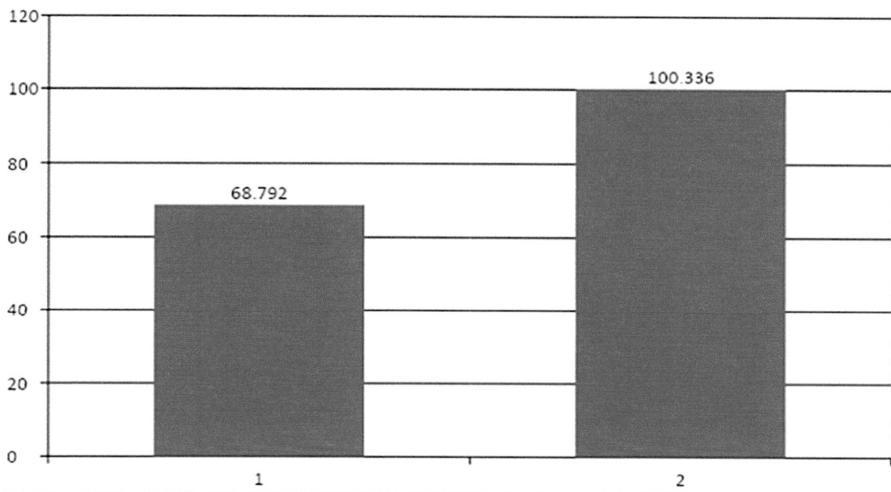


**Figure 11.15 Comparison of insulin levels of individuals with and without diabetes.**

**Table 11.8 Comparison of Body Mass Index (BMI) of Individuals with and without Diabetes**

| | *Body Mass Indwex (BMI)* | |
|---|---|---|
| | *No Diabetes* | *Diabetes* |
| N | 500 | 268 |
| Mean | 30.304 | 35.143 |
| Std. deviation | 7.690 | 7.263 |
| Std. error mean | 0.344 | 0.444 |
| Mean difference | –4.838 | |
| t′ | 8.472 | |
| p value | 0.000 | |

### *11.3.3.7 Diabetes pedigree function*

Table 11.9 compares the diabetes pedigree function of individuals with and without diabetes.

Table 11.9 and Figure 11.17 show that the mean diabetes pedigree function score of the individuals without diabetes is 0.430 and with diabetes it is 0.551. The

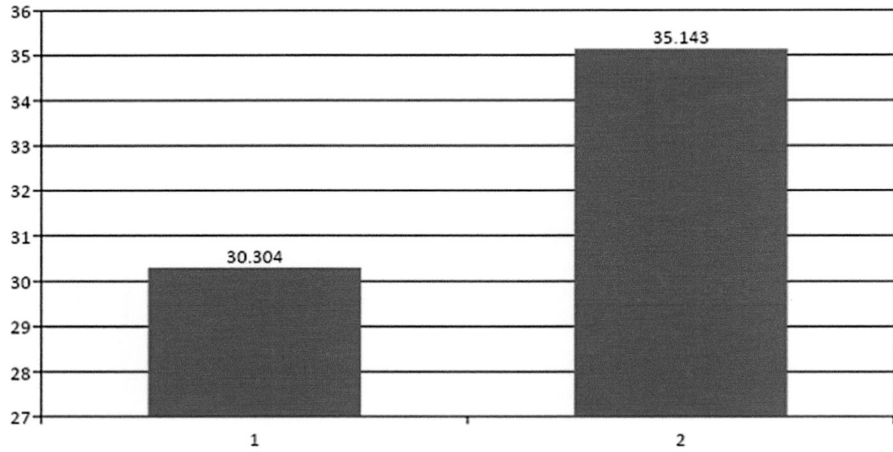


**Figure 11.16 Comparison of Body Mass Index (BMI) of individuals with and without diabetes.**

**Table 11.9 Comparison of Diabetes Pedigree Function of Individuals with and without Diabetes**

| | *Diabetes Pedigree Function* | |
|---|---|---|
| | *No Diabetes* | *Diabetes* |
| N | 500 | 268 |
| Mean | 0.430 | 0.551 |
| Std. deviation | 0.299 | 0.372 |
| Std. error mean | 0.013 | 0.023 |
| Mean difference | −0.121 | |
| t′ | 4.886 | |
| p value | 0.000 | |

mean difference is found to be 0.121 and the t-value is found to be 4.886, which is significant at 0.01 level ($p < 0.01$). It infers that there is a significant difference in the diabetes pedigree function scores of individuals with and without diabetes. Furthermore, the mean score shows that persons with diabetes have significantly higher diabetes pedigree function scores than those without diabetes.

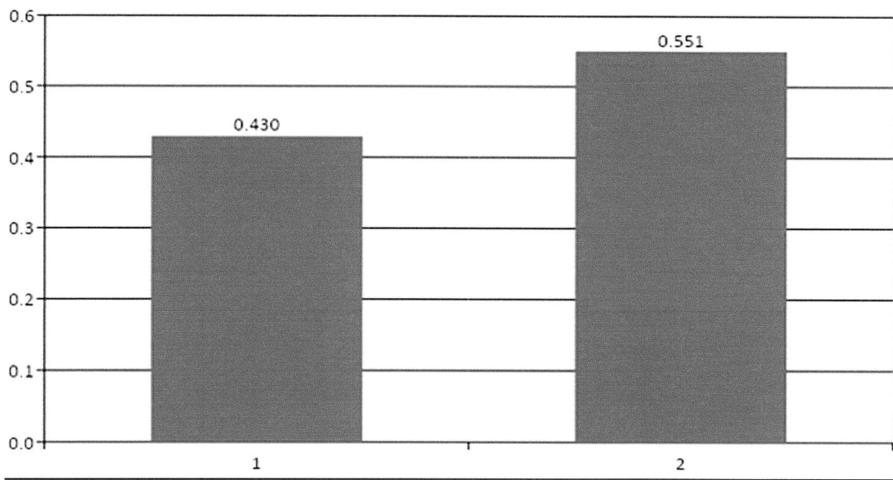


**Figure 11.17 Comparison of diabetes pedigree function of individuals with and without diabetes.**

**Table 11.10 Comparison of Age (in Years) of Individuals with and without Diabetes**

| | *Age* | |
|---|---|---|
| | *No Diabetes* | *Diabetes* |
| N | 500 | 268 |
| Mean | 31.190 | 37.067 |
| Std. deviation | 11.668 | 10.968 |
| Std. error mean | 0.522 | 0.670 |
| Mean difference | –5.877 | |
| t′ | 6.793 | |
| p value | 0.000 | |

## *11.3.3.8 Age*

Table 11.10 compares the ages (in years) of individuals with and without diabetes.

Table 11.10 and Figure 11.18 show that the mean age of the individuals without diabetes is 31.190 and that of those with diabetes is 37.067. The mean difference is found to be 5.877 and the t-value is found to be 6.793, which is significant at 0.01

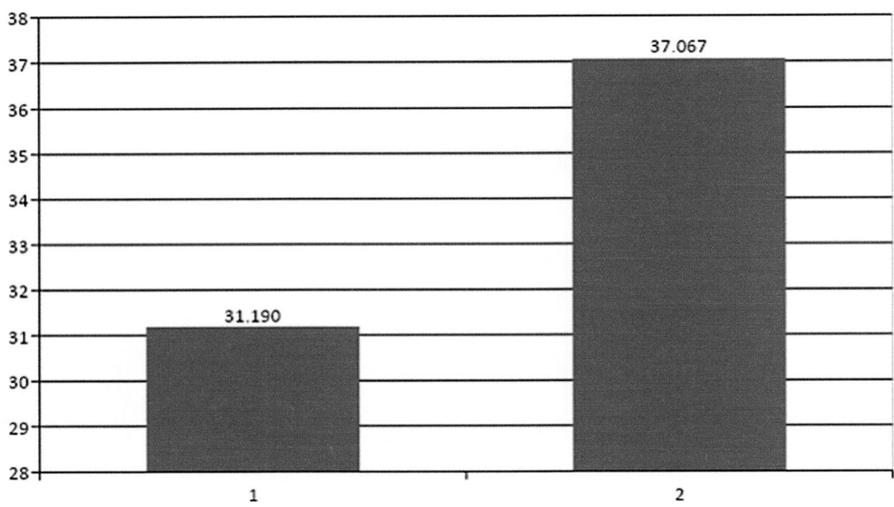


**Figure 11.18 Comparison of Age (in years) of individuals with and without diabetes.**

level (p s 0.01). It infers that there is a significant difference in the age of individuals with and without diabetes. Furthermore, the mean score shows that the persons with diabetes are significantly older than those without diabetes.

## 11.4 Machine Learning Algorithms

### *11.4.1 Random forest algorithm*

One of the popular machine learning algorithms based on the supervised learning technique is random forest. Initially random samples are selected from the given dataset and are referred to as bootstrap data. Thereafter, multiple decision trees are constructed through selected random samples and prediction results are acquired from every decision tree. For every predicted result voting is performed, and finally the prediction result with the highest votes is selected. The main advantage of using random forest is that it runs efficiently even for large datasets without compromising accuracy.

### *11.4.2 XGBoost algorithm*

This is a machine learning algorithm based on decision trees that uses a gradient boosting framework. It is often used for unstructured data. XGBoost improves on the base gradient boosting framework through parallelized building of decision trees and tree pruning using the DFS approach. It also handles missing data efficiently; however, our dataset does not have any missing data.

### *11.4.3 Support vector machine (SVM)*

One of the most popular supervised learning algorithms, which is used for both regression and classification problems, is SVM. It is generally used for image classification, face detection, handwriting detection and many other use cases. The data points, represented in spaces, are mapped in such a way that data points are separated into different categories by a wide gap.

### *11.4.4 Artificial neural network (ANN)*

In an ANN, the neurons are connected to one another in distinct network layers, like a human brain. These neurons are known as nodes. Different activation functions are used in different layers. The most commonly used optimization method is gradient descent. The task is performed in two phases: forward propagation and backward propagation. The movement from the input layer to the output layer is forward propagation, whereas the movement from the output layer to the input layer is backward propagation.

## 11.5 Result and Analysis

The random forest classifier performed classification on the test dataset, which was regarded as unseen data. The model was never trained on this data before. The model was fitted with the dependent variable and the test was run on the default parameters, producing an accuracy of 81.168%. Figures 11.19 and 11.20 show the confusion matrix and ROC curve resulting from this model.

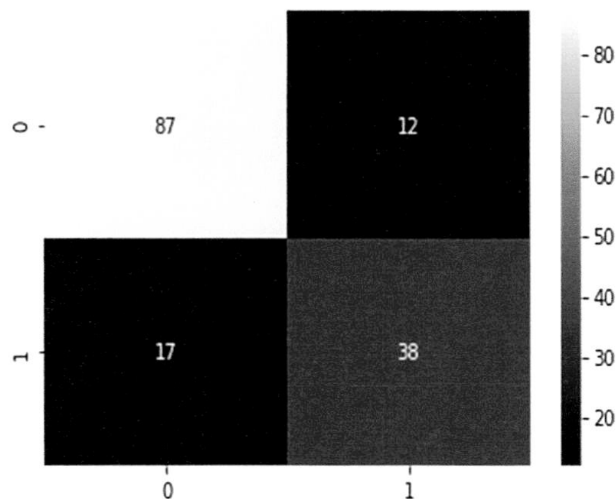


**Figure 11.19 Confusion matrix of random forest classifier.**

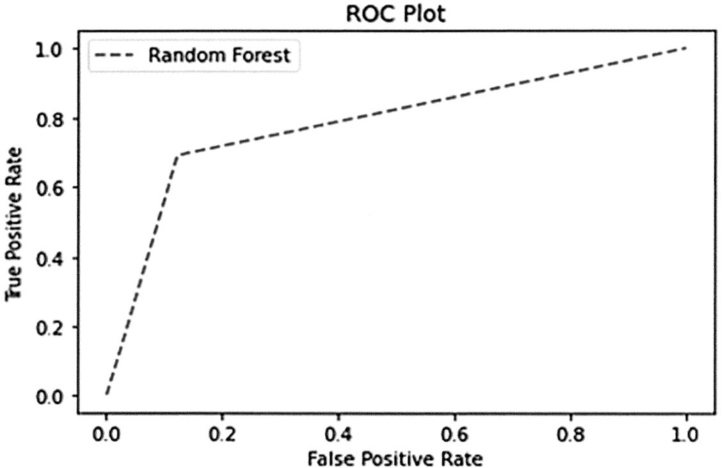


**Figure 11.20 ROC curve of random forest classifier.**

The SVM classifier performed classification on the test set, which was regarded as unseen data. The model was never trained on this data before. The dependent variable was encoded and feature scaling was performed. A linear kernel was used. The model was fitted with the dependent variable and the test was run on the default parameters which produced an accuracy of 82.467%. Figures 11.21 and 11.22 show the confusion matrix and ROC curve resulting from this model.

The XGBoost classifier performed classification on the test set, which was regarded as unseen data. The model was never trained on this data before. The dependent variable was encoded and the model fitted for classification. The model

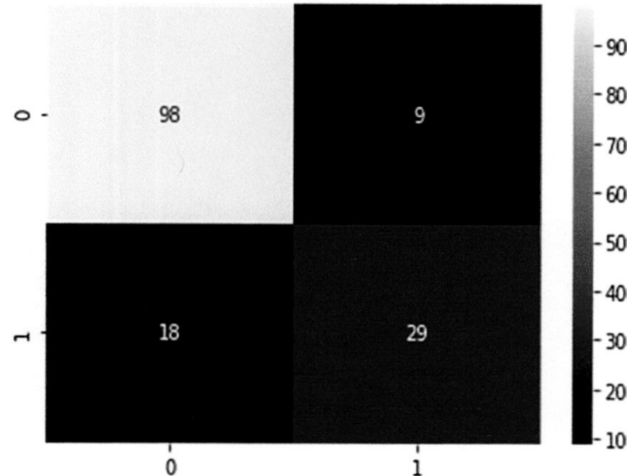


**Figure 11.21 Confusion matrix of SVM classifier.**

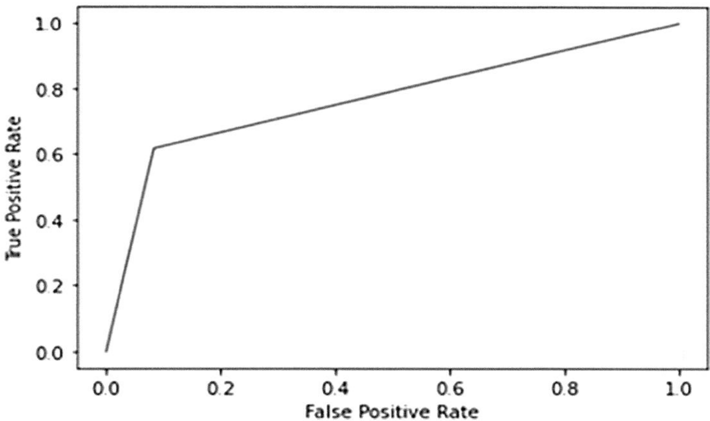


**Figure 11.22 ROC curve of SVM classifier.**

was fitted with the dependent variable and the test was run on the default parameters which produced an accuracy of 81.818%. Figures 11.23 and 11.24) show the confusion matrix and ROC curve resulting from this model.

The ANN was built to perform classification on the dataset, which was regarded as unseen data. The model was never trained on this data before. The 'relu' and 'sigmoid' activation functions were used. The 'Adam' optimizer and binary cross entropy loss was used. It was trained on 100 epochs having a batch size of 32. The model was fitted with the dependent variable and the test was run on the default

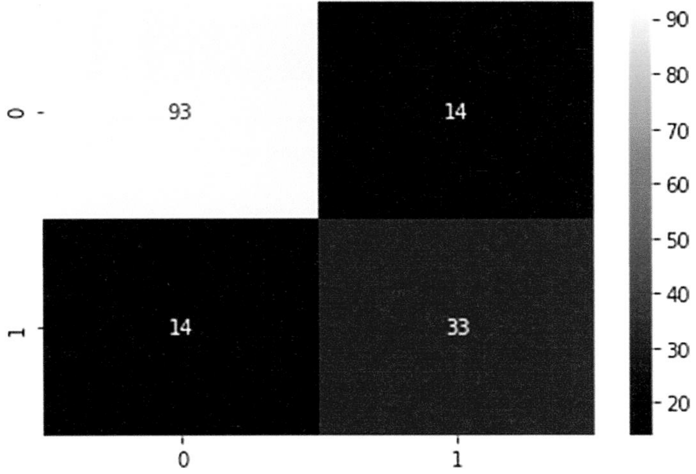


**Figure 11.23 Confusion matrix of XGBoost classifier.**

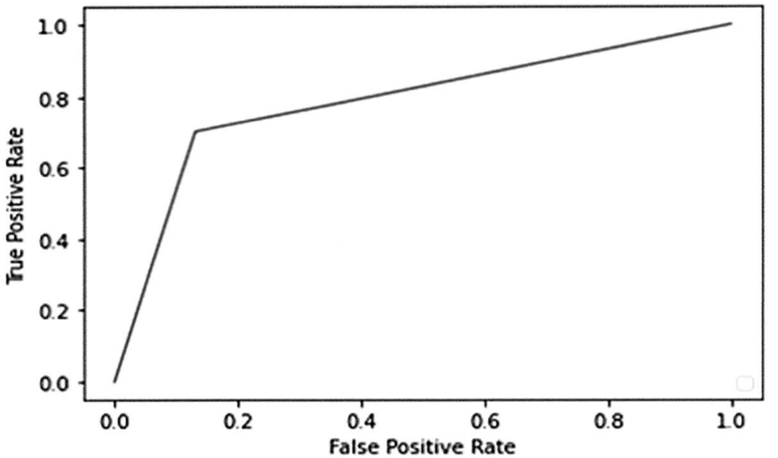


**Figure 11.24 ROC curve of XGBoost classifier.**

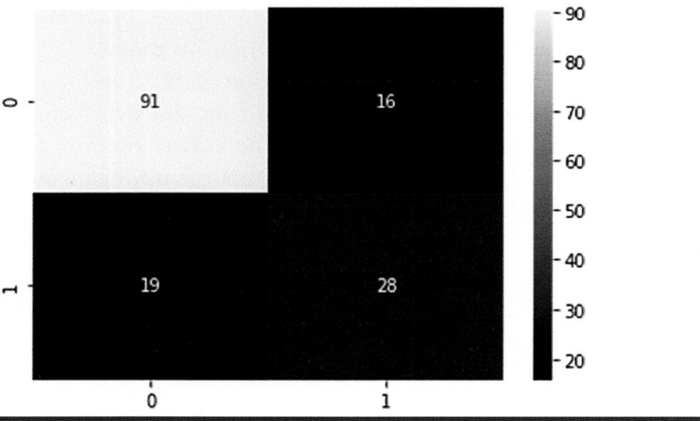


**Figure 11.25 Confusion matix of ANN classifier.**

parameters which produced an accuracy of 77.272%. Figures 11.25 and 11.26 show the confusion matrix and ROC curve resulting from this model.

The accuracy of selected classifier models is compared in Table 11.11.

The predicted indicators of the selected classifier models are depicted in Tables 11.12–11.15.

Table 11.12 shows the evaluation parameters of random forest model in which accuracy is 0.81168, precision is 0.76000, F1 score 0.72380, sensitivity (recall) is 0.69090 and the specificity is 0.87878. Table 11.3 also indicates the FPR as 0.12121, FNR as 0.30909, NPV as 0.85653, FDR as 0.24000 and the MCC as 0.58296 for the random forest model.

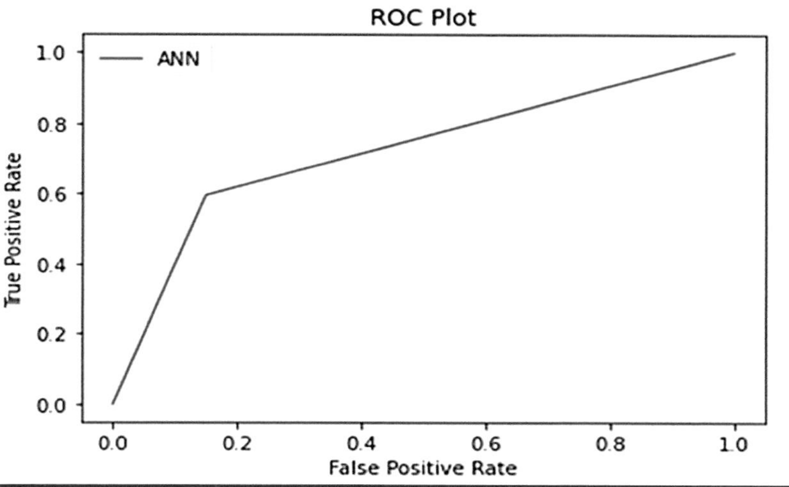


**Figure 11.26 ROC curve of ANN classifier.**

**Table 11.11 Accuracy of Selected Classifier Models**

| *Models* | *Accuracy (in %)* |
|---|---|
| **Random forest classifier** | 81.168 |
| **SVM classifier** | 82.467 |
| **XGBoost classifier** | 81.818 |
| **ANN classifier** | 72.272 |

**Table 11.12 Evaluation Parameters of Random Forest**

| *Accuracy* | *Precision* | *F1-Score* | *Sensitivity(Recall)* | *Specificity* |
|---|---|---|---|---|
| 0.81168 | 0.76000 | 0.72380 | 0.69090 | 0.87878 |
| FPR | FNR | NPV | FDR | MCC |
| 0.12121 | 0.30909 | 0.83653 | 0.24000 | 0.58296 |

Table 11.13 presents the evaluation parameters of SVM, in which accuracy is 0.82467, precision is 0.76315, F1 score 0.68235, sensitivity (recall) is 0.61702 and specificity is 0.91588.Table 11.3 also visualizes the FPR as 0.08411, FNR as 0.38297, NPV as 0.84482, FDR as 0.23684 and the MCC as 0.56921 for SVM.

**Table 11.13 Evaluation Parameters of SVM**

| *Accuracy* | *Precision* | *F1-Score* | *Sensitivity(Recall)* | *Specificity* |
|---|---|---|---|---|
| 0.82467 | 0.76315 | 0.68235 | 0.61702 | 0.91588 |
| FPR | FNR | NPV | FDR | MCC |
| 0.08411 | 0.38297 | 0.84482 | 0.23684 | 0.56921 |

**Table 11.14 Evaluation Parameters of XGBoost**

| *Accuracy* | *Precision* | *F1-Score* | *Sensitivity(Recall)* | *Specificity* |
|---|---|---|---|---|
| 0.81818 | 0.70212 | 0.70212 | 0.70212 | 0.86915 |
| FPR | FNR | NPV | FDR | MCC |
| 0.13084 | 0.29787 | 0.86915 | 0.29787 | 0.57128 |

**Table 11.15 Evaluation Parameters of ANN**

| *Accuracy* | *Precision* | *F1-Score* | *Sensitivity(Recall)* | *Specificity* |
|---|---|---|---|---|
| 0.77272 | 0.63636 | 0.61538 | 0.59574 | 0.85046 |
| FPR | FNR | NPV | FDR | MCC |
| 0.14953 | 0.40425 | 0.82727 | 0.36363 | 0.45484 |

Table 11.14 reflects the evaluation parameters of XGBoost, in which accuracy is 0.81818, precision is 0.70212, F1 score 0.70212, sensitivity (recall) is 0.70212 and specificity is 0.86915. Table 11.5 also represents the FPR as 0.13084, FNR as 0.29787, NPV as 0.86915, FDR as 0.29787 and the MCC as 0.57128 for XGBoost.

Table 11.15 explores the evaluation parameters of ANN in which accuracy is 0.77272, precision is 0.63636, F1 score 0.61538, the sensitivity (recall) is found to be 0.59574 and the specificity is 0.85046. The Table 11.5 also shows the FPR as 0.14953, FNR as 0.40425, NPV as 0.82727, FDR as 0.36363 and the MCC as 0.45484 for ANN.

## 11.6 Conclusion

This research work has compared the accuracy of different deep learning and machine learning classification models on the dataset provided for classifying patients as diabetic or non-diabetic. The SVM classifier showed the highest accuracy of 82.467%.

The model can be used by different medical organizations for rapid detection of diabetes so that the patient can be provided with further treatment.

## References


1. National Institute of Diabetes and Digestive and Kidney Diseases. https://www.niddk.nih.gov/health-information/diabetes/overview/what-is-diabetes (accessed 16-08-2021).
2. https://www.diabetesatlas.org/upload/resources/material/20200302_133351_IDFATLAS9e-final-web.pdf (accessed 19-08-2021).
3. https://www.who.int/india/Campaigns/and/events/world-diabetes-day#:~:text=Diabetes%20is%20a%20growing%20challenge,of%2020%20and%2070%20years (accessed 18-08-2021).
4. Kononenko, I. (2001). Machine Learning for Medical Diagnosis: History, State of the Art and Perspective. *Artificial Intelligence in Medicine*, 23(1), 89–109. https://doi.org/10.1016/s0933-3657(01)00077-x (accessed 19-08-2021).
5. Omodunbi, B. A., Okomba, N.S., Olaniyan, O.M., Esan, A., and Adewa, T. A. (2021). Development of a Diabetes Melitus Detection and Prediction Model Using Light Gradient Boosting Machine and K-Nearest Neighbour. *UNIOSUN Journal of Engineering and Environmental Sciences*, 3(1), 28–35.
6. Xue, J., Min, F., and Ma, F. (2020). Research on Diabetes Prediction Method Based on Machine Learning. *Journal of Physics: Conference Series*, 1684, 012062.
7. Swapna, G., Vinayakumar, R., and Soman, K.P. (2018). Diabetes Detection Using Deep Learning Algorithms. *ICT Express*, 4(4), 243–246.
8. Alić, B., Gurbeta, L., and Badnjević, A. (2017). Machine Learning Techniques for Classification of Diabetes and Cardiovascular Diseases. *2017 6th Mediterranean Conference on Embedded Computing (MECO)*, pp. 1–4. https://doi.org/10.1109/MECO.2017.7977152.
9. Santhanam, T., and Padmavathi, M.S. (2015). Application of K-Means and Genetic Algorithms for Dimension Reduction by Integrating SVM for Diabetes Diagnosis. *Procedia Computer Science*, 47, 76–83. https://doi.org/10.1016/j.procs.2015.03.185.
10. Iyer, A., Jeyalatha, S., and Sumbaly, R. (2015). Diagnosis of Diabetes Using Classification Mining Techniques. *International Journal of Data Mining & Knowledge Management Process*, 5, 1–14. https://doi.org/10.5121/ijdkp.2015.5101.
11. Islam, M., and Jahan, N. (2017). Prediction of Onset Diabetes using Machine Learning Techniques. *International Journal of Computer Applications*, 180, 7–11. https://doi.org/10.5120/ijca2017916020.
12. Soni, K. M., Gupta, A., and Jain, T. (2021).` Supervised Machine Learning Approaches for Breast Cancer Classification and a high performance Recurrent Neural Network. *2021 Third International Conference on Inventive Research in Computing Applications (ICIRCA)*, 1–7. https://doi.org/10.1109/ICIRCA51532.2021.9544630.
13. Jain, T., Jain, A., Hada, P. S., Kumar, H., Verma, V. K., and Patni, A. (2021). Machine Learning Techniques for Prediction of Mental Health. *2021 Third International Conference on Inventive Research in Computing Applications (ICIRCA)*, 1606–1613. https://doi.org/10.1109/ICIRCA51532.2021.9545061.

# Chapter 12

# Use of Machine Learning in Healthcare

Ishita Mehta and Arnaav Anand
*Manipal University, Jaipur, India*

## Contents

12.1 Introduction ....................................................................................237
12.2 Literature Survey..............................................................................240
    12.2.1 Learning Insulin–Glucose Dynamics in the Wild .......................242
    12.2.2 MRI-Based Diagnosis of Rotator Cuff Tears Using Deep Learning and Weighted Linear Combinations..................243
    12.2.3 Transferring Learning from Well Curated to Less Resourced Populations with HIV ...........................................................244
    12.2.4 Early Diagnosis of Epilepsy from EEG Data..............................245
    12.2.5 Evaluation of Doctor Interpretability of Generalized Additive Models with Interactions............................................246
12.3 Conclusion ......................................................................................248
References ..............................................................................................249

## 12.1 Introduction

The onset of the 21st century was a new beginning for an entirely new generation of technology, software, and computers. The amount of time, effort, money, and research that went into this new generation helped bring about massive advances in the field which had been of little relevance just a few years before. People started to focus on technologies like artificial intelligence, data science, machine learning,

DOI: 10.1201/9781003322597-12

and deep learning to help them with problems ranging from their day-to-day activities to solving complex problems in such fields as healthcare, medicine, agriculture, defense, and science.

The simplest definition of machine learning is a form of artificial intelligence where computers can be programmed in such a way that they can learn information and process data without the intervention of any human. Machine learning can also be described as a way by which a machine learns with the help of data. When a machine is supplied with data, it is first processed, and then interpreted to find underlying patterns and algorithms being used, in order to determine the correct relation between the pieces of data we have to hand.

This chapter focuses on the use of machine learning in the healthcare sector. Machine learning is now being widely used in various ways in medicine and healthcare, not only make the lives of healthcare workers easier, but to also help save millions of lives through ongoing research work in the field. The healthcare industry is one of the fastest growing and most extensively funded industries, with the US medical industry alone currently generating an annual revenue of nearly US$1.8 trillion. Developments are proceeding in healthcare more rapidly than in any other field, making the use of modern technologies like artificial intelligence even more important in progress towards a better and healthier future for future generations. This growing relationship between technology and healthcare gives us a glimpse into a future where millions of lives will be saved with the help of data, innovation, and analytics. While there is still a long way to go towards a future where everything in healthcare works with the help of AI, currently there are quite a few applications of ML in healthcare which are helping to save lives, maintain records, and diagnose patterns which can contribute to saving people from deadly diseases.

The applications mentioned below are among the important aspects of healthcare where machine learning is being applied extensively:

*Maintaining Health Records.* Maintaining and storing previous health records of patients has traditionally been difficult for both institutions and patients. Precious time and effort were often wasted searching for records which might no longer even exist. While smart devices have helped speed up the process of storing these data, it is still time-consuming to capture and safely store them for a longer period. But, with the help of document classification techniques in ML like vector machines and OCR engines for handwriting recognition, the process is starting to become straightforward, with all medical records being updated regularly on a cloud-based platform, accessible whenever needed.

*Manufacturing of Drugs and Vaccines.* If there was ever a question about the importance of continuous research and development of new drugs and vaccines, the COVID-19 pandemic ensured that no such doubt remained. With technologies like next-generation sequencing and precision medicine that aid in discovering alternate ways to treat multifactorial diseases, the prime clinical use of ML is in early-stage drug discovery. With the ability to identify patterns in data, unsupervised learning is an important part of this discovery process, which has so far helped find more suitable drugs to treat diseases including leukemia, pneumonia and malaria.

*Disease Identification and Diagnostics*. Some diseases and conditions are very hard to diagnose at an early stage, causing loss of life due to the delay in getting the right treatment. The prime example is early-stage detection of cancer. There are times when the exact location of tumorous cells is not detected until the cancer has reached a higher or a fatal stage. We can make use of technology to detect defective cells at an earlier stage. A prime example is IBM's Watson for Genomics, a technology that makes use of cognitive computing with genome-based tumor sequencing to enable diagnosis at an earlier stage when the chances of survival and full recovery of the patient are higher. In oncology, AI is being used to discover various therapeutic treatments. In mental health, PReDicT (Predicting Response to Depression Treatment) is trying to find a feasible way to diagnose and treat regular medical conditions which people often ignore.

*Medical Imaging*. Another important field in artificial intelligence is computer vision, a technology that makes use of both machine learning and deep learning to process various digital inputs, images, and videos. This technology is being used in various parts of the healthcare sector to create medical imagery – which is just a stepping stone to a world driven by AI-dominated diagnostic processes.

*Clinical Trials and Research Work*. The potential that ML has in the field of trials is yet to be fully reached, but the foundation is there to build towards a brighter future. The amount of time and money consumed during trials and research for any new drug sample to be passed for public usage is quite high. But with ML-based predictive analysis highlighting potential trials and their success rates, researchers can reach conclusions more quickly and with the data points marked, the process can also be made hassle-free.

*Prediction of Disease Outbreaks*. One of the most useful aspects of ML is its ability to make predictions from various data points and interpretations using various sources like social media, satellites, websites, etc. This is currently being used to make predictions and monitor the status of disease outbreaks in a particular region, the onset of an epidemic or even a pandemic, which can help in early detection and help stop the outbreak as early as possible. With the help of ANN, we can correlate all the relevant information and predict everything from a small outbreak of dengue to the spread of a new COVID variant at a global level. This technology is only going to grow as we move into the future, with Third-World countries being the biggest beneficiaries of potential preparation for medical emergencies.

*Radiotherapy Practices*. Radiotherapy is another field where ML plays a vital role. ML-based algorithms are mostly trained with the help of many samples, making it more reliable when it comes to the detection of lesions, tumors, cancer foci, etc. In medical image analysis, objects are classified in greater detail than with normal analysis. This technology assists with differentiating normal cells from cancerous ones and thus helps in the treatment of patients with radiation.

*Behavioral Modifications using ML.* Ever since the introduction of ML in the field of healthcare, much work has been done to identify and prevent the onset of disease at an early stage, which decreases the risk of it being fatal. With the help of data analytics that recognizes gestures and day-to-day habits of individuals, we can monitor any unconscious changes in the behavior or actions of the individual. This helps in finding and dealing with any abnormalities in due time.

*Making Personalized Treatment Plans.* A doctor treating a patient is working with a limited dataset. Treatment depends more on the generalized reaction to a medicine experienced by people with similar issues than on creating personalized treatment techniques for every person depending on how their body reacts. But with the help of ML, there is now a chance for personalized treatment for every person, depending on their long-term medical records. The development of several types of biosensors and health measurement devices is also well under way and will soon be available for public use to help every individual maintain up-to-date data about what suits them and what does not.

## 12.2 Literature Survey

With the enormous technological revolutions that have been taking place in recent years, machine learning has brought about a major impact on our lives by transforming all sectors including healthcare services, education, transport, food, entertainment, and many more.

The widespread adoption of machine learning algorithms happens to be the result of the availability of exceedingly large datasets and advances in computational strategies which contribute towards reducing overfitting, hence improving the generalization of trained models. These factors have been the key to speedy popularization and adoption of machine learning in almost every possible field we can think of. This, along with the increasing prevalence of interconnected devices or the internet of things (IoT), has created a rich infrastructure upon which to build predictive and automated systems.

Machine learning algorithms are broadly split into supervised and unsupervised learning. Both categories comprise a variety of algorithms that are used to implement mathematical models.

- Supervised learning comprises labeled training data. They mainly focus on classification and regression problems. Some examples of supervised learning algorithms are: random forest, decision trees, naïve Bayes models, and support vector machine (SVM).

- Unsupervised learning uses unlabeled data for model training. The most common algorithms for unsupervised learning are K-means clustering and deep learning.

With its rising importance in various industries, ML has enabled people to accomplish much more than before by collaborating with smart software. Such techniques can give rise to new possibilities for researchers and clinicians, allowing them to make more advanced decisions to benefit mankind. With a greater amount of investment in AI taking place in the past five years than ever before in the history of the healthcare sector, the amount of research and development going on has also increased at an exponential rate. This makes it even more important to examine research work and proposed models.

The growing popularity of artificial intelligence in the field of healthcare has caused a large percentage of the population to become aware of its true potential. AI can enhance the efficiency and effectiveness of our healthcare ecosystem and is thus rapidly becoming one of the most important advances in biomedical discovery, clinical research, medical diagnostics/devices, and precision medicine.

The three main applications of ML in healthcare are medical imaging, natural language processing of medical documents, and genetic information.

First, ML algorithms are applied in medical imaging like magnetic resonance imaging (MRI), computerized axial tomography (CAT scans), and ultrasound (US) imaging to predict images which may indicate a serious medical issue.

The second application is natural language processing of medical documents. The amount of existing physical medical records in hospitals makes the documentation process slow and tedious. This calls for the development of algorithms that can usefully interpret electronic medical records (EMR) to save time and improve efficiency.

The third machine learning application encompasses the use of human genetics to predict diseases and find their cause. With the explosion of genetic data, the attempt to recognize meaningful information about how genetics may influence human health is now at the forefront of many research endeavors. Understanding how complex diseases may manifest and how genetics may affect an individual person's risk can help in preventative healthcare.

Though the idolization of AI as the superior diagnostic platform seems appealing, several unique challenges have impeded progress. With the increasing efficiency of AI algorithms and the increasing dependency on AI systems in the healthcare industry, its legitimacy is often questioned and is a topic for debate.

Among the issues that have been addressed are quality and quantity of data; access to and use of EMR; transparency of the system in contrast to the entire clinical workflow; and the impact of bias on system outputs. Addressing these barriers prior to widespread implementation will allow research to continue to its full potential by learning lessons from previous experiences and realizing the full capability of MI in healthcare settings, while avoiding pitfalls that are easily intensified due to the inherently intimate nature of health and healthcare. At present, thorough scrutiny of AI systems is recommended, with providers being cautious of over-reliance on their efficacy to treat patients.

The following sections discuss real-life applications of machine learning in health care.

### 12.2.1 Learning Insulin–Glucose Dynamics in the Wild

In their paper, Andrew C. Miller, Nicholas J. Foti and Emily Fox have proposed a fusion between physiological and statistical models of insulin–glucose dynamics for predicting future glucose values in a Type 1 diabetic patient, using real-world management data consisting of continuous glucose monitors (CGM), insulin pumps, and carbohydrate logs.

Physiological simulators like UVA/Padova are not flexible enough to be able to model real-world data with disturbance and noise. However, this fused model inherits realistic inductive biases from the physiological model and the flexibility and predictive power of modern machine learning sequence methods.

A unified approach was proposed by fusing two distinct components: a structured UVA/Padova simulator and a deep state-space model, which we call the Deep T1D Simulator (DTD-Sim). The DTD-Sim model uses a multi-layer perceptron with two hidden layers of size 128 with rectified linear unit (relu) nonlinearities (Figure 12.1).

The DTD-Sim model is formally specified as:

$$z0 \sim \mathrm{N}\left(\mu 0, \Sigma 0\right) \text{ initial latent state} \tag{12.1}$$

$$zt \sim Azt - 1 + Bat + Q\,1/2\,\epsilon t, \epsilon t \sim \mathrm{N}\left(0,\ \mathrm{I}\right) \text{ latent temporal dynamics} \tag{12.2}$$

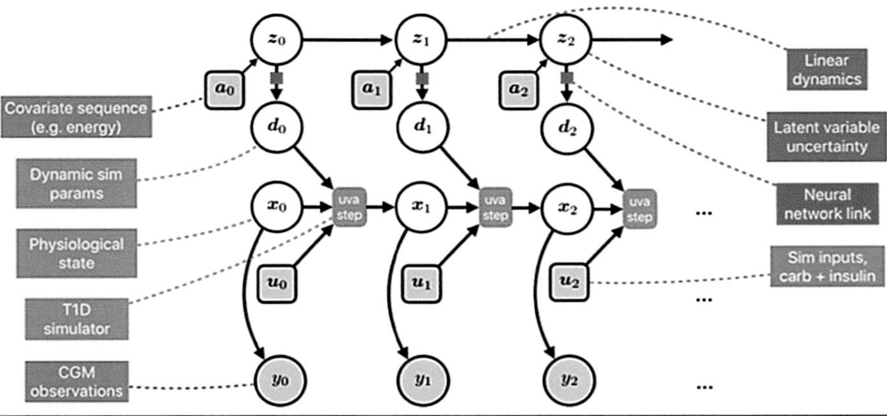


**Figure 12.1 Graphical depiction of the DTD-Sim model.**

$$dt = NN\phi(zt)\ \text{dynamic simulator params} \tag{12.3}$$

$$xt = UVA - step\left(xt - 1, dt, ut, s, \Delta t\right)\ \text{T1D simulator} \tag{12.4}$$

$$yt \sim N\left(CGM\left(xt, s\right), \sigma 2\right)\ \text{CGM observation} \tag{12.5}$$

where zt ∈ R D, dt ∈ R K, xt ∈ R 13, ut ∈ R J, and s ∈ R J.

Certain areas of improvement have been highlighted, including incorporating a direct model of noise in both the observation of meals and their overall mass, which could improve forecasts, as well as including additional input sequences to the DTD-Sim.

While the authors do not claim that their model entirely solves glucose forecasting for T1D management, this model can better describe long-term architecture in real-world T1D data.

### *12.2.2 MRI-Based Diagnosis of Rotator Cuff Tears Using Deep Learning and Weighted Linear Combinations*

In their paper, the authors Mijung Kim, Ho-min Park, Jae Yoon Kim, Seong Hwan Kim, Sofie Van Hoeke and Wesley De Neve have proposed a computational approach towards rotator cuff tear (RCT) diagnosis, a common condition among middle-aged and elderly populations. Diagnosing an RCT requires the availability of shoulder MRI and proton density-weighted imaging, which is both time-consuming and expensive. A computational approach has therefore been introduced which uses a weighted linear combination (WLC) layer, in combination with a deep CNN, to make the most of the available 3-D MRI data and weighted cross-entropy loss to attenuate class imbalance scenarios.

After the last convolutional layer, all FC layers are removed from the VGG-16 backbone and individual slices in the MRI scan acquire an embedding function. The last feature maps are flattened by installing global average pooling (GAP) layers. Overfitting is reduced by installing dropout layers before and after the GAP layer (Figure 12.2).

Every output is given as an input to a WLC gφ, where θ and φ are the weights. If x denotes MRI scan, then x ∈ R16 × 224 × 224 × 3. fθ denotes the embedding function, consisting of the first 13 layers of VGG-16. Then,

$$g\varphi(x) = GAP\left(f\theta(x)\right)T \cdot w\varphi.$$

By obtaining the highest m-AUC score (98%) and the highest specificity value, the proposed model outperformed all baselines, and proved to be robust. The use of a CNN with a WLC layer can accomplish higher diagnostic efficiency than human

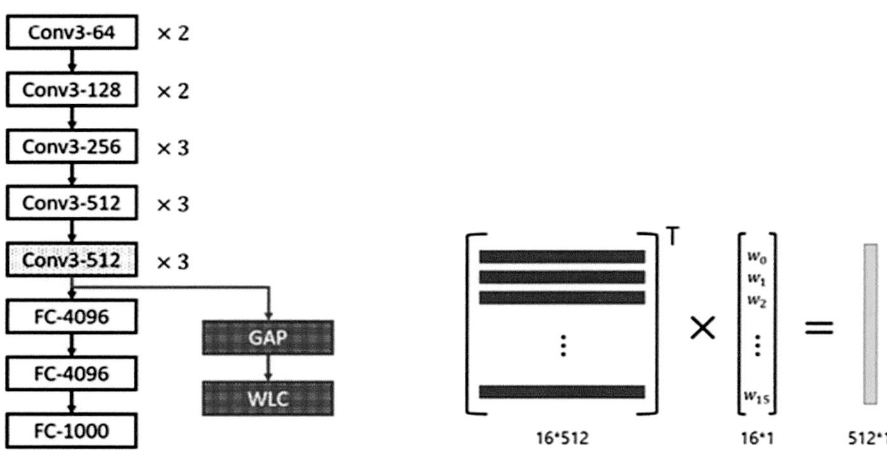


**Figure 12.2 Network architecture and weighted linear combination.**

annotators when carrying out computational diagnosis of RCTs in 3-D MRI scans. The approach was also successful in making a distinction among low-grade partial-thickness (thickness below 50%), high-grade partial-thickness (thickness above 50%), and full thickness RCTs.

### *12.2.3 Transferring Learning from Well Curated to Less Resourced Populations with HIV*

Sonali Parbhoo, Mario Wieser, Volker Roth and Finale Doshi-Velez have proposed an approach for reasoning about the consequences of a series of intercessions for HIV therapy selection in areas where genetic sequence data is not readily available at the time of testing – particularly in regions like Africa, where lack of readily accessible technology makes it harder to monitor the virus. This work aims to identify symptoms for the predicted patient and suggest treatment that may be missing.

Given patient data X from two cohorts, πtransfer (transfer policy) provides treatment based on compressed information from the European patients. Πlocal (local policy) searches for patients with the most similarity from the African cohort and provides relevant treatments. A mixed policy πe of treatments T is produced from the mixture of experts (Figure 12.3).

It was inferred that while locally trained baselines and transfer-based baselines do not perform well individually, high rewards are achieved using a mixture of experts.

This paper tackles the challenge of HIV therapies being less effective in regions experiencing high heterogeneity of the virus, and immense genetic sequencing costs, by applying a novel mixture-of-experts approach. A transfer expert was trained to identify relevant information that could be sent across populations. If the transfer

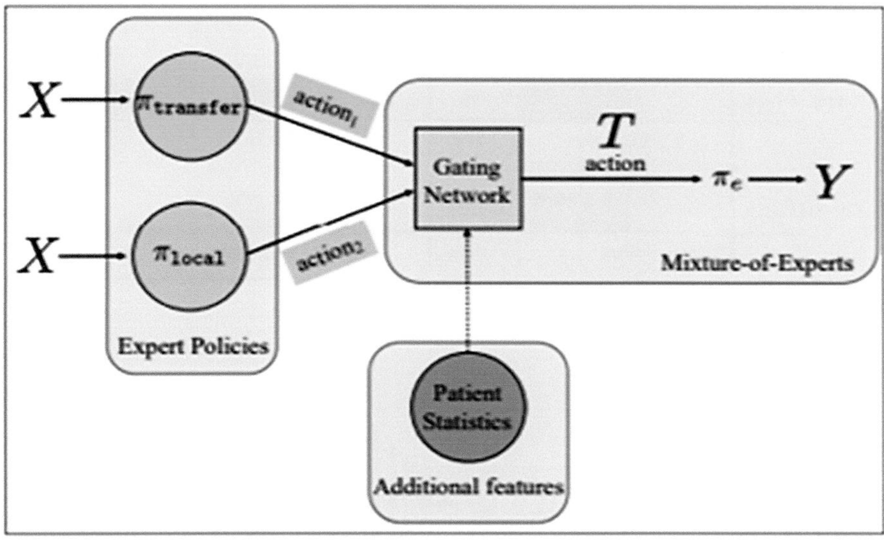


**Figure 12.3 HIV therapy selection through various cohorts.**

was not feasible, a local expert was trained to identify effects among the population useful for deducing patient outcomes. The given approach can be applied in scenarios where measurements are missing, and where one wishes to evaluate current treatment guidelines across different populations.

There is no real method of inspecting the validity of an important assumption that is made in this paper – the fact that confounding factors may be measured. Performances of various policies were evaluated using various types of off-policy evaluations, which can lead to high variance. The simplicity of the gating network used to apply the transfer and local experts is also one of the limitations of this paper.

### 12.2.4 Early Diagnosis of Epilepsy from EEG Data

Authors Jochen Triesch, Sebastian Bauer, Valentin Neubert, Lara Sophie Costard, Felix Rosenow and Diyuan Lu have explored whether deep learning techniques can detect epileptogenesis (EPG), a common neurological disorder, from intracranial electroencephalography (EEG) recordings days/weeks before the occurrence of any seizures. Continuous EEG recordings were obtained from a rodent model of mesial temporal lobe epilepsy with hippocampal sclerosis (mTLE-HS), till the first spontaneous seizure (FSS) took place. Epilepsy was induced by electrical perforant pathway stimulation (PPS). The samples recorded before PPS define the baseline (BL) class, whereas the samples recorded after the PPS but prior to the occurrence of the FSS form a class called the epileptogenesis (EPG) class. In this paper, a deep learning framework is proposed to classify EPG vs. BL by training on raw EEG data (Figure 12.4).

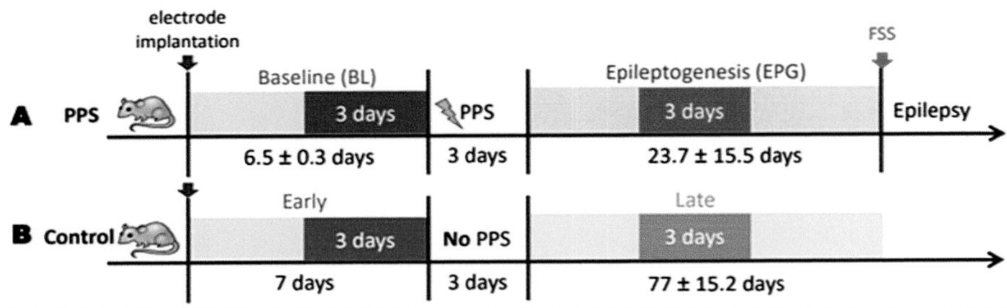


Figure 12.4 **Comparative analysis of EPG and BL.**

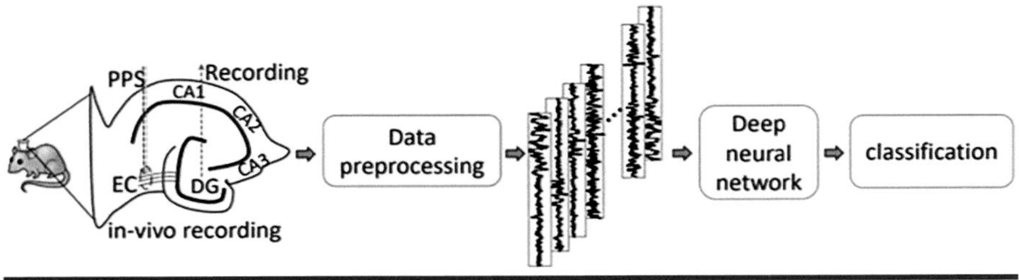


Figure 12.5 **Data processing and classification process.**

Since a major portion of normal brain EEG patterns are also present in the EPG phase, predictions are made from a longer time interval (e.g., 60 minutes) and combined through linear aggregation. The main aim is to detect whether a brain is likely to develop epilepsy before the occurrence of FSS. If this is made possible days/weeks before the FSS, it would enable interventions that could reduce or even arrest the growth of the disease before any spontaneous seizures take place (Figure 12.5).

This model is a deep neural network (DNN) with 33 convolutional layers with residual connections. The pre-activation from one layer is connected with the input of another previous layer through the residual connection, skipping numerous layers in between. Non-linear activation is then applied to the sum to evaluate the next layer's input. The collection of computations between a residual connection is called a ResBlock. With the flattened feature maps as input, the SoftMax layer is given as output and a probability distribution is returned over the two possible classes.

### *12.2.5 Evaluation of Doctor Interpretability of Generalized Additive Models with Interactions*

In their paper, Stefan Hegselmann, Thomas Volkert, Hendrik Ohlenburg, Antje Gottschalk, Martin Dugas and Christian Ertmer have presented various types of machine learning algorithms and how they can be useful for recognizing patterns that can be applied in medical imaging.

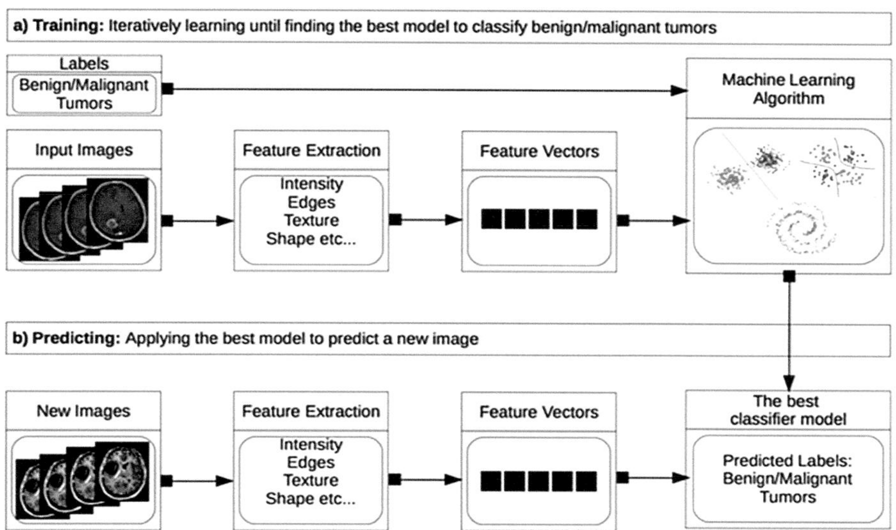


**Figure 12.6 Training and prediction of the model.**

The various training techniques are elaborated upon using the example of separating the regions on a brain image into tumor (malignant or benign) versus normal (non-diseased) tissue. For supervised learning, brain tumor images would be labeled as benign or malignant, and the algorithm would have to classify the unseen images (test images) into these two categories based on the trained data. In unsupervised learning, images are classified, without any information about these groups being explicitly provided. Reinforcement learning consists of a classifier trained using labeled data, but later provided with unlabeled data to further improve the classification by characterizing this data in a better manner (Figure 12.6).

In an example of 70/30 cross-validation, to separate brain tumor from normal brain tissue, CT images obtained with and without contrast material are used as input. With 100 input vectors from white matter and 100 input vectors from tumor, these vectors were sequenced such that the first value is the mean CT attenuation of the ROI on the non–contrast material-enhanced image, and the second value is the mean attenuation of the ROI on the contrast material-enhanced image. Enhancing the tumor will have higher attenuation on the contrast-enhanced images. The variance in attenuation will be calculated and used as the third feature in the vector. 70 normal brain tissue ROIs and 70 tumor ROIs are sent as input to the machine learning algorithm system, which will assign random weights to each of the four features. If the sum is greater than 0, the algorithm system will identify the ROI as tumor; otherwise, the ROI will be identified as normal brain tissue. The weights are continuously adjusted by the system until there is no more improvement in accuracy. Prediction accuracy is then evaluated for the remaining 30 examples of each normal brain tissue ROI and each tumor ROI. A different group of 70 tumor ROIs and 70 normal tissue ROIs are now trained in a new network to determine the accuracy of the algorithm. This process is repeated several times to derive a mean accuracy for this algorithm.

Various types of machine learning algorithms, especially those involving neural networks, k-nearest neighbors, SVMs, decision trees, naïve Bayes algorithm, deep learning, and their applications are discussed in this paper.

The authors state that with technological advances over the years, today's machine learning techniques are highly beneficial and robust. Understanding ML tools is critical to applying them in the most efficient manner. It is also crucial for us to engage in areas of research to provide the best medical care to patients in the future.

## 12.3 Conclusion

The research papers discussed highlight the importance of machine learning in healthcare, and how it helps patients in many ways. The increasing applications of AI in the healthcare industry gives us a brief glimpse of a future where treatments and innovation work hand in hand to help patients in an effective manner. Such techniques have helped the healthcare industry in every way possible. From helping radiologists to make smart decisions when reviewing CT, MRI, and PET images to maintaining a better record of a patient's medical history and their response to different treatment methods to predicting the outbreak of diseases and preparing for them in advance. All these things are possible today due to advances in the field of machine learning going hand in hand with the development of the healthcare sector. The performance of ML algorithms has also proved to be a good indicator of the fact that the future is going to be dominated by artificial intelligence, where the work done by a piece of code or an algorithm is as important as that of any medicine.

From offering quality control services to improving patient care at health care facilities, technology is changing the way we operate as human beings in the professional sphere. It is evident that recent advances in technology are allowing healthcare specialists to adopt smart healthcare practices in a cost-effective manner. It has also made a significant contribution to improving patient safety by alerting clinicians to patterns or signals that they may have missed. It is important to realize the tremendous potential that artificial intelligence holds and the changes it can bring in the healthcare sector. With the massive financial investment coming into the healthcare industry, it is becoming quite clear that the future of this industry depends on how well it can incorporate AI in its day-to-day activities. While there is a long way to go to reach a period where everything is dependent on AI, if the research and development currently going on are anything to go by, then we are well on the way to reaching a situation where AI officially takes over the day-to-day activities of not only a medical professional, but also a normal person in general.

The recent COVID-19 pandemic showed how vulnerable our medical system is when there is a sudden outbreak of a deadly disease. This pandemic has not only emphasized the importance of having a well-tuned prediction model pointing towards future outbreaks that can be a danger to our society, but has also helped accelerate the process of data collection, processing, and identification exponentially. The existence of well-tuned data sets, identification of important behavioural patterns, detection and diagnostics of muscle injuries, location of cancerous cells, and maintenance of up-to-date medical records are just a few of the uses of machine learning in the medical field, but each of these individually has the potential to save millions of valuable lives across the globe. With all these things in mind, we can safely say that the future lies in the hands of artificial intelligence and machine learning.

## References

1. Miller, A. C., Foti, N. J., and Fox, E. (2020, September). Learning Insulin-Glucose Dynamics in the Wild. In *Machine Learning for Healthcare Conference* (pp. 172–197). PMLR.
2. Kim, M., Park, H. M., Kim, J. Y., Kim, S. H., Hoeke, S., and De Neve, W. (2020, September). MRI-Based Diagnosis of Rotator Cuff Tears Using Deep Learning and Weighted Linear Combinations. In *Machine Learning for Healthcare Conference* (pp. 292–308). PMLR.
3. Parbhoo, S., Wieser, M., Roth, V., and Doshi-Velez, F. (2020, September). Transfer Learning from Well-Curated to Less-Resourced Populations with HIV. In *Machine Learning for Healthcare Conference* (pp. 589–609). PMLR.
4. Lu, D., Bauer, S., Neubert, V., Costard, L. S., Rosenow, F., and Triesch, J. (2020, September). Towards Early Diagnosis of Epilepsy from EEG Data. In *Machine Learning for Healthcare Conference* (pp. 80–96). PMLR.
5. Hegselmann, S., Volkert, T., Ohlenburg, H., Gottschalk, A., Dugas, M., and Ertmer, C. (2020, September). An Evaluation of the Doctor-Interpretability of Generalized Additive Models with Interactions. In *Machine Learning for Healthcare Conference* (pp. 46–79). PMLR.

# Index


A

accomplishments, 174
accountable, 92
accuracy, 8, 15, 18, 23, 29, 31, 32, 35, 43, 46, 53, 55, 56, 62-76, 78-84, 88, 105, 113, 115, 118, 134, 147, 149, 150, 163, 164, 175, 187, 191, 193, 214, 218-220, 222, 240–246, 247, 248
adaboost, 165
africa, 52, 54, 244
agent-based, 125, 132, 133
amplifier, 174
anatomization, 71
annealing, 134
architecture, 22, 31, 45, 75, 90, 92, 102, 104, 105, 126, 127, 129, 143, 154, 161, 167, 176, 181, 201, 203, 243, 244

B

backbone, 167, 243
bacterial, 134, 196
bottleneck, 161, 194
brain-inspired, 174, 183
brain–machine, 174

C

cambridge, 157, 195
cancer, 26, 36, 47, 84, 85, 130, 136, 137, 148, 149, 155, 157, 161, 164, 165, 168, 179–181, 247, 251
cardiac, 62, 107
cardiology, 8, 62
cardiovascular, 5, 7, 73–75, 84, 183, 202, 247
cell, 57, 58, 107, 145, 169, 181
cloud, 40, 93, 95, 97, 109, 137, 142, 151, 174, 177, 194, 213
clustering, 18, 21, 23, 31, 35, 36, 134, 147, 163, 168, 253
clusters, 20
cmos, 187, 188
cnn, 22, 26, 28, 30–32, 114, 115, 136, 144, 166, 193, 215, 219, 243
convolution, 188
convolutional, 14, 22, 26, 28–30, 32, 35, 49, 70, 71, 109, 113–115, 130, 132, 136, 144, 155, 160, 166, 179, 180, 183, 188, 215, 219, 243, 246
coronavirus, 106, 112, 129, 132, 133, 139, 153, 200, 204, 206, 207, 210–212
covid-19, 1, 5, 7, 8, 88, 106, 111–127, 129-133, 144, 147, 153, 155, 156, 162, 172, 173, 175, 182, 200, 206, 207, 210–212, 215, 238, 249
ct-scan, 48
cyber, 94, 100, 108, 109, 152, 215
cyberattacks, 94

D

decrease, 37, 40, 115
default, 241–243
defect, 37, 101, 103
defective, 251
defects, 101
defense, 178, 188, 238
define, 52, 245
defined, 24, 48, 62, 63, 169, 218, 221
defines, 48, 95
diabetes, 1, 5–9, 51–57, 59, 61–65, 67–71, 153, 155, 164, 215, 217–221, 223, 225–241, 243, 245, 247

diabetic, 53, 66, 69, 156, 180, 219, 220, 224, 254
diffusion, 19

E

edge, 15–17, 19, 20, 25, 39, 42, 43, 107, 132
edge-based, 21
emr, 174, 253
epidemiological, 116

F

f1-score, 223, 245, 246
feed-forward, 58, 166
firefly, 134
fuzzy, 18, 21–23, 30, 31, 51, 53, 56, 59–61, 70, 71, 109, 130, 188, 215
fuzzy-based, 214

G

ga, 68, 134
gradient, 32, 76, 116, 145, 167, 188, 219, 240, 241, 247
gradients, 19
greywolf, 134

H

heatmap, 224
histograms, 224
hybridization, 23, 31

I

influenced, 19
intel, 9, 35, 44, 89, 97, 137, 204, 206
intelligence, 1, 5, 7–9, 13–15, 17, 19, 21, 23, 25, 27, 29, 31, 33, 35, 36, 49, 52, 55, 71, 84, 85, 86, 87, 89, 92, 109, 112, 116, 130–132, 135, 136, 141–143, 153, 155, 159–162, 167, 169, 172, 173, 174, 176, 178–184, 196, 201, 204, 207, 214, 215, 247, 248, 249–251, 253
iot, 1, 6–8, 87–99, 106, 107, 109, 137, 157, 174, 187, 194–196, 199–207, 209–213, 215, 252
iot-based, 7, 195, 199, 202, 207, 210, 212, 213

K

k-means, 21, 35, 220, 247, 253
k-nearest, 14, 53, 62, 114, 131, 159, 164, 219, 247, 248
knn, 53, 62, 75, 114, 116, 159, 164, 219

L

learning-based, 22, 24, 116, 131, 132, 155, 161, 174, 183
leukemia, 251

M

malaria, 251
mapreduce, 141, 148
mation, 40, 100, 147, 150, 203
matrix, 77, 78, 80, 82, 171, 180, 218, 221, 224, 225, 230, 241–244
models, 1, 5, 7, 8, 20, 26, 32, 42, 46–49, 52, 56–58, 84, 93, 97, 101, 103, 105, 111, 112, 114, 117, 120, 121, 124, 125, 130, 132, 137, 138, 144, 145, 150, 153, 159, 161, 163, 165–167, 169, 171, 173, 174, 175, 177–179, 181, 183, 184, 188, 193, 219–221, 244–246, 249, 252–254

N

naïve, 53, 62, 78–83, 114, 131, 220, 252
nature-inspired, 150
neural, 14, 18, 20, 22, 26–30, 32, 34, 35, 46, 49, 51, 53, 55–58, 70, 71, 84, 85, 89, 109, 113–116, 130–132, 134, 136, 144, 155, 156, 160, 161, 165, 166, 173, 174, 179, 181, 183, 184, 188, 215, 218, 219, 241, 246, 247, 248
neuro-fuzzy, 53, 70
neurological, 174, 245
noisy, 15, 17, 220
npv, 218, 224, 244–246
optimization, 21, 26, 28, 33, 46, 53, 58, 59, 70, 102–104, 130, 134, 147, 160, 167, 168, 173, 241

P

pandemic, 8, 106, 112, 115, 117, 121, 125–127, 129, 130, 139, 153, 155, 173, 175, 200, 204, 207, 210, 238, 249, 251
pipelines, 90

pneumonia, 112, 131, 202, 251
predictions, 1, 78–80, 82, 83, 110, 116, 121, 148, 163, 221, 223, 224, 246, 251
pre-trained, 105, 114, 115
protein, 8, 113, 134, 160, 165, 167–172, 180, 181, 183
protocol, 188, 213
pso, 134
radiological, 173
regression, 32, 42, 48, 51, 53, 56, 58, 59, 62, 63, 67, 68, 71, 81, 114, 116, 121, 136, 159, 162, 163, 165, 180, 191, 192, 220, 241, 252

R

regular, 42, 69, 95, 204, 251
rnn, 32, 53, 62, 136, 144, 145, 166, 181, 224
robots, 89, 90, 100, 105, 117

S

science, 9, 14, 34, 46, 48, 56, 57, 63, 70, 84, 132, 137, 153, 154, 156, 157, 167, 175, 179–181, 183, 184, 194–196, 201, 238, 247, 249
security, 49, 71, 84, 87, 94–97, 100, 103, 107, 109, 131, 142, 144, 160, 162, 174, 178, 181, 207, 213, 215
segmentation, 13, 14, 16, 18–24, 26–31, 34, 35, 43, 131, 134, 145, 155, 156, 161, 166, 179, 180, 182
simulation, 43, 46, 101, 105, 117, 121, 123–128, 133
smartphone, 66, 118, 132, 214
softmax, 114, 246
software, 17, 49, 88, 90, 95, 100, 102–104, 109, 131, 133, 137, 164, 194, 249, 253
spread, 8, 69, 106, 111, 113, 115, 117, 118, 120, 121, 132, 141, 193, 206, 207, 210, 212, 251
statistical, 41–43, 47, 49, 58, 62, 71, 99, 121, 147, 168, 172, 174, 181, 190, 194, 219, 254
stress, 174, 189, 194, 196, 203
supervised, 33, 55, 58, 76, 84, 85, 116, 159, 162–164, 176, 219, 240, 241, 247, 252
svm, 9, 53, 56, 58, 59, 75, 113, 114, 116, 165, 174, 218–220, 224, 241–243, 245–247, 252
synthetic, 108, 190

T

telemammography, 157
tele-mammography, 149
telemedicine, 200, 206, 210, 212, 213
thermographic, 189
thermography, 174, 189, 195
thingspeak, 205
threshold, 57, 58, 165, 202
thresholding, 19, 134
tolerance, 52, 59, 67, 221
trained, 75, 76, 101, 114, 115, 161, 163, 166, 193, 221, 241–245, 247, 248, 251, 252
training, 20, 22, 30, 32, 33, 41, 42, 58, 76, 95, 114, 161–163, 165, 168, 176, 178, 180, 220, 245, 247, 252, 253
transparency, 106, 160, 169, 177, 253
treatment, 7, 8, 14, 26, 54, 69, 97, 104, 106, 134, 136, 137, 140, 144, 148, 152, 160, 162, 165, 169, 173, 178, 200, 201, 219, 244, 245, 247, 248, 251, 252
tree-based, 165
t-score, 37
tumor, 30, 34–36, 49, 71, 85, 132, 165, 173, 247, 248, 251

U

ultrasound, 173, 253
unstructured, 137, 140, 141, 144, 148, 150, 160, 174, 240
unsupervised, 21, 33, 55, 58, 140, 159, 162–164, 175, 247, 251–253

V

vaccination, 111, 112, 124–127, 129, 133
vaccination_rate, 126, 127
valuable, 139, 140, 249
variety, 1, 7, 21, 24, 97, 103–105, 137–142, 144, 145, 148, 151, 165, 169, 173, 175, 189, 252
viruses/diseases, 120
visualization, 19, 48, 204, 215

W

wavelet, 203
wearable, 106, 107, 157, 177, 200, 203, 205, 206, 212
weights, 32, 57, 58, 243, 247
wifi, 86, 118, 203

wi-fi, 107
wired, 93, 190, 204
wireless, 93, 94, 154, 155, 188, 190, 196, 203, 204, 207, 212–215
wolf, 70
workers, 105, 117, 141, 145, 148, 206, 212, 238
workflow, 174, 253
workload, 54
worse, 116, 137
worst, 93, 126
worst-case, 127
worthiness, 100

## X

xgboost, 8, 73, 76, 77, 113, 218, 220, 240, 242–246
x-ray, 14, 37–43, 46–49, 97, 113, 114, 130, 147, 162, 172, 173
x-rays, 8, 111, 114

## Z

zigbee, 118, 188, 203, 214
z-score, 163